Breathing Race
into the Machine

T0321405

Breathing Race
into the Machine

The Surprising Career of the Spirometer
from Plantation to Genetics

Lundy Braun

University of Minnesota Press
Minneapolis · London

The publication of this book was assisted by a bequest from Josiah H. Chase to honor his parents, Ellen Rankin Chase and Josiah Hook Chase.

Portions of chapters 1 and 2 were previously published as "Spirometry, Measurement, and Race in the Nineteenth Century," *Journal of the History of Medicine and Allied Sciences* 60 (2005): 135–69.

Published by the University of Minnesota Press
111 Third Avenue South, Suite 290
Minneapolis, MN 55401-2520
http://www.upress.umn.edu

LIBRARY OF CONGRESS CATALOGING-IN-PUBLICATION DATA
Braun, Lundy, author.
   Breathing race into the machine : the surprising career of the spirometer from plantation to genetics / Lundy Braun.
   Includes bibliographical references and index.
   ISBN 978-0-8166-8357-4 (hc : alk. paper)
   ISBN 978-0-8166-8359-8 (pb : alk. paper)
   I. Title. [DNLM: 1. Spirometry—history. 2. Spirometry—instrumentation. 3. African Continental Ancestry Group. 4. European Continental Ancestry Group. 5. History, 19th Century. 6. History, 20th Century. 7. Lung—physiology. 8. Pneumoconiosis—etiology. 9. Racism—history. WB 284] RC773
616.2'44—dc23
2013032948

Printed in the United States of America on acid-free paper

The University of Minnesota is an equal-opportunity educator and employer.

30 29 28 27 26 25 24   10 9 8 7 6 5 4 3 2

To my sister Martha

1951–1979

Contents

Acknowledgments

This book represents the culmination of my journey from the laboratory to the archive that began in the late 1990s after I read an article in
my local newspaper about race correction of pulmonary function in an
asbestos class-action lawsuit. Having just joined the Race in Science
and Medicine Workshop at MIT, organized by Evelynn Hammonds,
I was intrigued by the idea of "correcting" for race. A conversation
with my good friend David Kern, a wonderfully thoughtful physician
in occupational medicine, revealed that race correction was standard
practice in pulmonary medicine. In his usual meticulous fashion
David assembled key articles on the topic for me to read. What I
initially conceptualized as a short article became a long but truly
enjoyable excursion in the history of race and lung-function testing.

The encouragement of friends and colleagues on three continents
made the process of researching and writing this book a pleasure. I
offer the usual caveat that I alone am responsible for the interpretation of this history. My sincere appreciation goes to colleagues at
Brown University. I have been fortunate that the structure at Brown
allowed me to cross disciplinary (and epistemological) boundaries
that are usually difficult to navigate. In the Department of Pathology and Laboratory Medicine, I thank Agnes Kane, my chair; Kim
Boekelheide; and my former chair, Nelson Fausto (who, sadly, did
not live to read this book), for unflagging support and encouragement
over the years when it would have been much easier on the department if I did my job in a more conventional way. Special thanks go
to my colleagues in Africana studies, especially Lewis Gordon, who
in 2001 invited me to join the Department of Africana Studies, and
subsequent chairs Tony Bogues, Tricia Rose, and Corey Walker, who
provided important intellectual support for this work. Anne Fausto-
Sterling organized the Science and Technology Studies program just
as I was making the shift from basic science to historical research.

Her intellectual generosity and that of other faculty members in STS were critical to the evolution of this study.

I am deeply grateful to those who took time out of their busy schedules to read drafts of one or more chapters: Rina Bliss, Molly Braun, Merlin Chowkwanyun, Anne Fausto-Sterling, Françoise Hamlin, Agnes Kane, David Kern, Sophie Kisting, Nancy Jacobs, Miriam Reumann, Susan Reverby, Joan Richards, Samuel Roberts, David Rosner, and Amy Slaton. Their comments enriched the manuscript—and made the process more interactive and fun. In addition to her famously quick turnarounds on copy, Susan deserves special mention for support and advice as the project evolved. That this project became a book is largely due to Keith Wailoo, who first suggested at a conference in 2006 that I consider the idea. Miriam, Merlin, David, and Molly were truly heroic in reading and commenting on the entire manuscript. I thank Peter Braun for his legal insight on the asbestos case.

Friends and colleagues in South Africa played a critical role in the development of this project. In particular, Neville Alexander, Eugene Caincross, Sophie Kisting, and Karen Press were gracious in helping me appreciate South Africa's complex history and the brutal legacy of a racialized mining system. Neville's vision of and sacrifices for a more just future hover over this book; I am deeply saddened by his death. Sophie stands out for her remarkable insight. She took an immediate interest in the project and helped to arrange interviews with South Africans involved in the debate over reference standards and several seminars at an early stage of this project. The work of Jonny Myers was a constant inspiration. Tony Davies was remarkably generous with his time answering e-mails and helping me locate valuable documents from the Pneumoconiosis Research Unit.

I conducted a large number of interviews with physicians and activists in the United States, South Africa, and Britain. Although they will remain anonymous under the terms of my human subjects' approval, I am grateful for their time and interest in discussing this complicated topic. I gained valuable insights over the years from many participants, especially the organizer, Evelynn Hammonds, in the Race in Science and Medicine Workshop, first held at MIT and then Harvard; the Race Seminar in Cape Town; the RACEGEN listserv; and numerous seminars and talks. I thank Kay Dickersin and Melanie Wolfgang for their patient collaboration on the incredibly grueling systematic review, which informs sections of this book.

I was fortunate to be the recipient of several grants that gave me precious time and funding to work on this project: a professional development grant from the National Science Foundation, a National Science Foundation Scholar Award, a Royce Teaching Fellowship, and a Salomon grant from Brown University.

Librarians in South Africa, the United States, and South Wales were extraordinarily gracious with their time and knowledge. Special mention goes to the staff at Amherst College, Brown University's John Hay Library, the National Library of South Africa, and to Sian Williams of the fabulous South Wales Coal Miners Library. Diana Wall from Museum Africa and Rosemary Soper of the Archie Cochrane Archives went way beyond the call of duty in searching their collections for suitable images.

Thank you to Jason Weidemann and members of the editorial, production, and marketing staff at the University of Minnesota Press. The expert copyediting of Roxanne Willis, David Thorstad, and Nancy Sauro made this a more readable book. I thank David Luljak for his meticulous indexing and Beth Mellor for the maps.

I deeply appreciate the sage comments, advice, and encouragement I received from the two reviewers of this book, Troy Duster and Steven Epstein.

Finally, I express my love and gratitude to Lucia, Catherine, and John Trimbur for their patience with what became my strange and lengthy obsession with something as esoteric as lung function. They each read and edited drafts of chapters—John more drafts than he cares to recall. John quietly endured my sense of a vacation to mines in South Africa, South Wales, the United States, and Canada. (Sorry, I don't anticipate this will change.)

Measuring Vital Capacity

> Precision carries immense weight in the twentieth
> century . . . It connotes trustworthiness and elegance
> in the actions or products of humans and machines.
> Precision is everything that ambiguity, uncertainty,
> messiness, and unreliability are not. It is responsible,
> nonemotional, objective, and scientific. It shows
> quality . . . These values of precision have become
> part of our heritage.
>
> M. NORTON WISE
> *The Values of Precision*

On March 25, 1999, the front page of the *Baltimore Sun* featured a startling headline, "Racial Basis for Asbestos Lawsuits? Owens Corning Seeks More Stringent Standards for Blacks." According to the article, the American insulation manufacturer Owens Corning was engaged in another legal maneuver to limit disability claims. This time it would be more difficult for African Americans in Baltimore to qualify for compensation.[1]

Home to former shipyards and Bethlehem Steel's plant at Sparrow's Point, Baltimore had been the site of endless legal wrangling in a massive lawsuit against asbestos manufacturers for decades. Over the years, lawyers for Owens Corning made numerous attempts to delay proceedings and many verdicts went against the defendants.[2] But, invoking a racial basis for disability assessment represented a troubling twist in the legal landscape. How, at the dawn of the twenty-first century, could there be a racial basis for legal redress in the United States?

Plaintiffs would soon learn that Owens Corning's motion rested on a long-standing belief among pulmonologists that racial groups—particularly "blacks" and "whites"—differed in the capacity and the function of their lungs. In fact, the idea of difference is so widely accepted that manufacturers program race and ethnic "correction" into the spirometer, the instrument that measures lung function.[3]

The company's motion to apply the practice of "race correction" in this contentious case surprised workers. The effects of asbestos exposure were among the most heavily debated health issues in U.S. courts during the twentieth century. Many former asbestos workers in Baltimore were on the inactive docket, suffering at home from asbestosis, mesothelioma, and lung cancer, their physical condition—and lung function—deteriorating steadily. At the time Owens Corning presented its motion, approximately fifteen thousand cases were waiting to be heard in Baltimore. In making race the central issue with which to limit disability claims, this deeply divisive case suddenly became even more contentious. The authority of science was at stake.

In a letter to the *Sun,* Jim Fite, an asbestos activist with the White Lung Association, angrily wrote that the "idea that blacks (once the court has decided what that is) should require a higher level of disability rating to qualify for compensation is vulgar and discriminatory. To maintain that there is any scientific justification to this nonsense is more 'science' by corporate donations."[4] Anthony Bradford, a former worker for Bethlehem Steel, vehemently decried the practice: "I would say this is a low point in the system that you're going to make a rule based on race, of an African-American's lungs not being equal to a white person's lungs. . . . But it doesn't surprise me. When you have a racist viewpoint I guess you can get a doctor to say anything."[5]

Owens Corning's tactic to limit disability claims was not only legally clever; it was also scientifically grounded. Race-specific criteria for impairment were consistent with the guidelines of the American Thoracic Society (ATS), one of the most authoritative associations in pulmonary medicine. Had the company's motion been successful, black workers would have had to demonstrate lower lung function and worse clinical symptoms than white workers before receiving compensation for asbestos-induced disease.[6] To the surprise of courtroom observers, Maryland Circuit Court Judge Joseph H. H. Kaplan denied the motion by Owens Corning in an oral ruling.[7] Race correction would not be allowed in this particular case, at least for the time being.

Beyond the fractious medicolegal issues related to compensation, this case made public a long-standing—but rarely examined—history of racial assumptions informing the theories and practices of lung function research. In this case, cultural notions of race became embedded in the architecture of an apparently ordinary instrument that purports to measure lung function. Had lawyers for Owens Corning researched this history (which they probably did), they would have uncovered a large scientific literature detailing racial difference in lung function, with white norms higher than almost all other racial and ethnic groups.[8] They might also have located occasional attempts to contest this idea. Not surprisingly, company lawyers based their legal argument on the consensus view, as articulated by the ATS and the American Medical Association, that blacks have lower lung function than whites. In a legal deposition, a leading pulmonary specialist defended the mainstream view that average values differ in blacks and whites.[9]

This book explores the central historical question behind these debates: how did the idea that the lungs of blacks were different from the lungs of whites develop? The belief in racially distinctive lungs was a "racial project," enmeshed in an industrial capitalist system that emerged concurrently with enthusiasm for precision instruments, measurement, and statistical analysis—increasingly reductive frameworks for understanding respiratory physiology—and problematic notions of race.[10] These dynamics enhanced the epistemic authority of comparative scientific analyses of racial "traits," while the spirometer and the social and scientific beliefs embedded in it traveled across time and space.

The idea of racial difference in lung capacity cannot be dismissed as "pseudo-," "junk," or "bad" science, or as the work of scientists with explicitly racist intent. On the contrary, the practice of "race correction" or "ethnic adjustment" is a historical product of mainstream, prominent, and mostly well-intentioned scientists. Elite professional societies and consensus panels have long sanctioned—and promoted—race correction, though official statements often cautioned that the "causes of differences were unclear."[11] Science produced with the spirometer was thus "normal." Only rarely in the history of spirometric measurement were the racial meanings ascribed to lung capacity questioned. For the last century, debate has centered on technical issues, such as operator error, subject compliance, procedure, cutoffs for normal, and standardization of the hardware and software that control the spirometer's operation without critically examining the underlying meanings of racial difference.[12]

To Correct or Not to Correct?

At the center of this story is the spirometer, now widely used in a range of biomedical contexts. When first developed in the mid-nineteenth century, the spirometer was primarily a tool of experimental physiologists. In the twentieth century, pulmonary specialists began using the instrument to diagnose and monitor disease. Primary care practitioners worldwide routinely use the spirometer in their offices. The UK Biobank selected spirometric measurements as a key indicator of overall health.[13] Public health specialists view spirometry's potential as comparable to that of blood pressure in general health assessments.[14] In China, schoolchildren's report cards record vital capacity and supposed declines in vital capacity have triggered national anxieties over physical fitness.[15] Since 2010, World Spirometry Day, a "fitness and respiratory health" campaign of international respiratory societies, has promoted spirometry.[16] Yet most patients would not recognize the name of the machine.

To be clinically useful, the numbers generated by the spirometer must be interpreted in relation to reference standards or values— also called prediction equations—obtained from "normal," "healthy," or "representative" populations. Such standards are routinely "corrected" or "adjusted" by the instrument for gender, height, age—and race or ethnicity. Adjusted lung function measurements are widely used in research investigations for clinical diagnosis of pulmonary diseases; medical surveillance of industrial workers; preemployment physical examinations; and disability assessments.[17] By 1990, approximately half of pulmonary training programs in the United States and Canada adjusted for race or ethnicity.[18] European respiratory societies have endorsed adjustment since the 1990s.[19] The medical and public health implications of race correction are thus immense.

American scientists conducted the first study of racial difference. By the early twentieth century, studies across the globe were reporting differences in lung function by race, ethnicity, nation, or geographic region. Although race and ethnicity were not explicitly defined in most of these studies, groups variably referred to as "non-Caucasians," "nonwhites," or "non-Europeans" were thought to have lower lung capacity than "whites/Caucasians," "Europeans," or "Westerners."[20] The available evidence indicates that low lung function is associated with poor health outcomes.[21] Yet, as this book discusses, whether observed differences represent variation or pathology has plagued interpretation of lung function values.[22]

The majority of these studies—most emanating from the United States—chronicle difference between blacks and whites. Textbooks in pulmonary and occupational medicine describe race correction as standard practice. Race correction is taught to medical students and fellows as scientific fact. As one specialist explained, "I was taught as a pulmonary fellow that African Americans tend to have smaller lungs so therefore one should use a different set of predicted [equations] so that we didn't overdiagnose restrictive lung disease."[23] Although explanations vary, innate biological and genetic differences have been consistent frames in the scientific literature.

There are two methods used to "correct" or "adjust" for race and ethnicity, both rooted in a paradigm of difference. Until recently, the most common method of race correction—referred to as proportionate adjustment—involved a reduction of the predicted "white" norm, usually by 10 to 15 percent for groups labeled "black" and 4 to 6 percent for groups labeled "Asian." The alternative approach—distinct from a "correction factor" in not explicitly setting up "white" values as normative—employs population-specific standards. In this case, the operator of the machine assigns an individual to a racial group and then compares their values to standards derived from studies of lung function in the purportedly same group. Like proportionate adjustment, this method of race correction also assumes difference based on group membership. The most recent guidelines of the Joint Working Party of the ATS/European Respiratory Society (ERS), published in 2005, recommend the use of race- and ethnic-specific reference values, depending on their availability.[24]

Since the 1920s, pulmonary researchers have developed standards specific to populations. But organizing studies sufficiently large to be scientifically credible is costly and time-consuming, a luxury only possible for investigators in resource-rich countries. Additionally, this work assumes the constitution of groups to be straightforward and their composition homogeneous—or homogeneous enough. In the late 1970s, statistician Charles Rossiter from South Wales and pulmonologist Hans Weill from New Orleans first proposed applying a fixed scaling factor of 13.2 percent for black lung function values; their simple method of correcting by a specified percentage became a more pragmatic option.[25] Until spirometers were computerized, the calculations necessary for correction were done manually. With computerization, crude though it initially was, correction factors were directly—and invisibly—programmed into the spirometer. All specifications, correction factors, and interpretations are now contained on small chips and built seamlessly into the equipment. The entire process is so fully automated that users are often unaware that, in selecting a patient's race, they are activating a "correction process." Clicking a mouse or pushing a button is all that is required to operationalize race correction.[26]

For the user to gain detailed information on either the standards or the method of correction, now buried in complex electronics, requires considerable work. Specification sheets must be located in busy and crowded offices and hospitals, manufacturers consulted directly, or Web sites searched, layer by layer. In my own research it was time-consuming and difficult to locate precise information about race or ethnic correction on manufacturer Web sites. Many of the physicians and operators I talked to did not know what standards they used. In some offices, the specification sheets had been misplaced; in other offices, a variety of spirometers were used—each programmed with different standards.

FIGURE 1.
A spirometer in a primary care physician's office, showing switch for race and sex correction, 2009.
Author's personal collection.

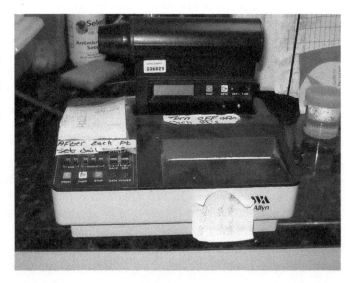

This is a complicated situation that did not arise by accident, from technical error, or because of confusion on the part of developers and users. Rather, the current situation is the product of a long and largely unexamined history during which scientists relinquished knowledge of the body to precision instruments, obscuring the social nature of the categories employed, the decisions made during instrument design, and the ambiguities of disease processes.[27] For workers' compensation, manufacturers' and operators' pragmatic decisions regarding reference standards are especially consequential, both epistemologically and financially. As illustrated in the Baltimore case, race correction makes it more difficult for black workers to qualify for compensation.[28] In addition to demonstrating its discriminatory impact on black workers, this book analyzes how race correction reinforces—and buries—the idea of "naturally occurring" differences in lung function in ways that are difficult to unmask.

Respiratory disease and disability assessments are especially important in occupational medicine. Here, too, U.S. guidelines for correction are a patchwork of population-specific standards and correction factors. In 1978, the U.S. Cotton Standards, used in many occupational settings, mandated the use of a race correction factor. The American College of Occupational and Environmental Medicine (ACOEM) now recommends population-specific standards from the American-based National Health and Nutrition Examination Survey (NHANES III) for all workers, with one exception. For cotton-exposed workers, a correction factor remains a statutory requirement. The only groups for whom standards are available from NHANES III, however, are "Caucasians," African Americans, and Hispanics. This leaves correction factors as the default for other groups. For Asians (defined as Chinese, Japanese, Indian, and Pakistani), the guidelines recommend a correction factor "to account for the larger thoracic cages observed in Caucasians when compared to Asians of the same age, height, and gender."[29] In Europe, on the other hand, correction factors are used routinely, according to the guidelines of the ERS. Most guidelines recommend self-identification as a means of defining race.

Lowering the standard of normal by a set percentage for people of color can have a discriminatory outcome in compensation cases. Yet, the picture is more complicated if we look beyond medicine and compensation to assessing eligibility for work, that is, in preemployment physical examinations. Writing in 1991, pulmonologist Yossef

Aelony cautioned, "the failure to use ethnic/racial norms . . . adversely and unfairly affects job opportunities for healthy Asian and black workers. . . . Ignoring these differences can no longer be excused."[30]

More recently, in a guest editorial for the *Journal of Health Care for the Poor and Underserved*, physicians Roscoe Young and Jean Ford of Columbia University stated, "the use of predicted normal standards for pulmonary function tests derived from majority populations to test minorities is unjust." To avoid clinical mismanagement and "exclusionary hiring practices," they urged further study of "homogenous racial and ethnic groups."[31]

While the mechanical operations of the spirometer are now routine, the racialization of spirometric measurement (that is, the process by which concepts of race as innate difference got attached to and embedded in the instrument and the entity it purports to measure) has had a dynamic history, one linked both to changing social and political contexts and technical innovation. As this book shows, the outcome of spirometric measurement was historically contingent. Interest in spirometry would disappear from one domain only to appear in another. Early spirometers were elegantly designed precision instruments, but as large, unwieldy, and complicated machines, they were difficult for clinicians to use. Over time, numerical determinations became increasingly complex, requiring the assistance of statisticians for interpretation. Newer spirometers, popular among general practitioners, are small and portable, entailing limited technical expertise to operate and making the underlying processes increasingly invisible.

Beyond setting a discriminatory standard for compensation, race correction also raises important historical and theoretical questions about the ways in which cultural assumptions about race and ethnicity inform and are informed by "normal" or routine scientific and technological practices. This book argues that describing and sanctioning difference while leaving the causes and meanings of any disparities unexplained is deeply problematic. In other words, the ideology of racial difference is inseparable from its explanatory framework. Whether through proportionate adjustment or population-specific standards, the practice of race correction places spirometric measurement in a long history of scientific projects that divide socially constructed racial and ethnic groups along biological lines. Such efforts have political consequences, despite the best intentions of individual researchers. This book explores the emergence and unintended consequences of a racialized understanding of lung function.

Race, Technology, and Precision Instruments

Over the past several decades, scholars of science and technology studies (STS) have explored the socio-technoscientific processes by which scientific knowledge is produced.[32] As STS scholars David Skinner and Paul Rosen argued in 2001, race has been an understudied topic in STS. Rather than simply refuting past racial science, they called for further research into the emergence of new forms of race and racism. Otherwise, "new discoveries could reopen the debate about racial difference."[33] This is, of course, precisely what has happened in the twenty-first century, as genomics produced new forms of racial science that built on—rather than challenged—race-based models.[34] As sociologist Troy Duster famously declared, the concept of race in science was "buried alive."[35] In recent years, a growing number of STS scholars have begun to explore the role of technoscience in the revitalization of the concept of race.

Historian Keith Wailoo's *Drawing Blood: Technology and Disease Identity in Twentieth-Century America* stands out as a seminal contribution to the history of race as it intersects with technology.[36] Exploring various technological innovations—Victor Emmel's blood test in 1917, electrophoresis at midcentury, and mass screening tests in the 1960s and 1970s—Wailoo demonstrates how sickle cell became an iconic marker of biological difference, considered unique to people of African descent. Once established in the scientific and popular imaginations, sickle cell disease continued to serve as a signpost guiding the search for difference lurking in the genetic material of black bodies. *Breathing Race into the Machine* builds on Wailoo's study by examining the complex and contradictory historical processes by which differences, such as race, class, and gender, actually get embedded into the very architecture of scientific instruments.[37]

In the nineteenth and early twentieth century, scientists mobilized measuring devices to dissect the finer details of difference—occupation, social class, twin status, age, gender—and race. Accordingly, deterministic models focused on groups suffused the technical knowledge produced by phrenologists, nutritional scientists, psychometricians, and anthropometrists in this period.[38] Writing about

IQ testing in the early-twentieth-century United States, historian Hamilton Cravens observes, "technical knowledge seemed to reflect and to sustain deeper assumptions about social mobility and stratification that were fully integrated into social structures and cultural perceptions of the nation at large."[39]

Some racial projects were discredited, and others disappeared as they were replaced by new paradigms. Still others, though discredited, reemerged in different contexts. Perhaps the most famous example is the nineteenth-century obsession with measuring skulls and ordering these measurements hierarchically. In the *Mismeasure of Man,* Stephen Jay Gould argues that Samuel Morton's bias against African Americans distorted his measurements.[40]

For reasons that I address, the history of race and lung capacity measurements has largely escaped critical examination. The few historians who have studied the spirometer and the entity it purports to measure have not addressed the role of race, class, and gender in the history of its invention, uptake, and dissemination.[41] Beyond bias, I argue that social assumptions of racial difference shaped the design and interpretation of lung function measurements. Placing race, class, and gender at the center of the story, this book asks: By what historical processes did racial discourses get attached to and embedded in the spirometer, such that a hierarchy of difference was established? How and why have these processes been obscured? What explains the tenacity of the association between race and lung capacity? What accounts for the persistence of the belief in difference?

The spirometer first emerged as a tool to probe the lungs of workers in the socioscientific context of mid-nineteenth-century Britain. By this time, quantification was an important feature of technological devices, but cultural enthusiasm for precision instruments was relatively recent. Only in the late eighteenth century, according to historian of science Norton Wise, did precision instruments and numbers become highly valued in international commerce, state apparatuses, developing industries, chemistry, and physics.[42] In the United States, mid-nineteenth-century debates over the optimal way to estimate the force and power of turbines with the dynamometer embodied the epistemic tensions over the scientific approach to "exact" measurement, which would come to displace craft-based technical knowledge. (Anthropometry studies, including a large post–Civil War study by Benjamin A. Gould, as discussed in chapter 2 used dynamometers.) At stake were the "kinds of technical knowledge that mattered" and who could produce that knowledge—self-trained mechanics or scientifically trained experts.[43] With imperial expansion, technological tools assumed enhanced epistemic authority as markers of civilized societies and their hierarchical ranking.[44]

The drive for precision and accuracy profoundly influenced knowledge-making practices in the biological sciences. In the emerging field of experimental physiology scientists drew on newly developed precision instruments to probe the inner processes of the body with a previously unimaginable exactitude. Hermann Helmholt's visual depictions of muscle contraction with the graphical method, for example, brought new meanings to precision, physiology, and the body.[45]

Central to the cultural and scientific appeal of precision instruments were the numbers they generated, the graphical and tabular representations they made possible, and—as this book shows—the ranking of social groups they produced. Empirical validation through measurement enhanced the authority of technical instruments to produce reliable, valid, reproducible, and what came to count as "objective" knowledge in the mid-nineteenth century.[46] Difference became a fact of nature, the social decisions that went into the development of measuring devices obscured.[47] In generating numerical readings, the spirometer promised to capture—and to order—the abstract, invisible entity of lung capacity. Statistical techniques (such as race correction) could "smooth out" the messy reality of individual and social group variability. Although statistical efforts to erase the wide variability in lung function were unsuccessful, they were successful in masking the uncertainties rooted in measurement, allowing for innate explanations for racial difference to flourish.[48] The spirometer conveyed a sense of authority and trustworthiness, thus positioning the instrument to adjudicate societal debates. As this book argues, the social, political, and scientific processes by which spirometric measurement produced and obscured knowledge about the messiness of human variation were integral to the racialization of the instrument.

The racialization of the spirometer did not, however, emerge fully formed. A central point of this book is that race became a key organizing principle of spirometry *in dialogue with* other categories of difference—including occupation, social class, gender, and disability—whose cultural salience changed over time and place. As spirometric measurement moved between various social worlds, it incorporated new social meanings, both continuous and discontinuous with earlier ones. Whiteness has, however, "historically come at a price."[49]

In the nineteenth century, the use of the spirometer extended well beyond medicine. Initially linked to industrialization, it was deployed not only to diagnose disease, but also to measure vague yet culturally resonant qualities such as vitality, fitness, efficiency, and well-being, mostly of male working-class bodies. By the second half of the century, anthropometrists were adding lung capacity measurements to their growing armamentarium. Some predicted its utility for life insurance assessments. Initially concerned with white males, physical educators considered lung capacity a marker of vigor and vitality. The spirometer's potential for surveillance of labor—whether police, military, or industrial—was key to its initial appeal. In the twentieth century, medical and industrial uses would converge, as the spirometer was deployed to adjudicate the politically divisive issues of disability and compensation for work-related disease in which race and class were intertwined.

Moving across different sociopolitical, scientific, and national domains, the spirometer was an astonishingly flexible device. During its constant readaptation to new spheres, it gained legitimacy as a tool to probe the secrets of nature. Indeed, the credibility of this device—and its mobility—were mutually reinforcing. As its epistemological relevance faded in one domain, it was taken up, adapted, and investigated in another. In the process, an industry for the manufacture of the spirometer emerged. As the material infrastructure to support lung capacity measurements developed, the entity produced by the spirometer became "real," credible, mobile—and racialized. Why was this device so extraordinarily flexible? To what can we attribute the authority that allowed knowledge of vital capacity to travel so rapidly across the world? And why did spirometry allow for such sweeping claims about bodies—all with little contestation?

Outline of Chapters

This book tracks several key moments in the history of spirometric measurement. Examining the transnational exchanges of spirometric knowledge among Britain, the United States, and South Africa, three countries whose knowledge networks were central to the racialization of spirometry in the English-speaking world, I explore how and why the spirometer became enmeshed in social debates over industrialization, labor, and especially race. Emphasizing the social *and* scientific context of "invention," the material dimensions of the instrument, the evolving infrastructure for its manufacture, and innovations such as portability, I follow the racialization of spirometric measurement through its transnational travels during the nineteenth and twentieth centuries. I conclude with an examination of the racial context of spirometry in twenty-first-century biomedicine.

My purpose is not to write a comprehensive history of the spirometer. There are many aspects of the instrument—such as its role as a medical device in the establishment of pulmonology as a medical subspecialty—that I mention only briefly. I could have placed much more emphasis on the manufacturing industry that arose around the spirometer, a fascinating project in itself. Because of the long history of globalization of American notions of race and the vast Anglo-American spirometry industry, this book follows the processes of racialization within and across three English-speaking social worlds. Although I briefly mention the travels of the spirometer to other European countries, such as Germany, and to Asia, including China and India, an examination of how spirometric measurement intersects with race in the non-English-speaking world remains an important area for further study.

Chapter 1 begins in mid-nineteenth-century Britain, at a moment of growing cultural enthusiasm for precision instruments, innovation in statistical analysis of biological phenomena, and acute social and political anxieties about unruly working-class bodies. In this context, John Hutchinson, a University College, London-trained physician and medical innovator, built a new spirometer that he demonstrated to learned London societies. Although credited with inventing the spirometer, Hutchinson's work is best understood as the adaption to large-scale population studies of a device that physiologists had used in the laboratory since the seventeenth century.

Hutchinson's rigorous methods of analysis and categories of classification reflected mid-nineteenth-century concerns. By assembling large sample sizes, visually representing data in tables and graphs, and categorizing information hierarchically according to male occupations, Hutchinson positioned himself to make sweeping scientific and social claims for the spirometer that were readily communicated to other scientists. In reporting the correlation between height and lung capacity, Hutchinson claimed that the spirometer revealed laws of nature. He promoted the spirometer's potential for monitoring the fitness of the police and armed forces, screening of life insurance candidates, and diagnosing tuberculosis. Although the possibility of managing tuberculosis, the great scourge of nineteenth-century Britain, interested scientists at the time, practitioners were more ambivalent about medical technologies, and uptake of spirometry in medicine was fitful and uneven.

Authorized by elite scientists, in the United States, spirometric measurement was deployed in contentious debates about race, freedom, and human worth. As chapter 2 shows, knowledge of Hutchinson's work traveled quickly throughout the Continent and across the Atlantic, where physicians and statisticians marshaled spirometry's power to mark black bodies as fundamentally flawed. Whether on the plantations of the American South or on the battlefields of a bloody Civil War, race replaced occupation as the organizing principle of spirometric measurement. This chapter argues that the deployment of the spirometer to quantify racial difference enhanced the instrument's credibility.

Samuel Cartwright, Southern physician and slave owner, was an early adopter of the spirometer. Later, Benjamin Apthorp Gould, working for the United States Sanitary Commission, published a seminal anthropometric study (still cited by present-day pulmonary researchers) in which he devoted an entire chapter to the lower lung capacity of black soldiers as compared to whites. Explicitly choosing to classify subjects by race and nativity, rather than occupation, Gould "let the facts speak for themselves"—and loudly did they speak. Thirty years after Gould's study, Frederick Hoffman, later chief statistician for Prudential Life Insurance Company, singled out Gould's chapter in his 1896 racist diatribe *Race Traits and Tendencies of the American Negro* to question who was manly and civilized and therefore entitled to freedom. Despite vigorous contestation by leading black intellectuals W. E. B. DuBois and Kelly Miller, the hierarchy of lung capacities established at this moment in history became scientific fact. Finding its way into Charles Darwin's *Descent of Man and Selection in Relation to Sex,* by the mid-nineteenth century the notion of innate racial differences in lung capacity was firmly established through a constellation of overlapping and mutually reinforcing socioscientific theories and practices.

Spirometric measurement provides insight into the mutually

constitutive projects of producing whiteness and blackness in the United States. In chapter 3, I track the uptake and use of lung capacity measurements as anthropometric variables in the white middle-class domains of physical culture and physical education. While Gould drew on anthropometry to compare black and white bodies, describing and producing the contours of both whiteness and blackness, physical educators, on the other hand, eschewed direct racial comparisons, drawing on anthropometry to craft the potentialities of an Anglo-Saxon race. Beginning with the work of Edward Hitchcock at Amherst College, physical educators measured lung capacity with fastidious detail on thousands of middle-class college students, defining and monitoring fitness and working through prevailing cultural anxieties about Anglo-Saxon manhood and womanhood. Continuous technological innovation with the spirometer supported this vast enterprise. By the end of the century, a large infrastructure for the manufacture of the spirometer had developed, positioning the device to be adapted to an array of medical uses in the early twentieth century.

Chapter 4 analyzes the social contexts in which spirometric measurements were deployed in Victorian and Edwardian Britain. With the growth of the industrial working class, bodies were simultaneously a source of wealth and disorder. Drawing on principles of science, the language of improving the physical and moral condition of the "racial stock" framed the fitness movement in Britain. At the turn of the century, fears of national decline and race degeneracy intensified. In the aftermath of the South African War (1899–1902), vague notions of "physical culture" merged with the technocratic national efficiency movement. In such a climate, the idea of "efficiency" as something that could be measured and quantified had a receptive audience.

Linking vital capacity—crudely estimated by chest measurements—to labor, physical educators such as Oxford's Archibald MacLaren carried out anthropometric studies on the bodies of the English male elite at midcentury. In the hands of the technically talented Francis Galton, spirometric measurement later became a refined scientific endeavor with explicit social goals. Attuned to imperial concerns and fearful of national degeneration, Galton promoted mass anthropometry to mark, monitor, and rank the efficiency of the "race." The indefatigable Galton delivered on his promise by combining simple measurements, which included "breathing capacity," into a single test for "bodily efficiency." Funds were insufficient for bodily efficiency to become a component of civil-service examinations and interest in this device as a measure of fitness died out. But the spirometer remained on the move.

Chapter 5 travels back to spirometry's biomedical beginnings to examine the transnational projects of standardization and knowledge exchanges among physician-scientists in the United States, Britain, and South Africa in the early twentieth century. Emphasizing the dynamic interplay between technological innovation, social context, and racialization, this chapter addresses the significance of local standardization projects to global ideas of innate difference in lung capacity. In the United States, hospital-based physician-scientists interested in respiratory disease turned to the spirometer in their efforts to place their practice on a scientific foundation. In Britain and South Africa, innovation with the spirometer centered on its utility as a screening tool for the air force and as a marker of fitness and vitality. Carnegie Foundation researchers working on the "poor white problem" in South Africa also drew on vital capacity measurements. Through philanthropic health programs of the Rockefeller Foundation, both in China and in the American South, researchers again applied spirometry to the topic of racial difference. By the end of the 1920s, the idea of racial difference in lung capacity had become scientific "fact," laying the foundation for future transnational race-based research.

Chapters 6 and 7 return to the context of occupation to examine the relationship among technological innovation with the spirometer, social crises over work-related disease and disability, and race. From the coal mines of South Wales to the gold mines of South Africa, workers, industry, and governments looked to the spirometer to adjudicate workers' compensation, a historic compromise among labor, capital, and the state. As an instrument already linked discursively and materially to problems of vitality, efficiency, and the fitness to work and fight, the spirometer seemed ideally positioned to mediate conflicts between worker and employer. Government researchers at the Pneumoconiosis Research Unit (PRU) in South Wales, established by the Medical Research Council after World War II, honed the instrument for this important task. Out of this local context grew transnational collaboration between a PRU scientist and an American physician that produced the statistical technique of race correction.

As detailed in chapter 7, labor strife helped to establish a PRU in

Johannesburg, South Africa. Racialized systems of labor prevailed and spirometric measurement focused on white bodies until the late 1960s when comparative research began. The white Mine Workers Union, embattled with the state over compensation for occupational silicosis since the early twentieth century, helped to bring spirometry into state surveillance mechanisms for occupational disease and compensation negotiations. Lacking similar statutory rights to medical surveillance, black miners were not examined spirometrically. This chapter shows how, in a local context that excluded blacks from medical care, the spirometer came to embody whiteness, just as it did in the domain of physical education, but for very different historical reasons.

In tracking the uptake, dissemination, and use of spirometric measurement across time and place, *Breathing Race into the Machine* demonstrates that racialization of spirometric measurement was not inevitable. The spirometer was deployed in a variety of ways for many different reasons over time and space. During the course of its travels, this tool gained legitimacy as an arbiter of scientific truth. Consequently, when the spirometer was applied to race, it made the idea of racial difference difficult to contest and dislodge. The question of inevitability is a crucial political and scientific point. If racialization was not inevitable, it is possible to change racialized thinking about the device. Popular and scientific ideas of race, and their intersections with notions of fitness, vitality, and efficiency, are mutually reinforcing. Teasing apart how social assumptions about race and racism work in scientific practice can provide us with the insight to craft alternative narratives. As genetic explanations for lung function gain momentum in this era of "race-based medicine," the need to open a space for alternative narratives becomes more pressing. The hierarchical ordering of lung capacity along racial lines, dating from the mid-nineteenth century, should alert us to a problem in our way of seeing, knowing, and studying the health significance of this anthropometric measure.

When presenting this work, I am often asked "Are the differences real?" "What are we to do?" or "Aren't we damned if we do and damned if we don't?" This book does not attempt to answer these questions directly. Instead, it suggests that we should be asking different questions, questions that probe how and why spirometry became racialized, questions that are attuned to paths not taken, questions that examine possibilities not pursued.

"Inventing" the Spirometer
Working-Class Bodies in Victorian England

Arguments about the constitution of medical
knowledge were arguments, very often public,
about the organization of society. Medical men
and others built into their models of the body and
disease prescriptions for maintaining or changing
the social order.

CHRISTOPHER LAWRENCE
Medicine in the Making of
Modern Britain, 1700–1920

With a landed aristocracy in crisis, labor in turmoil, and the
specter of revolution across the English Channel still poignant for
the ruling classes, the first half of the nineteenth century in England was a period of acute cultural anxiety. The industrial economy
was expanding, but so were urbanization and overcrowding. As approximately one-eighth of England's population crowded into London in the 1830s, bourgeois urbanites came ever closer to epidemic
diseases rampant among the unruly working class.

Disease, however, was not just restricted to the seemingly degenerate bodies and lax morals of the lower classes. As literary critic
Bruce Haley observes, "throughout much of the Victorian period
. . . it was difficult ever to feel comfortable about the state of one's
health."[1] Urban pollution, respiratory afflictions, and other "filth diseases," from which no one, regardless of class, could wholly escape,
haunted the popular psyche.[2] The laissez-faire state's response was

contradictory: while parliamentary legislation regulated factory conditions, sanitation, and slum clearance, the liberal bourgeoisie's commitment to minimal government intervention in industry and commerce tempered reform.[3]

For the visionary middle classes, a productive labor force was central to the prosperity of the nation. As anxieties over health mounted, the British state began collecting data to police disease-ridden bodies of the lower classes more systematically. Beginning in the 1830s, reformers were busy developing statistical methodologies to document a working class physically (and morally) debilitated by poor nutrition, long hours in hazardous factories, and squalid living conditions.[4] Secretary to the new Poor Law Commission Edwin Chadwick's famed 1842 *Report on the Sanitary Conditions of the Labouring Population* laid bare the public health crisis emerging in the cities of England.

Liberal and radical social reformers framed their polemics about public health around vague notions of vitality, physique, constitution, and degeneration. Whether in Victorian novels or reformers' tracts, anxiety over the vitality of uncontrollable masses living in squalid slums and laboring in dangerous and unregulated factories pervades accounts of urban life in England. In recounting the chaotic living and working conditions of the laboring classes, Friedrich Engels lamented the "mental and physical lassitude and low vitality" and "marked relaxation of all vital energies" generated by overcrowded housing and factory work.[5] According to historian Anthony Wohl, workers' physical ailments signaled their particular occupation, be it "potters' asthma," "matchmakers' necrosis," "black spit," or the pervasive social threat, "phthisis."[6]

With its potential for policing the body, on which industrialization had placed brutal new demands, the spirometer emerged as a device to monitor vital processes, capacities, fitness to work, and disease. It was not inevitable that spirometric measurement would perform such broad social and technoscientific functions. Rather, spirometric measurement of what would be termed "vital capacity" became, in the words of historian Lorraine Daston, a culturally salient "scientific object" for historically contingent reasons.[7] With this in mind, I ask: How did anxieties about industrialization get embedded in the spirometer and the entity it purported to measure? Why did other monitoring devices, such as the inspirator and the stethometer disappear, whereas the spirometer lived on?[8]

This chapter explores the discursive and material processes by which socioscientific claims about the spirometer and vital capacity gained epistemic authority in nineteenth-century Britain, such that its virtues would quickly travel the world over. Specifically, I examine how British physician-scientist John Hutchinson's work on vital capacity of the lungs intersects with three aspects of emerging Victorian science: (1) the state of physiology and medicine; (2) societal fascination with precision instruments and instrument making; and (3) the institutionalization and professionalization of statistics, with its attendant innovations in the presentation and analysis of scientific "facts." Finally, I consider the transnational pathways by which knowledge claims about spirometry circulated worldwide, laying the foundation for its racialization.

A Matter of Priority

John Hutchinson (1811–61) is typically credited by both his contemporaries and modern pulmonologists with "inventing" the spirometer. Born of a distinguished middle-class family of farmers, parish clerks, and "gentlefolk" in the coal-mining region of Newcastle-on-Tyne, Hutchinson's coal merchant father introduced him to the problem of mine ventilation as a young man. We can only speculate whether these underground excursions made Hutchinson aware of respiratory diseases afflicting coal miners. We do know that he was drawn to a career in medicine, and initiated his medical studies in London in the 1830s at the newly established University College. Over the next fifteen years, the physician-scientist assumed a variety of positions: as surgeon to the Southhampton Dispensary, as physician for the Britannia Life Assurance Company, and as assistant physician at the recently opened Brompton Hospital for Consumption and Diseases of the Chest in 1850.[9] Inspired perhaps by his experience in collieries and his work with an insurance company, Hutchinson brought his interests in mechanical engineering, medicine, statistics, and physiology to bear on the mechanics of respiration as it related to scientific research, health, and public policy.

Beginning in 1844, Hutchinson started presenting his research findings and the elegant apparatus he designed and built to the venerable London Society of Arts and the Statistical Society of London. He also published several papers in rapid succession in influential journals. Notably, Hutchinson was the first to coin the term "spirometer," to name the entity it measured "vital capacity," to adapt the instrument for quantitative studies in large groups, and to present measurement data in tabular and graphical form. On the basis of this work, Robert Bentley Todd, Fellow of the Royal College of Physicians, invited him to write the entry on the thorax for the prestigious *Cyclopaedia of Anatomy and Physiology*.[10] Hutchinson's status as inventor is remarkable in that he only published for eight years, after which he abandoned scientific research and left England for Australia.[11]

Variably referred to as a pneumatic apparatus, pulmometer, breathing machine, breath-meter, breath-measurer, or air-holder, the life histories of the spirometer are more complex than the notion of a single invention conveys. For centuries, researchers experimented with devices that measured the volume of air in the lungs; a few even anticipated its potential as a marker of disease.[12] Beginning with John Alphonso Borelli in the 1680s, experimentalists struggled to define the precise volume of air inspired and expired and the concept of normal or "standard" lung capacity.[13] R. Menzies described placing subjects into a hogshead filled with water to determine the amount of water displaced during respiration.[14] Tackling the nature of disease, the best means of cure, and the mechanical effects of respiration on the lungs, physician Edmund Goodwyn's experiments—mostly on living animals—included measuring lung volumes in human cadavers with a simple device he called a "pneumatic vessel."[15] For Goodwyn, however, the goal of "establish[ing] a medium" volume of lung capacity remained elusive.

Brainchild of physician Thomas Beddoes, the Pneumatic Institution was established at Clifton in 1798. The Institution was a technologically innovative site of research on the therapeutic properties of gases, especially when the pioneering chemist Humphry Davy was director. Working with Beddoes, Davy, and inventor James Watt, the chemist William Clayfield constructed the "mercurial airholder and breathing machine."[16] This device, adapted from Watt's gasometer, was a cutting-edge apparatus for measuring lung capacity.[17]

Featuring glass cylinders, brass arms, a mercury seal, and a system of weights to force air through mercury and stopcock modifications to enhance precision, Davy's celebrated *Researches, Chemical and Philosophical; Chiefly concerning Nitrous Oxide, or Diphlogisticated Nitrous Air, and Its Respiration*, published in 1800, featured Clayfield's elegant apparatus (Figure 2). Davy considered the search for a standard lung capacity useless. His own lung capacity, he observed, was "most probably below the medium."[18] Although Davy

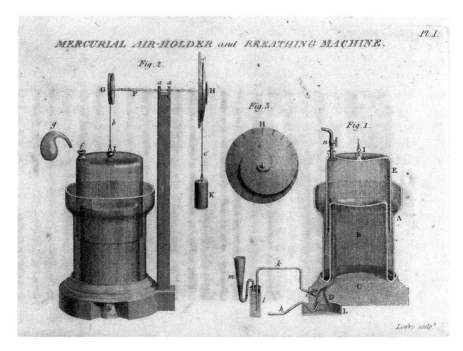

FIGURE 2. **Clayfield's Mercurial Air-Holder and Breathing Machine.**
From Humphry Davy, *Researches, Chemical and Philosophical: Chiefly concerning Nitrous Oxide or Dephlogisticated Nitrous Air and Its Respiration* (London: J. Johnson, St. Paul's Churchyard, 1800).

was not to pursue work with the "mercurial air-holder and breathing machine," he claimed its potential was "capable of more extensive application than any other."[19] Other experimentalists, such as Johannes Purkinje, continued to innovate with the spirometer to study the physiology of respiration.[20]

E. Kentish was likely the first to apply this type of technology—in his case, a device he called the pulmometer—when he published on its use in the diagnosis of disease in 1814; he also began relating lung capacity to the concept of physical fitness.[21] Kentish's health studies were soon followed by those of physician and provincial reformer Charles Turner Thackrah (1795–1833), who used the pulmometer to conduct a pioneering health survey to chronicle the bodily damage of industrial processes on workers, professionals, merchants, and gentlemen in England.[22] In his widely acclaimed book, *The Effects of Arts, Trades, and Professions, and of Civic States and Habits of Living, on Health and Longevity: With Suggestions for the Removal of Many of the Agents Which Produce Disease, and Shorten the Duration of Life*, Thackrah reported on lung capacity measurements of flax workers, soldiers, and shoemakers, relating changes in lung capacity to disease.[23] Thus, by the time Hutchinson began his work, the instrument we now know as the spirometer had an established place both in the experimental study of normal respiration and in surveys of respiratory disease. Despite continued innovation, the definition of "average" or "normal" lung capacity remained unresolved, limiting the clinical utility of the spirometer.

Thackrah's work caught Hutchinson's attention. Praising Thackrah's "industry and accuracy," Hutchinson continued with systematic study of the spirometer's potential for experimental investigation of the mechanics of lung function, diagnosis of pulmonary disease, and assessment of physical fitness.[24] Importantly, he combined his observations with statistics to probe general laws of nature, a major preoccupation of Victorian scientists and intellectuals. To do this, Hutchinson built what he called a "pneumatic apparatus," part of a larger "breathing machine," to measure the lung capacity of men categorized by occupational, social, and bodily status, including fire-brigade men, wrestlers, gentlemen, and a "well-made" dwarf (Figure 3). He presented and performed his empirical work in the tradition of testimonials to the London Society of Arts in May 1844, and weeks later, to the Statistical Society of London.[25] An inquisitive but sympathetic audience crowded the Statistical Society, staying long into the night to discuss Hutchinson's "highly interesting and laborious researches" and the instrument he named the "spiro-meter."[26]

According to Hutchinson, the spirometer's most significant contribution was to reveal a "rule," a general law of nature that demonstrated a

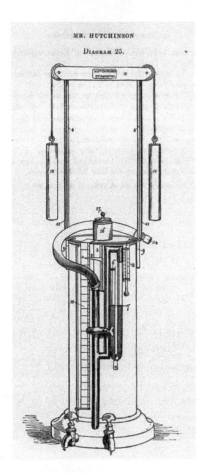

FIGURE 3. **Hutchinson's spirometer.**
From John Hutchinson, *Medico-Chirurgical Transactions* 29 (1846).

uniform relationship between lung capacity and height. Studying 1,200 men, a large sample size even by today's standards, he marveled that "so beautifully regular is the increase of capacity with the height, that the curve or continuous line in the above diagram will be seen to ascend with nearly perfect regularity."[27] Such scientific findings promised to resolve centuries of uncertainty over what—and whose—lung capacity was "normal."

Given his early interest in mine ventilation, Hutchinson likely had prior technical experience with equipment for measuring gases.[28] Like earlier investigators, his apparatus was based on devices widely used in gasworks, and its technical features were of great interest to Hutchinson.[29] In his first lecture to the Society of Arts, Hutchinson's apparatus was displayed prominently on a table. His paper published in the *Transactions of the Society for the Encouragement of Arts, Manufactures, and Commerce* emphasized the technological aspects of the machine rather than its measurements.[30] After these early reports, however, there is scant mention of the details of the apparatus. Measurement assumed priority.

Although we are most familiar with the spirometer, Hutchinson's "pneumatic apparatus" was actually composed of two separate precision instruments. These devices purported to assess distinct aspects of lung function—and of "vitality": the solid brass "breathing machine" measured the volume of the lungs, and an "inspirator" drew on the strength of the muscles to measure what Hutchinson called "respiratory power." For lung capacity measurements, study subjects were directed to inspire deeply and then to exhale through a flexible tube connected to a receiver. The receiver, an inverted graduated cylinder placed in another cylinder filled with water, was delicately balanced by weights attached to cords and pulleys. As air was expelled, the receiver would rise, and the volume of air exhaled was quantified in cubic inches on a scale. The mean of three separate measurements determined an individual's vital capacity. The device used to measure the strength of the intercostals muscles on inspiration and expiration was similar to a thermometer. The elevation of a column of mercury produced by each respiratory action was measured in inches, the numbers then organized into six categories, ranging from "weak" to "very extraordinary."

By the time Hutchinson spoke to the Statistical Society, he had already rationalized the naming of his "breathing machine." Calling it the "spirometer," a name not used by any previous investigators, would contribute to his status as inventor. According to W. H. Bodkin (in the chair), "other names have been given to it [the breathing machine], as 'stethometer,' or 'pulmometer;' but as the stethoscope is sometimes strangely miscalled, and as those who have been submitted to its application have been said to have been 'stereotyped,' the author thought it better to denominate this machine by some more intelligible appellation."[31] Although earlier publications included no illustrations, Hutchinson's 1846 monograph contained four illustrations of the spirometer and detailed instructions in the text for its use. Hutchinson ardently promoted the spirometer in London's professional circles. His advocacy, however, centered on the instrument as a tool for early diagnosis of tuberculosis and for life insurance assessments, rather than a device for physiological experimentation. Ultimately, the spirometer would prove consequential in all three domains.

Following his first two public demonstrations, Hutchinson published his research in the *Journal of the Statistical Society* and a 115-page monograph in the *Medico-Chirurgical Transactions* (the journal of the Royal Medical and Chirurgical Society of London), in which he expanded his theories of the capacity, power, and movement of the lungs.[32] Touted as "one of the most brilliant papers ever read before the Society," Hutchinson's report conceptualized the lungs as a perfectly proportioned and tightly regulated machine, powered by the thoracic muscles.[33] Although "ambiguously treated" by previous researchers, Hutchinson argued that the lungs' mechanisms and function could be understood experimentally.

With the help of this new, refined instrument, "lung capacity" became a discrete entity that could be measured, quantified, and ranked. A crucial early step in making spirometric measurement credible was to use the machine to divide the "quantity of air in the chest" into distinct spaces. Representing these spaces in visually striking diagrams, Hutchinson identified four separate compartments, each with its own "peculiar character": residual air, the amount of air remaining in the lungs after maximal expiration; reserve air, the amount of air remaining in the lungs after "gentle expiration"; breathing air, the amount of air required for "the ordinary gentle inspiration and expiration"; and complemental air, the amount of air available during strenuous exertion (Figure 4). According to Hutchinson, the last three divisions—reserve air, breathing air, and complemental air—were not static, but rather the product of carefully synchronized, machinelike movements of air into and out of the lungs. These movements were the result of the action of the chest muscles and under "the control of the will." Considering three of these divisions essential to life, he collapsed them into a single entity, which he named, for the first time, "vital capacity."[34] With Hutchinson's instrument, what had been formerly diffuse, ambiguously functional invisible spaces would now become visually distinct and measureable compartments that described, presumably with precision, the functioning of a vital organ system.

Had Hutchinson been the first to label the compartment of the lungs with a precision instrument, his status as "inventor" of the spirometer would be understandable. He was not, however, the only researcher studying the compartments of the lung at midcentury. In 1843, Julius Jeffreys (1800–1877), a well-known inventor and former medical officer in India, brought the experience of Europeans in the colonies to the study of the structure, function, chemical composition, and capacity of the lungs.[35] Insisting that knowledge of different climes and different races was essential to physiologists' understanding of the "functions and power of the various parts of the human body," Jeffreys, like Hutchinson, considered studies of lung capacity important both for the science of physiology and for medical therapeutics.[36] To address the oversights and inaccuracies

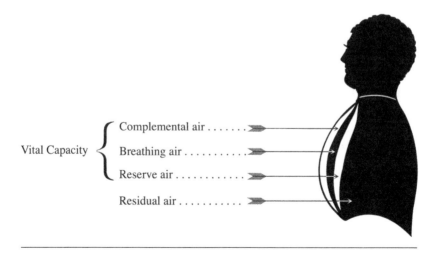

FIGURE 4. **The division of air in the lungs according to Hutchinson.**
From John Hutchinson, *Medico-Chirurgical Transactions* 29 (1846).

of previous experimenters, such as Thackrah, Jeffreys constructed an unnamed apparatus to identify four volumes of the lungs. To illustrate their functional significance in respiration, he labeled them residual air, supplementary air, the breath, and complementary air.

Despite Jeffreys's cutting-edge studies, Hutchinson is credited with identifying the discrete components of lung capacity. Nowhere in Hutchinson's thoroughly referenced publications does he cite Jeffreys directly. Some prominent textbook authors, such as William B. Carpenter, noted Jeffreys's contribution along with Hutchinson's, but others, such as William Senhouse Kirkes, single out Hutchinson's role in naming vital capacity, ignoring Jeffreys's work.[37]

There are several possible explanations for Jeffreys's obscurity. First, his approach to lung function was rooted in the anatomical tradition, a perspective that was losing ground with the rise of physiology. "The contents of the chest," he asserted, "must be studied collectively, as a compound of vital, chemical, and pneumatic operations, all acting in concert, and harmony."[38] Also, Jeffreys glossed over the technical features of his machine. The only reference to the apparatus was to its "accuracy."[39] Moreover, with a small sample size and large individual variability, the meaning of Jeffreys's lung capacity measurements was unclear. Finally, a charge of plagiarism by provincial physician George Calvert Holland, featured in the *Lancet,* undoubtedly undermined Jeffreys's credibility.[40]

That Hutchinson was not the first to study lung capacity, to "invent" the spirometer, to describe and name distinct compartments in the lungs, or even to use an instrument like the spirometer in large studies raises several questions: Why was Hutchinson's reputation as sole inventor of the spirometer so widely accepted? Why were scientists at the time—and for centuries to come—so receptive to Hutchinson's findings? How, in other words, did spirometric measurement become a credible "scientific object"?

In the next section, I will show how Hutchinson's narrow focus on the machinelike dimensions of the lungs and the functional significance of vital capacity and respiratory power; his large sample sizes, extensive statistics, tables, and graphs; his demonstrations of the spirometer; and his advocacy of the "rule" that height and vital capacity have a constant relationship placed him squarely at the forefront of what would become scientific medicine. In Hutchinson's hands, vital processes of the lungs would be defined with scientific precision.

Physiology and Medicine in Mid-Nineteenth-Century Britain

When Hutchinson conducted his research in the 1840s, British physiology was stagnant. Locked in a rigid conceptualization of the relationship between structure and function, physiology struggled to separate from anatomy and to establish itself as the foundational subject in medicine. Debates over vitalism, that is, the existence of a separate life principle, versus mechanism, in which life processes were reduced to immutable physicochemical laws, persisted in Britain, coexisting uneasily with experimentalism. The majority of medical schools in Britain evolved from hospitals, not universities, thus establishing medicine on a weak intellectual foundation. Until the late 1870s, there were no physiology journals or professional physiology societies in Britain. The lack of funding for laboratory research in Britain compounded these problems. Whereas professional research was emerging on the Continent, research in Britain was still primarily a gentlemanly avocation.

What we might now consider a multidisciplinary approach to scientific inquiry shaped Hutchinson's experimentation with the spirometer. His work linked the spirometer with two powerful traditions in nineteenth-century medicine: pathologic anatomy, which centered on anatomical diagnoses after death, and experimental physiology, which focused on functional changes in the living.[41] Letting the facts speak for themselves, he deftly avoided controversies (most likely unintentionally), including philosophical ones over vital principles, mechanism, the existence of a soul, and materialism. Since he didn't work with animals, Hutchinson managed to avoid the wrath of vocal antivivisectionists.

Focusing narrowly on vital capacity, Hutchinson simply ignored Jeffreys. For Hutchinson, previous work on the compartments of the lungs was chaotic. "Owing to the various terms used to designate the different divisions of respiration," he writes, "I have found it difficult to separate this division from the chaos of physical experiments hitherto made upon the lungs. And what I have gathered from them is of little value, not being connected with any other observations upon the human frame."[42] When Hutchinson deployed the spirometer to comment on a particularly contentious debate between Swiss naturalist Albrecht von Haller and professor of medicine at Jena Georg Erhard Hamberger over the role of the intercostals muscles in respiration, he did so within the narrow confines of the structure-function approach dominant in British physiology.

Just as Hutchinson negotiated the anatomical and physiological traditions, he also skillfully bridged scientific and clinical medicine. As an experimentalist, Hutchinson focused on probing the mechanics—not the histological and anatomical structure—of the lungs. Hutchinson and his supporters often repeated that his "rule" was a product of the experimental method, not speculation. While recounting Hutchinson's studies to the Royal Medical and Chirurgical Society, for example, respiratory specialist Dr. Cursham reports that

> Some very curious results arrived at by Mr. Hutchinson, might be adduced, to show the great importance, in a science like medicine, of our being guided by observation alone; for although they are not inconsistent with any known principles, they are very different from the conclusions at which we should have arrived by a priori speculation; such, for instance, is the law that the quantity of air which can be expired bears but little relation to the girth of the thorax, but is influenced mainly by the height of the individual.[43]

As a physician, Hutchinson integrated experimental physiology with anatomy and microscopic examination of lung tissue to understand the relationship between disease and vital capacity. He also produced beautiful casts of the anatomy of the lungs at death, which he displayed in his publications. In so doing, he respected, rather than rejected, contemporary physiologists who still adhered to an anatomical paradigm.

In 1846, Hutchinson replaced the conventional term "lung capacity" with the vague term "vital capacity." The reasons for this move are unclear. Other than a footnote to *The Spirometer, the Stethoscope, and the Scale-Balance,* in which he commented that "according to physiological nomenclature, perhaps the term *vital capacity* may be objectionable; but we adopt it for want of a better term, it being the largest volume of air which can be displaced by any movement of the living body, and may therefore be termed the *vital volume* or the vital capacity," Hutchinson never offered an explanation for the new nomenclature.[44] Yet, the language of vital capacity evoked the dynamic and life-supporting nature of respiration as opposed to the fixed and static anatomical structure of the lung. In contrast to the nebulous invocations of a "vital principle," Hutchinson's "vitality" acquired a material basis, grounded in observable facts and accessible through experiment. Through the spirometer, vital capacity and height were bound together by natural law; the relationship could be measured, compared, diagrammed, graphed, and organized into tables. The living process of breathing could be understood in mechanical terms.

Although we have no written indication that Hutchinson was a committed antivitalist, his conviction that the organized action of physical forces, which could be measured with precise instrumentation, explained lung function allied him with materialists in British experimental physiology for whom structure and function were inseparable.[45] While the boundary between science and theology was still being negotiated, the strident vitalism–materialism debates had died down, and the notion of a vital principle was losing its explanatory power. Yet, vague notions consistent with the operations of a vital principle—including "forces," "capacity," "vital energies," and "powers"—pervade Hutchinson's descriptions of lung function.[46] Thus, vitalistic concepts that embodied popular anxieties over the pernicious effects of industrialization on workers' "vitality" and "vigor" may have informed Hutchinson's renaming of the entity under study.[47] Although Hutchinson is a minor figure in the history of physiology, his investigations of lung capacity defined spirometry and shaped future clinical practice. This enduring legacy stems in part from making the science of spirometry legible to old and new.

Precision Instruments and the "Quantifying Spirit"

Over time, the development of precision instruments would transform—and order—bodily functions and chemical reactions. In improving on the senses, these devices ostensibly would elucidate the physicochemical laws governing living processes and materialize them through measurement. As part of the "quantifying spirit" emerging in the late eighteenth century in Britain, there was growing interest in the technical features of measuring tools like the spirometer.[48] Physicians frequently either made the instruments themselves or hired assistants to work with them. By 1861, London was a major site of manufacture for precision instruments, including the spirometer.[49]

Despite this enthusiasm, the incorporation of technology into clinical medicine was slow and uneven. At midcentury, clinical practice still relied on physical examinations and medical histories, rather than machine-assisted diagnosis of disease. Physicians were overworked, and few had expertise in using precision instruments. Debates over the changing nature of medicine emphasized the importance of clinical experience.[50] Although exciting for experimentalists, manually recording measurements was time-consuming, making instruments like the spirometer daunting for physicians. In the absence of already-established norms, the many observations needed to interpret variability in healthy people were unrealistic in the clinical context, limiting the utility of spirometric measurement.[51]

Another barrier to clinicians' adoption of the spirometer was its lack of portability. Hutchinson's spirometer was large and unwieldy, and not suitable for the cramped quarters of a physician's office or for house calls. The device required a large amount of water, and the need to close the stopcock immediately at the end of expiration was difficult for an untrained operator to manage. In his 1844 report on Hutchinson's lecture to the Statistical Society, Sykes emphasized that "the apparatus might be rendered portable; a simple Indian-rubber bag might be employed to bring home an observation of capacity on an individual, and the breath might then be measured by the breath-meter at home."[52]

In an 1869 lecture at the Annual Meeting of the British Medical Association, physician W. P. Bain credits Hutchinson as the "brilliant" inventor of the spirometer but laments the general failure to use it in the early diagnosis of phthisis. "His physiological views were very extensively adopted, and they are now standard in all works on physiology. But how have we benefited by these discoveries? In the treatises on medicine at this day, they seem to be entirely ignored. . . . Dr. Guy, in speaking of respiration, treats very fully of the spirometer; and yet, when he treats on the diagnosis of phthisis, not a word is spoken of its practical value." He attributes these shortcomings to "the bulk, the weight, the consequent want of portability, and general complex arrangements of stopcocks and valves."[53] For some physicians, the spirometer could be "one of the most excellent diagnostic helps in diseases of the chest."[54]

Growing fascination with precision instrumentation coexisted with anxiety about the role of instrumentation in medicine. According to the *British Medical Journal,* "It is not difficult to foresee the time when the prescribing chemist will be a thing of the past. There will, in fact, be no need for him: his shope will be crowded with penny-in-the-slot machines, by the use of which the patient's weight will be taken, his eyesight tested, his urine examined, his vital capacity ascertained, his muscle power measured so that it can be made up by an assistant."[55]

Notwithstanding these concerns, the spirometer continued to engage the imagination of innovators, instrument makers, and entrepreneurs. In a monograph published in 1852, the year he left England for Australia, Hutchinson called attention to recent technological innovations: the Jappaned spirometer, which enclosed weights in tubes, and the Dial-face spirometer, which enclosed the entire apparatus in a stylish mahogany case. While stressing its ease of use since "it is not merely a measuring gasometer," the monograph also addressed the difficulty of "correct" manufacture and recommended spirometers made by the firms of Mr. Ewart and the Mathematical Instrument Makers, Negretti and Zambra, both of London, for physicians' offices or life insurance companies.[56]

By the 1870s, several different models of the spirometer were commercially available. With a surge of patent applications in the 1880s, the total reached twenty-seven by the end of the century.[57] Innovations included coin operation, increased portability, reduced cost, glass cylinders, and improved accuracy.[58] In 1870, London innovator Robert Mann Lowne (1844–1928) applied to the British Office of the Commissioners of Patents for a patent on a fan-wheel spirometer.[59] Lowne went on to become a scientific instrument maker of some renown, in the tradition of craft-based manufacture.[60] By the late 1870s, Lowne had solved the problems of portability and cost, and his spirometer was distributed, along with other apparatuses for anthropometric studies, by the London firm Hawksley. As one advertisement in a popular manual on anthropometry noted, "the instrument [spirometer] is very portable and sensitive," and, at £5 10s, it was priced similarly to other anthropometric instruments.[61] New versions of spirometers continued to be featured in medical journals over the next few decades.[62]

"An Avalanche of Numbers":
Categories and the Institutionalization of Statistics

The first three decades of the nineteenth century were years of cultural enthusiasm for counting—what Ian Hacking calls "an avalanche of numbers."[63] During this period, quantification became a privileged form of producing knowledge about society. In the 1830s, statistical societies professionalized this enthusiasm for numbers— though not without tension and outright contestation. Initially excluded from the British Association for the Advancement of Science, statistics was embroiled in debates over its legitimacy as an objective, value-free science, distinct from the domain of politics. Its utility in public health, politics, and economics initially undermined its claims to objectivity. For a variety of reasons—including the emergence of the "tabular form" of representation—statistics became accepted as a science, although debates continued over whether it was a science in its own right or primarily a method in service to other sciences.[64]

The reformers of this period drew on and contributed to the emergence of statistics in a project that Mary Poovey terms "disaggregating" a social domain, separate from but related to the political and economic spheres. This process of "making a social body" real was central to the consolidation of the apparatuses and power of the modern British nation-state, placing industrial workers—and the casual poor, in particular—under the gaze of middle-class reformers and requiring new systems and tools of surveillance.[65] By producing numbers and representing them as unmediated facts, statistics offered a tool whose epistemic authority was enhanced by the experimental methods and instrumentation of the natural sciences.

Medical statistics, a branch of statistics distinct from public health, was in its infancy when Hutchinson was conducting his research. The large volume of numerical determinations (ten thousand "facts" by his own estimation) replaced a priori speculation with empirical observation. The ways in which he categorized, represented, and analyzed these numbers impressed contemporary scientists, placing him squarely in the mainstream of this emerging field. The 1849 entry on "medical statistics" in the *Cyclopaedia of Anatomy and Physiology* articulates the growing centrality of numbers to the science of medicine:

> There is no science which has not sooner or later discovered the absolute necessity of resorting to figures as measures and standards of comparison; nor is there any sufficient reason why physiology and medicine should claim an exemption denied to every other branch of human knowledge. On the contrary, they belong in an especial manner to the class of sciences which may hope to derive the greatest benefit from the use of numbers. . . . The absolute necessity of observation and experiment towards the improvement of the science and art of medicine, in the widest acceptation of those terms, may, therefore, be safely taken for granted. The only points upon which any serious difference of opinion or divergence of practice exists, are the degree of care and accuracy which should be brought to bear on individual observations and experiments, the properties which fit single facts to be thrown into groups or

classes; the language which ought to be employed in expressing the general results of such classifications; and the number of facts which, being so grouped or classified, may be required to establish a general proposition.[66]

To Hutchinson's esteemed London audience, observation, experiment, exact measurement, and visual depiction of physiological phenomena, all enhanced by instruments of precision, signaled progress in science and medicine.

Medical statistics grounded Hutchinson's empirical work. Unlike investigations of the chemical composition of the air, in which "one experiment established the chemical law," Hutchinson claimed, "thousands are required to determine the physiological question."[67] Most striking to contemporaries (and most significant to his legacy) was Hutchinson's claim that these thousands of facts revealed a "conspicuous" relationship between vital capacity and height. From this relationship one could discern the "rule" that "'for every inch of height (from 5 ft. to 6 ft.), eight additional cubic inches of air, at 60°, are given out by a forced expiration.'"[68] Testing this rule and exploring its mathematical details was a huge undertaking, one that would occupy researchers for the next century and a half.

With large numbers, moreover, it would be possible to determine a "healthy standard," a critical step to demarcating abnormality. So enamored was Hutchinson of the "rule" that any deviation raised the specter of disease. Between his 1844 and 1846 reports, he increased his sample from 1,151 to 4,000 people. Informed by the Belgian mathematician Adolphe Quetelet, who first proposed the notion that anthropometric measurements followed the laws of chance, Hutchinson attempted to establish laws by correlating vital capacity with a variety of "collateral observations" of height, weight, and chest size, which he then arranged into a series of tables.[69] With this data he constructed tables of lung capacity measurements that made the spirometer more authoritative than previous pulmometers.[70]

As already noted, apparatuses and tables were two central elements of practice that authorized Hutchinson's empirical work. To these we must add a third element—people. The use of dwarfs and giants in his demonstrations and publications is of particular interest. Along with other "curiosities"—such as dancers and singers—dwarfs and giants were exhibited at fashionable parties in the 1840s and frequently used in scientific study.[71] Hutchinson's demonstrations with these "curiosities" placed him in the mainstream of medical statistics.[72]

Hutchinson identified Robinson, the dwarf, and Randall, the giant, by name in several published reports. In the early 1840s, Hutchinson examined Freeman, the American giant who traveled to Britain for prize fights, before a big fight and later as he languished and died from tuberculosis. The deterioration of Freeman's vital capacity during his struggle with tuberculosis illustrated the connection Hutchinson sought to make between vital capacity and disease. Exhibiting dwarfs and giants in scientific demonstrations was not simply an exercise in exotification. As "extreme values," they had an acknowledged place in statistical methods and theory. According to Guy, extreme values, which had been understudied, were a critical test of "numerical theories." Averages represented "probabilities," whereas extreme values represented "possibilities." Including dwarfs and giants, who represented deviations from the typical form, further rationalized the correlation between height and vital capacity. Through the typical form, "chaos and confusion became order and regularity, and hence resulted the beautiful law."[73]

As the credibility of statistics grew, the authority of narrative description diminished. As Poovey points out, however, the process of legitimizing "figures of arithmetic" as opposed to "figures of speech" was slow, uneven, and not absolute.[74] In Thackrah's writings, for example, lung function measurements were less important to assessing health than stethoscope-assisted physical examinations or interviews with workers. With only two mortality tables, statistical analysis remained marginal to this narrative of workers' health experiences. Thackrah did not elaborate on lung capacity, ascribe any particular meaning to measurements of lung capacity, or make explicit comparisons between different groups of workers. Similarly, few diagrams, tables, or figures and limited mathematical analysis of lung volumes appeared in Jeffreys's largely textual argument. In contrast, Hutchinson's work featured tables, graphs, and visual images, replacing earlier stories of individual people's health experiences. Hutchinson did not, however, completely jettison narrative. In deploying extensive description as well as numbers to support his claims, he successfully negotiated the social controversies around statistics at midcentury.

Hutchinson's publications made extensive use of tables, graphs, elaborate images of the instrument, and drawings of the lungs with their component parts, several of which continue to be printed in textbooks. He was a skilled draftsman and apparently drew the near-photographic images himself.[75] In one of his earliest presentations to the Statistical Society, Hutchinson papered the walls with tables and distributed copies to members of the audience.[76] In his publications, he presented data in both tabular and graphic form, as physiologists had begun to do.[77] Although his statistics were rudimentary, Hutchinson's use of a precision instrument that appeared observer-independent and value-free heightened their credibility.

Statistical methods, however, could not resolve the ambiguity inherent in the variability of lung capacity measurements. Averages produced with large numbers masked the unpredictability of biological processes. Despite this messiness, the belief in the existence of a rule—a natural law defining the relationship between vital capacity and height—was strong. The problem of a normal standard would haunt the technology for another century and a half, but the idea of a rule lived on.

"Collateral Observations"

Numbers, of course, have no meaning in and of themselves. As Hacking points out, "counting is hungry for categories."[78] In the case of the spirometer, numbers acquired meaning through the sociopolitical projects of categorizing people and linking "collateral observations" to these categories. One notable feature of Hutchinson's statistical analyses was the prominence of occupational categories as a framework for organizing data generated with the instrument.

Thackrah was the first to deploy occupational categories in a spirometric study of the "problem" of industrial workers and their diseased bodies. As one of the generation of liberal reformers anxious about the "condition of England," Thackrah's empirical study of the industrial working class was important. In 1816, after training at Guy's hospital in London, Thackrah returned to Leeds, a rapidly industrializing, prosperous northern town known for its dyeing houses, woolen mills, and flax-spinning factories. After settling in Leeds, he cared for poor patients through the Workhouse Board, trained private students in surgery and apothecary, lectured at the Philosophical Hall, taught anatomy and surgery at the new Leeds School of Medicine, and began studying the health effects of manufacturing industries.[79] By organizing his treatise on work-related disease according to occupation, Thackrah cast working-class bodies as objects of scientific study and of social reform. Through his studies, a wider scientific audience became aware of the pulmometer, a version of the spirometer. Thackrah was not alone in focusing on occupation. William Farr, director-general of the newly formed General Register's Office, would soon create a system for recording mortality rates by occupation. Occupation as an organizing principle of scientific investigation was a sign of the times.

Hutchinson's use of occupational categories to analyze his data remained important long after he ceased research.[80] The occupational categories that he analyzed are "of particular note."[81] Unlike Thackrah, Hutchinson's main interest was not to probe the bodies of the industrial working classes. Rather, Hutchinson's project was to establish a standard of health drawing on representatives of "robust physicality"—specifically the police and armed forces, two groups that Continental anthropometrists routinely measured. Healthy military men and a smaller number of pugilists formed comparison groups to the presumably less healthy classes—of artisans, paupers, gentlemen, and "girls." Not surprisingly, bodies of the police and pugilists were good specimens with high lung capacity; artisans were "a very poor set of men"; gentlemen were "very low in power."[82]

That Hutchinson would select these occupational groups is not surprising. At midcentury, military men represented ideals of physical fitness. Yet, the reliability and efficiency of the armed and police forces in the face of social chaos was a source of anxiety to the nascent British empire.[83] In *The Condition of the Working Class in England,* Engels notes the problem of finding adults fit for military service.[84] An effective police force was only established in London in the late 1830s to combat rampant theft from warehouses, markets, docks, and railways. The language and practices of science distanced Hutchinson from the raging political debates over public health and social reform; however, embedded in the selection of men of the armed forces as standards of health were growing cultural anxieties over bodily degeneration, the nation-state, and empire, all themes that would reach a fever pitch toward the end of the century.

In the first—and probably most significant—table, Hutchinson presented to London societies mean measurements of vital capacity for men in each work category, but he only made crude comparisons among these categories in relation to one another. Hutchinson believed that, beyond creating a healthy "standard," the spirometer also held great promise for making comparative judgments, of individuals and groups. He explicitly promoted the instrument not only for the selection of men for the police force, fire brigades, and various branches of the military, but also for the inspection of prisoners and for the screening of life insurance applicants. With even more variables to be considered in the future, he opined, "we should then see more clearly than we do at present, what trade, occupation, or locality, was most conducive or deleterious to life and health."[85] Supplementing statistical probabilities and expert judgment with more precise biological predictors of health promised to assist the unstable insurance industry in its quest to manage risk profitably with minimal government intervention.[86]

Hutchinson was most concerned with the condition of male bodies. Whether because of their "peculiar costume" or "costal breathing," the bodies of women were aberrant, peripheral to his main conclusions. The invisibility of women in Hutchinson's demonstrations, published tables, analyses, and discussions is striking. In his paper on respiratory power, women warranted only a brief mention. When women are present, they—like dwarfs and giants—embodied biological difference and abnormality. For example, although he claimed to have examined vital capacity in twenty-six "girls" (a mere 0.12 percent of the total sample), Hutchinson presented little data on females in his monograph. The only data on women comes from a small experiment in which he estimated the vital capacity of six female and fourteen male cadavers by measuring their "conformation and general dimensions" and applying the "rule" derived from living males.[87] (Despite the fact that all six dead women had a higher vital capacity than five of the dead men, an 1879 British medical text asserted that "the vital capacity of women is much less than that of men.")[88] While discussing respiratory movements, Hutchinson claimed females were more limited than males because their "costal breathing is a provision against those periods when the abdomen contains the gravid uterus," not because of their "peculiar costume."[89] In later work, he saw no theoretical reason why the vital capacity of females might differ from that of men. Although the topic required more investigation, it was vital capacity in males that would hold the attention of Hutchinson and many future researchers.

As mentioned earlier, in emphasizing the spirometer's utility for early diagnosis of phthisis, this type of research was part of a medical world that was beginning to see itself as scientific—and numerical precision was nothing if not scientific. The potential of spirometry for early diagnosis of phthisis was important to the promotion of the device. Yet, of Hutchinson's very large sample size, only 2.8 percent of people were classified as diseased. These small numbers, however, did not prevent him from making a bold claim—that a precise 16 percent decline in vital capacity marked phthisis. Although some writers were skeptical, by linking a numerical figure with the spirometer, he underscored the promise of this new technology to distinguish health from disease with precision—and to manage the leading cause of death in industrial Britain.

The general laws of nature fascinated Hutchinson, but as a physician working for an insurance company, he framed this pursuit in public health policy terms. He begins his first major publication in 1844 by stating that, "if in the present day there is one subject pre-eminently engaging the public mind, it appears to be the best means of preserving the public health. And if any one among the various divisions of that subject can be ranked before another on the score of utility, it should seem to be, that regarding the effects produced on individual health by particular occupations." He continued: "I would also respectfully invite the attention of prison inspectors to this apparatus. Let every man that enters prison be tested on entering, and again on leaving; a comparison of the two observations will determine his loss or gain in health and strength. Also I solicit the attention of those who examine for insurance offices; since even non-professional men can make these experiments with certainty. . . . And, lastly, I would recommend it to the consideration of all who inquire into the effect of employments upon health; for by it I have shown how low the printers and the artisans rank in that respect."[90] Although Hutchinson anticipated the cultural work of spirometry, the task of developing "normal" standards, organizing occupations into a rigid hierarchy, and exploiting the instrument to mediate the scientific and social worlds would be left to twentieth-century researchers.[91]

Transnational Exchanges of Spirometric Knowledge

Knowledge of spirometry spread transnationally, as scientific journals translated and published reports of Hutchinson's public demonstrations and textbook authors promoted his findings.[92] Between 1844 and 1861, when Hutchinson died at the age of fifty, at least sixteen published abstracts or translations of his work on spirometry appeared in Britain and on the Continent. A full translation of his paper in *Medico-Chirurgical Transactions* was published in Germany, where researchers were particularly interested in the diagnostic potential of vital capacity in respiratory disease.[93] Technologically oriented physicians in the United States—many of whom were trained at German universities where physiology and instrumentation to support it flourished—engaged the technology to help diagnose tuberculosis.[94] In an 1847 letter to the editor of the *Boston Medical and Surgical Journal,* a reader referred to Hutchinson's "unique and very valuable" *Medico-Chirurgical Transactions* paper:

> If there has not been any extended notice of this paper by our journals, it has occurred to me that it would be not unacceptable to give it such an one at least as would arrest the attention of those in our profession who interest themselves in its advancement; the number of whom, "on this side of the water," I am led to believe is not small.[95]

By the 1850s, in the United States, as in Britain, skepticism among practitioners tempered enthusiasm for the instrument in early diagnosis of latent phthisis.[96] Using a spirometer similar in design to Hutchinson's, William Pepper, a private practitioner in Philadelphia, conducted his own empirical investigations on a series of twenty-seven men from various occupations who had been admitted to Pennsylvania Hospital. Pepper acknowledged that the instrument could sometimes be useful in detecting tuberculosis but concluded: "we are more liable to be misled by the spirometer than by the stethoscope."[97] On the basis of an even larger series, Dr. E. Andrews noted in 1854 that "this instrument cannot be relied on for diagnosis except where the previous vital capacity of the individual is known."[98]

Despite some physicians' reservations, the spirometer's accuracy, ease of use, and modifications for mass screening opened a market niche in North America. Dr. S. Weir Mitchell, most famous for his treatment of neurasthenia, the rest cure for women, and the collection of statistics "of the native born white race in North America," adapted a dry gasometer to survey the pulmonary capacity of five hundred men. Along with a craniometer, he exhibited this small (14" H x 11" W) instrument at a meeting of the Academy of Natural Sciences of Philadelphia in 1858. Apparently, there was sufficient interest in making such measurements that Messrs. Code and Hopper, manufacturers of gas meters in Philadelphia, made large numbers of the instruments, which were sold for eight to ten dollars, nearly half the price of other spirometers on the market. Still a complicated device, this new version did reduce friction and made more accurate measurements (Figure 5).[99] In 1862, a Dr. Bowman from Montreal published detailed specifications for a technically simpler spirometer constructed with two tin containers similar to a stovepipe.[100]

Along with scientific journals and presentations at professional meetings, textbooks facilitated transnational exchanges of knowledge about spirometric measurement. In the first edition of his widely circulated textbook *Principles of Human Physiology, with Their Chief Applications to Pathology, Hygiene, and Forensic Medicine,* renowned textbook writer William Carpenter, professor of medical jurisprudence at the University of London, drew attention to the variability in lung capacity measurements.[101] By the third edition, published in 1846, Carpenter acknowledged Hutchinson's work on the relationship between height and lung capacity. Subsequent editions in Britain and the United States continued to highlight Hutchinson's contributions, engaging with the American debate over whether muscular power was a determinant of vital capacity.[102] Given Carpenter's stated goal only to "select the most important and the most stable—not rashly introducing changes inconsistent with usually-received views," the inclusion of Hutchinson's research so soon after its publication is significant.[103] To Carpenter, Hutchinson's investigations offered the possibility of resolving centuries of uncertainty over the meaning of average values.

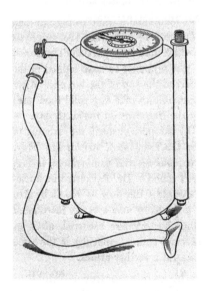

FIGURE 5. **The spirometer used by S. Weir Mitchell, 1859.**
From *Summary of the Transactions of the College of Physicians of Philadelphia.*

In physiology textbooks in this period, the object of interest is lung capacity, rather than the technological instrument used to measure this entity. Few textbooks illustrated the apparatus.[104] In contrast to physiology, textbooks of medicine tended to ignore lung capacity measurements until about 1876, when noted London medical educator John Syer Bristowe devoted a section in *A Treatise on the*

Theory and Practice of Medicine to spirometry. Bristowe emphasized the constant relationship between lung capacity and stature (Hutchinson's rule) and asserted its potential use for diagnosing lung disease. By the 1890s, spirometers the size of a watch were discussed in a U.S. medical textbook, although, according to one author, "there are many obstacles to the use of spirometers rendering them practically useless."[105] Thus, by the late 1800s, long after Hutchinson disappeared from the London scientific scene, spirometric measurement had an accepted place in physiology textbooks—and increasingly a place in medical textbooks—in Britain, the Continent, and North America. Hutchinson's reputation as inventor, experimentalist, and visionary scientific thinker was secure. According to historian Christopher Lawrence, "his life tables for the insurance companies and his spirometry readings [had become] tools for describing the population as a whole, for constituting the normal but also for situating each individual in relation to it."[106]

As the social and scientific meanings of spirometric measurements were being negotiated, uptake of the technology by medical practitioners in both Britain and the United States proceeded in fits and starts. There was little consensus on the appropriate relationship between medical judgment and numbers produced by machines. The resources for new medical technologies in British hospitals were limited.[107] Although mentioned in textbooks, it is unlikely that physicians outside of London encountered the spirometer in their training, further limiting its use in clinical diagnosis. In terms of respiratory disease, the identification of the tubercle bacillus and the discovery of X-ray imaging in the late nineteenth century offered more promise in the early diagnosis of phthisis than measurements of vital capacity. Indeed, spirometry would not influence patient care in Europe or North America until the early twentieth century—and even then its clinical utility would remain uncertain and contested. Despite this lack of enthusiasm for spirometry among medical practitioners, the technology would flourish in two spaces where its strengths were transferable: life insurance and the emerging science of anthropometry. Both sites provided opportunities for transnational innovation and experimentation and for enhancing the legitimacy of spirometric measurement as a scientific object.

Indeed, Hutchinson's occupation as a physician for a life insurance company, an emerging transnational industry, likely influenced his experimental investigations with the spirometer. He often wrote enthusiastically about the device's utility for life insurance assessments. In his last publication, *The Spirometer, the Stethsocope, and the Scale-Balance,* Hutchinson provided a physician's testimonial to benefits of the device for insurance: "I now never examine a person for life-assurance without trying him on the Spirometer, and feel persuaded, if it were generally used, many lives would be refused which are now taken."[108]

Conclusion

During the second half of the nineteenth century, spirometric measurement emerged as a credible scientific object. In this same period, the metropolitian bourgeoisie was preoccupied with both working-class bodies and, increasingly, the "varieties of mankind." Although anthropometrists were eagerly measuring and comparing physicial traits of Europeans to non-Europeans, there were no explicit attempts to compare lung capacity by racial group in Britain in this period. Yet, race hovered over the technology. Toward the end of the century, vital capacity measurements, as ordered and ranked through the frame of occupation (social class) and gender, would be deployed in debates over national efficiency and race deterioration. Charles Darwin would affirm racial differences in lung capacity. But Darwin did not turn to Britain to make his claims. Rather, it was the American context, where physicians working on plantations in the South and anthropometrists studying soldiers at the end of the Civil War used the instrument, that caught his attention. In the racially polarized context of the United States, notions of ranked difference in vital capacity would be extended from occupation and gender to race.

Black Lungs and White Lungs
The Science of White Supremacy in the Nineteenth-Century United States

We are never so steeped in the past
as when we pretend not to be.

> MICHEL-ROLPH TROUILLOT
> *Silencing the Past: Power and the*
> *Production of History*

Slavery had established a measure of man and a
ranking of life and worth that has yet to be undone.

> SAIDIYA HARTMAN
> *Lose Your Mother*

Coincident with its transnational dissemination, spirometric measurement became racialized across the Atlantic in the "natural laboratory" of the United States. As in Britain, the spirometer would travel across the distinct but sometimes overlapping domains of statistics, anthropometry, medicine, and life insurance, shaping technological innovation and producing new "truths" about the lungs of black people. Such nineteenth-century racial "truths" would frame thinking about difference in ways that persist in the twenty-first century.

The notion that blacks had weaker lungs than whites had a special place in the early American psyche. The first articulation of this view can be found in Thomas Jefferson's "Notes on the State of Virginia." For Jefferson, there were many physical distinctions between the races, including "a difference in the structure of the pulmonary apparatus . . . the principal regulator of animal heat." In rendering "them more tolerant of heat and less so of cold, than the whites," Jefferson's theories provided a rich foundation to speculate about the natural conditioning of blacks for agricultural labor—on the plantations of the southern United States.[1]

Jefferson's larger argument that blacks were a race apart reflected Enlightenment thinking on the North American continent. Although environmental explanations for racial differences were widespread among natural philosophers, hierarchical notions of race were built into classification systems, by thinkers like Linnaeus and later Blumenbach. As this chapter will show, however, such ideas did not go uncontested, even as they evolved and hardened.

The Science of White Supremacy

By the mid-nineteenth century, the use of science to support white supremacy was becoming more systematic. On the basis of skull measurements, leading scientists, such as physician Samuel Morton, made sweeping claims about innate intelligence and morality.[2] Northerners supported polygenist interpretations of racial origins, while Southern physicians deployed science to defend the institution of slavery. Less well known, however, is the positioning of respiratory biology, as a defining marker of physiological difference, in these debates.

As early as 1851, Southern physician and plantation owner and strident apologist for slavery Samuel Cartwright (1793–1863) argued that disease must be understood through the lens of "anatomical and physiological difference." Incorporating (and reinforcing) assumptions of physiological, mental, and moral difference in a widely cited article in the *New Orleans Medical and Surgical Journal*, Cartwright cataloged numerous racial "peculiarities," concluding that blacks were best suited to manual labor—specifically, to compulsory labor under control of the whites. Without specifically mentioning the spirometer, alongside many well-known absurdities such as drapetomania (slaves' compulsion to run away), Cartwright described racial differences in the respiratory system and their implications for labor. According to Cartwright, if left free, the lungs of blacks cannot "vitalize the blood." Incompletely vitalized blood was a racial characteristic that produced "lack of vitality," cured only by forced labor.[3]

By the following year, Cartwright connected precision instrumentation to Jefferson's natural philosophical theories to support his claims. To the skeptical question posed by Dr. C. R. Hall of Torquay, England, *"How is it ascertained that negroes consume less oxygen than white people?"* Cartwright responded: "I answer, by the spirometer." With the precision of a spirometer of his own design, Cartwright purported to show that "the expansibility of the lungs is considerably less in the black than the white race of similar size, age and habit." With the spirometer he could define the deficit quantitatively, leaving no question that difference represented pathology. "The deficiency in the negro," Cartwright wrote, "may be safely estimated at 20 percent." Foreshadowing arguments for race correction in the twentieth and twenty-first centuries, Cartwright cautioned that "to judge the negro by spirometric observations made on the white man, would indicate, in the former a morbid condition when none existed."[4] As the deficient respiratory apparatus affected "hebetude of mind and body," lower oxygen consumption had far-reaching consequences for labor. The authority of whites over Negroes was both a necessity and "a blessing."[5] Pointing to Jefferson's observations on "pulmonary apparatus of the negro," Cartwright claimed that difference was both anatomical and physiological."[6]

The prolific Cartwright was a leading pro-slavery theorist. Although his racist theories are offensive to most modern readers, he was not a fringe thinker at midcentury. Apprenticed to the eminent Benjamin Rush as a young man, Cartwright attended medical school in Maryland and Pennsylvania. Traveling to Europe in 1837, he gained a cosmopolitan sophistication evident in his theorizing. His use of a cutting-edge precision instrument elevated his status as a scientist. (To my knowledge, he produced the first published account of the spirometer in the United States.)

As historian Mia Bay writes in *The White Image in the Black Mind,* faced with the onslaught of an increasingly "scientific" racism, black intellectuals such as John Rock, James McCune Smith, and Frederick Douglass, mounted critiques rooted in a commitment to the essential unity of humankind. Drawing on eighteenth-century environmentalism, scriptural evidence, and historical understandings, they questioned racial distinctions. They published manifestos, abolitionist tracts, books, and essays; they preached in churches; and they gave public lectures to build a case for racial equality—albeit contradictory and sometimes tentative. According to Bay,

> the lack of emphasis on color in the racial thought of both unlettered
> and educated black Americans suggests that the preoccupation

with the corporeal character of black people that so distinguishes the racial ideology of white Americans was not the inevitable response of one physically different population to another, as scholarship on white American racial thought sometime seems to suggest. Rather than being a natural response to racial difference, the disdain white Americans expressed toward the color and physical being of black people reflects one of the ways in which this dominant group's racial ideology served to explain the subordination of black people as the natural condition of the black race.[7]

Free black David Walker, for example, called for a new ethnology: "'We and the world wish to see the charges of Mr. Jefferson refuted by the blacks *themselves,* according to their chance; for we must remember that what whites have written respecting this subject, is other men's labours and did not emanate from blacks.'"[8] Yet, as Bay notes, black ethnology was "to some degree, ensnared by the idea of race even as [it] sought to refute racism's insult to their humanity.... Equality *does not easily coexist with difference or separation.*"[9]

Physician James McCune Smith (1811–65), a contemporary of Cartwright's and the first African American to receive a medical degree, was an important figure in countering notions of innate black inferiority. Denied entry to American universities, McCune Smith received both his undergraduate and medical degrees at the University of Glasgow. Son of a prosperous New York merchant father and a slave mother, he was a successful practitioner, active abolitionist, respected statistical expert, and prolific writer opposed to colonization movements. Informed by climatological theories, McCune Smith located backwardness in both extremely hot and extremely cold climates, emphasizing the essential unity of humankind.

On the eve of the Civil War, McCune Smith published "Civilization: Its Dependence on Physical Circumstances," in the inaugural issue of *Anglo-African Magazine.* Drawing on Quetelet's notion of the "average man," he linked "advanced civilization" to mental and physical vigor, both of which he considered geographically changeable. As a physiological mediator between the external and the internal environment, McCune Smith viewed the respiratory system as an environmentally sensitive index of physical vigor. While noting that "the dark races in hot climates have flattened chests, from the relatively less exercise or expansion of their lungs in breathing," McCune Smith argued that blacks gained physical vigor when transported from tropical to temperate climates.[10] "This Afric-American race, are not only far superior in physical symmetry and development to the pure African now found on the coast, but actually equal in these respects the white race of Old Dominion, who have never lived in any but a temperate clime."[11] According to McCune Smith, the most advanced civilizations were those whose populations were mixed.

Anthropometry and the United States Sanitary Commission

The centrality of war to technological innovation is a consistent theme in the history of spirometry. Repeatedly, social anxieties about the physical fitness of soldiers were resolved through science and anthropometric measurement. A massive anthropmetric study of soldiers at the end of the Civil War was a turning point in the science of race difference.[12] On the battlefields of a country divided by a bloody civil war, spirometric measurement gained further credibility as a marker of black/white difference.

In the wake of the early defeat of the Union army at the 1861 battle of Bull Run, President Lincoln authorized a group of prominent white intellectuals to create the United States Sanitary Commission to oversee relief efforts and improve hygienic conditions in the Union army. As members of an emerging class of experts seeking to organize U.S. society on a rational basis, the commission drew on an ideology of administrative efficiency. Commissioners recognized that, in addition to their philanthropic mission, the war presented a unique opportunity for statistical and anthropometric research. Underwritten by life insurance companies, research opportunities broadened as the military and naval service incorporated people of African descent.[13] Under the direction of the general secretary, Frederick Law Olmsted, in 1861 the commission undertook an ambitious two-part survey examining the physical and social characteristics of the volunteer army.

Olmsted was ideally positioned to carry out this work. Best known as a landscape architect, Olmsted had previously conducted a survey of the height, age, and nativity of one thousand laborers during his tenure as superintendent and architect-in-chief of Central Park in New York City.[14] Particularly interested in the effects of immigration on national character, Olmsted anticipated that these surveys would serve as "a sort of treatise on the established tendencies of the European races in the United States."[15] The commission shared his enthusiasm. Charles J. Stillé, the official historian for the commission, claimed that "the results arrived at by these examinations will probably afford the most important contribution of observations ever made in furtherance of 'anthropology,' or the science of man, considered in reference to his physical nature."[16] Until their resignations in 1863, Olmsted and the actuary Ezekiel Elliott oversaw the collection of data on the physical and social characteristics of eight thousand white soldiers, although the commission never analyzed or published the social statistics that so interested Olmsted.[17]

After Olmsted's departure, the board of commissioners appointed the esteemed Boston astronomer and president of the American Association for the Advancement of Science Benjamin Apthorp Gould (1824–96) actuary to the commission. In 1864, they asked him to conduct what would prove to be a seminal work in U.S. anthropometry. The first American to receive a Ph.D. in astronomy, Gould spent most of his career in Germany, the United States, and later Argentina, engaging in astronomical observations and analyzing massive amounts of data. In 1863, he was one of a small group of white scientists in Washington, D.C., who founded the National Academy of Sciences. As a renowned scientist and member of a prominent Boston family, imbued with the values of "precise measurement" through training in astronomy, Gould was a logical person to conduct this daunting survey.[18]

Focusing exclusively on physiological investigations, Gould used Olmsted's original questionnaire to guide inspectors' examinations of newly enlisted soldiers. However, the questionnaire had to be modified extensively to collect information on black soldiers who an ambivalent President Lincoln authorized in 1862 to serve in the Union army. Such a unique opportunity to measure the mental, moral, and physical dimension of racial difference, using modern precision instruments, was not lost on Gould, who matter-of-factly remarked, "the importance of such inspections [of black soldiers] need[ed] no comment."[19]

The product of this research—*Investigations in the Military and Anthropological Statistics of American Soldiers,* published after the Civil War in 1869—was a 613-page report. Filled with voluminous data on the physical characteristics of the men (stature, complexion, mean dimensions and proportions of the body and head, weight, respiration, pulse, pulmonary capacity, etc.), categorized according to nativity, age, and race, Gould expressed confidence that these statistics would "greatly surpass in amount all that has been previously gathered on the same subjects."[20] He wisely compensated for his lack of medical and anthropological expertise by consulting with "friends whose pursuits are of an anthropological or physiological nature."[21] These friends included the renowned Swiss natural philosopher Louis Agassiz of Harvard, member of the polygenist "American School of Ethnology" and fierce opponent of "amalgamation," whose interests in the "natural divisions of mankind" were already widely acknowledged.[22] With the assistance of these educated friends, Gould moved easily from counting stars to measuring people.

The commission had numerous specialized instruments made specifically for the survey, one of which was a spirometer. Despite the technical challenges of working with spirometers in the field, the decision to include spirometry in the survey was not surprising given the board's enthusiasm for science, measurement, and precision instrumentation. In contrast to Britain, where data was organized by occupation, in the United States, the classification systems of most interest were nativity and "race." The commission did collect data on occupation, but, unlike Hutchinson, Gould thought that the category would be too messy to analyze, so he limited his analyses to race and nativity.[23] For reasons that he did not articulate, Gould devoted an entire chapter to comparing aspects of lung physiology, most prominently lung capacity measurements. Unlike the majority of anthropometric measurements, he analyzed lung capacity *only* according to race, not national origin. In so doing, lung capacity in blacks, already demonstrated by Cartwright to be deficient, became a salient racial characteristic.

Expressing great admiration for the acknowledged pioneer in the field, Gould sought to extend Hutchinson's pioneering work with a larger sample size of 21,752 soldiers, sailors, students, and prisoners. Ever the meticulous researcher, Gould opened the chapter with two illustrations of "superior" spirometers, modeled on a gasometer built by the American Meter Company, suitable for conditions of war (Figure 6). The machine, its adaptability, and, most important, its precision captivated Gould and assured him of the credibility of the facts it would produce: "Far superior to the combrous and complicated apparatus hitherto employed for the same purpose," the spirometer was well adapted to the "rough usage" of the field, yet afforded "the highest degree of precision." He continued: "although

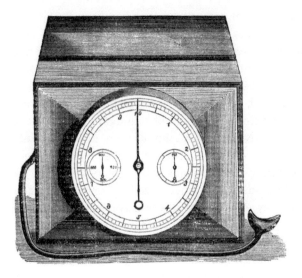

FIGURE 6.
Example of a spirometer used by fieldworkers in the U.S. Sanitary Commission's study of Union soldiers. From Benjamin Apthorp Gould, *Investigations in the Military and Anthropological Statistics of American Soldiers* (New York: Houghton, 1869).

there are of course many respects in which the experience now obtained would indicate important modifications of method, inquiries, and precautions, were this work to be repeated or continued, yet the instruments employed have given entire satisfaction and very few points have suggested themselves in which the apparatus could be clearly changed for the better."[24]

Comparing his findings to Hutchinson's, Gould displayed his "copious material" on the capacity of the lungs in relation to height, state of health, race, length of the body, circumference of the chest, play of the chest, and age. The first table, organized with elegant simplicity, laid the foundation for hierarchical notions of racial difference in lung capacity that survive to this day (Figure 7). Measuring lung capacity in cubic inches, obtaining a mean for each group, and arranging the data according to categories that dominated the popular (and scientific) imagination animated by civil war, Gould compared "White" soldiers, sailors, and students to what he labeled "Full Blacks," "Mulattoes," and "Indians"—under conditions of good health or "not in usual vigor." Depending on their state of "vigor," Gould reported that the lung capacity of "Full Blacks" was 6 to 12 percent lower than that of "Whites," and the lung capacity of "Mulattoes" was .023 percent lower than that of "Full Blacks." The measurements of "Indians" were equivalent to those of "Whites." Although Gould did not comment on the differences between "Full Blacks" and

"Mulattoes," a category only added to the U.S. Census in 1850, his discussion of the "inferior vitality" of the "Mulatto" clearly reflected mid-nineteenth-century cultural anxieties about race amalgamation. The differences in lung capacity in blacks and whites could not "fail to attract attention at first glance." Rather than comment further, though, Gould simply asserted that "its bearings are perhaps better manifested by the more detailed tabulations which will follow."[25] In what by now had become a common rhetorical move in science, Gould, like Hutchinson, let the "facts" speak for themselves. And they would continue to do so well into the twenty-first century.

Although they construct a compelling story about racial difference, the simplified tables in *Investigations* mask the messier reality of internal conflicts with the Office of the Secretary of War, Edwin Stanton, over access to data, incomplete information from harried examiners in the field, faulty equipment, setbacks owing to illness, and overwhelmed clerks slogging through voluminous data in Washington. Working at a feverish pace to publish, but nonetheless committed to accuracy, Lucius Brown, chief clerk in charge of data analysis, anxiously confided in Gould about lost data, discordant

TABLE I.

Average Capacity of Lungs.

	In usual Vigor		Not in usual Vigor		Total	
	No. Men	Cubic Inches	No. Men	Cubic Inches	No. Men	Cubic Inches
White Soldiers, Earlier Series .	4 837	175.655	1 915	155.699	6 752	169.995
White Soldiers, Later Series . .	8 895	187.868	1 541	166.321	10 436	184.686
Sailors	1 104	179.217	–	–	1 104	179.217
Students	288	204.382	–	–	288	204.382
Full Blacks	1 631	165.319	221	149.697	1 852	163.455
Mulattoes	671	161.635	138	145.428	809	158.870
Indians	504	185.058	7	179.286	511	184.978

FIGURE 7. **Summary table showing lung capacity measurements by race.**
From Benjamin Apthorp Gould, *Investigations in the Military and Anthropological Statistics of American Soldiers* (New York: Houghton, 1869).

results, and the difficulty of grouping data to give "satisfactory results." Regarding the Pulse and Respiration tables, Brown's anguish
about accurate categorization is manifest:

> The personal equation is evidently very large so that it is not pos-
> sible to compare the white and the colored races with any certainty
> of being right. The Full Blacks measured by Russell are unfortu-
> nately included with the Mixed Races as they were in the Spirom-
> etry tables but I have preferred that you should see the results
> as they now stand before making any attempts to correct or alter
> them. The colored men not in usual vigor are all together, never
> having been kept separate in the grouping.[26]

In response, Brown suggested that they "knock off about 60 of the
weak lunged."[27]

We can only speculate about the meaning of "satisfactory results"
and the precise methods Brown and Gould took to make them satisfactory. Ultimately, though, they published the data stripped of
messiness. In presenting a clear picture of whites having higher lung
capacity than blacks, white lung capacity became the standard of normal in the scientific imagination, both conceptually and empirically.

Racial assignment was not straightforward. Gould knew that
people did not fit into neat categories, as his detailed but confusing
revision of the original schedule made clear. He directed inspectors
to categorize soldiers according to their "stock," based on "appearance and statements of subject."[28] Otherwise they were to "state the
race, unless Caucasian, (as African, Malay, etc.); or if of mixed races,
and what" (226). He also instructed them to estimate "the proportion
of black blood" (although he gave no indication how this might be
identified or quantified). Using "the ordinary white private soldier
. . . as the standard of comparison," they were to assess the level of
intelligence—for blacks only (227).

Emphasizing his good intentions, Gould stated that "[s]trenuous
endeavors have been made to assort them [black soldiers] with more
nicety than has been found practicable, using various bases of classification. Three or more distinct races of negroes are to be found in
the Southern States, and these present themselves in every degree
and mode of admixture with one another and with the Indian and
white races" (297). But because "the different African races could
not be habitually distinguished from one another by our examiners,"
he proceeded to simply divide the "colored men" into two mutually

exclusive categories: "Full Blacks," in whom "no admixture of white or red ancestry was perceptible," and "Mixed Races" (297–98). Gould did not discuss the complexity of the category "White," even though he presented anthropometric data on white men by "Nativity."

From roughly 1840 to 1924, waves of Europeans immigrated to the eastern United States, first from Ireland, later from Southern and Eastern Europe. After the Civil War, "white" as a racial category became fragmented, as the state attempted to limit the rights of newcomers to citizenship. In the process, the black/white binary that prevailed prior to 1840 was partially undermined.[29] We see some of the instability of whiteness at work in Gould's classification of measurements by country of origin.[30] Yet, despite the disorder of immigration, lung capacity assessments, where black, white, mulatto, and Indians were the preferred categories, did not reflect the fragmentation of whiteness.

Other than vague references to "the effect of climate and soil upon the blacks," Gould avoided explicit explanations for racial differences in lung capacity. Instead, like Hutchinson, he let the facts—analyzed with statistical sophistication—speak for themselves. Not once did he address the comparability of conditions of life and labor of black and white soldiers. The majority of black soldiers in the survey had been enslaved on Southern plantations and suffered greatly as they flooded into Union camps. As has now been carefully documented, black soldiers in the Union army suffered a disproportionately high mortality rate, poor nutrition, and overcrowding in camps. They also received inferior medical care in the field and in segregated hospitals, and had higher rates of infectious diseases, such as malaria, yellow fever, typhoid fever, pneumonia, tuberculosis, and respiratory afflictions, some of which could affect lung function.[31]

Like Hutchinson, Quetelet strongly influenced Gould's belief that mathematical data, properly analyzed and interpreted, would reveal natural laws and biologically distinct "typical forms." Gould was so convinced of this unique opportunity for discovering "the type of humanity as well as the types of the several classes and races of man" that he rushed to increase the numbers of "colored soldiers" under study before they dispersed after the war. Upon completion of data collection, Gould sought to disseminate anthropometric measurement by distributing the apparatuses from the survey, including spirometers, among scientific and educational institutions in the United States.

According to Stillé, the work of the commission would be remembered for its contribution to "our permanent knowledge of physical laws, as well as to the maintenance of free institutions, to the perpetuation of American nationality."[32] African Americans, as revealed by natural law, were physiologically distinct racial types, low in the hierarchy of capacity and vitality, and outsiders to the American national project. Science and technology were central to promoting a racialized vision of the social, political, and economic order in the nineteenth-century United States.

"The Negro as a Soldier"

Although the Civil War studies helped to construct a scientific edifice for racialized bodies, scientific accounts of difference varied. While the Sanitary Commission focused on quantitative documentation of difference, a more complicated picture of physiology, racial difference, and human potential emerged from accounts of army surgeons who worked with black soldiers in the field. Abolitionist and surgeon for the Sanitary Commission Sanford B. Hunt questioned the model of difference promoted by men such as Samuel Morton, and concluded that the black soldier "has all the physical characteristics required [for military service], that his temperament adapts him [the soldier] to camp life and his morale conduced to this description. He is also brave and steady in action." With respect to pulmonary disease, though, Hunt accepted prevailing notions of greater susceptibility to tuberculosis and argued for more research on "measurements and the volume and the expansibility of the living thorax."[33]

Even more striking are the observations made during medical examinations on more than a million soldiers conducted by Jedediah H. Baxter (1837–90), chief medical officer of the Bureau of the War Department.[34] Like Gould, Baxter emphasized his mathematical expertise and use of the latest technologies, such as an "improved 'calculating engine.'"[35] Although the sample size was large, the measurements certifying fitness for military service were technically simple. In his report, Baxter included measurements of physical features, such as height, complexion, and color of the eyes and hair. He also noted the circumference of the chest—analyzed according to age, marital status, nativity, occupation, and race. Rather than employing the spirometer, the army surgeon's medical examinations estimated vital capacity by chest circumference at maximal inspiration and expiration—a method of assessment considered by

Hutchinson to be a reasonable approximation of spirometric mea-surement.[36] That he analyzed all variables in relation to chest cir-cumference highlights the importance of lung capacity as a marker of vitality and fitness.

Baxter's reservations about the precision of racial categories were more serious than Gould's. "The designation *'Colored Men,'*" he wrote, "intended to describe exclusively the negro and his hybrids, should not, perhaps, be admitted in scientific terminology on account of its obvious lack of precision, and its equal applicability to the ab-original inhabitants, as well as to more than one foreign race found among us."[37] Yet he too ignored the messiness, opting for common-sensical use of racial categories: "Usage . . . in the US has so confined the term to the single meaning, and the reports upon which these tables are based so constantly employ it," he concluded, "that it has been thought best to retain it." Once organized into tables, charts, and graphs, numbers took on the aura of scientific truth, thus mask-ing the ambiguities of classification.

Unlike Gould, Baxter found no racial differences in chest dimen-sions or pulmonary diseases. The mean chest circumferences of white and black soldiers were equivalent: 33.691 inches for black soldiers and 33.418 for white soldiers. Nor did chest expansion vary significantly by race or nativity: 3.232 inches for "colored" natives; 3.242 inches for white Americans; 3.272 for British Americans; 3.127 inches for English Americans; 3.208 inches for Irishmen; and 3.231 inches for Germans. Significantly, the rates of phthisis pulmonalis and general diseases of the respiratory system were lower among blacks than whites: for phthisis, 7.047/1000 cases for "colored" and 18.378/1000 for "whites"; and for respiratory disease, 4.22/1000 for "colored" and 10.142/1000 for "whites."[38]

Baxter's treatise contained both quantitative data and rich narra-tives describing the experience of army surgeons, the geography of the region, prevalent diseases, and causative agents of disease. He directed medical examiners to address "the physical qualifications of the colored race for military service" based on personal experi-ence. While contemporary stereotypes about race and race mixture pervade these evocative reports, they also convey a broad, if uneasy, consensus on the courage, strength, and soldierly qualities of black men. Reflecting ongoing debates over whether black recruits were fit for battle, some surgeons remarked on the intelligence of black soldiers. Especially intriguing are comments on chest development and capacity, which Gould found so deficient. A surgeon from New Hampshire pointed out, "of those presenting, the stature has been good, the development of the chest and muscles large. . . . I see no valid reason why they should not make efficient soldiers" (182). Another New England surgeon noted that the black soldier "possesses in general a sound and vigorous body, with a powerful development of the thorax and superior extremities" (237). To an examiner in West Virginia, "if bone and sinew, muscle, chest measurement, and general physique, are the criteria [the colored man] presents the greatest physical aptitude for military service" (370). Reporting from Kentucky, another surgeon asserted that "bodily, the negro is more strongly developed, and his lungs expand more freely" (394). Even more specifically, an Illinois examiner found that "in breadth and depth of chest, they have the advantage over other nationalities. They are, on the whole, a healthy and vigorous people" (433).

One possible explanation for the disparate accounts of racial difference in lung capacity presented by Gould and Baxter is sample selection. Gould's study was limited to volunteers, who were generally healthy, whereas Baxter's included volunteers, draftees, and regular soldiers, who varied in their physical condition. The rates of questionnaire completion might also have differed in Baxter's and Gould's samples. Another possible explanation is that Baxter and Gould situated themselves in similar, though distinct, epistemological traditions in science and medicine: Baxter was a physician, valuing direct experience and professional judgment, whereas Gould was a scientist, privileging experimentally derived, value-free data.[39] Limiting himself to quantitative data obtained with instrumentation and presented in tabular form, Gould constructed an uncomplicated narrative of profound difference between races. In contrast, relying both on quantitative data and qualitative accounts of army surgeons with direct field experience, Baxter found no evidence of physiological difference, predisposition to disease, or reduced "vigor." Where Gould's statistics erased the humanity of the people being measured, army surgeons—albeit grudgingly and informed by racist assumptions—were forced to acknowledge black recruits as human beings who were participating as active agents in their struggle for freedom. Thus, at this critical moment in U.S. history, when former or escaped slaves, fighting in an uneasy alliance with Northern whites, were engaged in "a general strike" against the plantation system, views of racial difference—whether physical, moral, or intellectual—were more fluid than later in the century.[40]

A Harvard professor and member of prestigious U.S. scientific societies, Gould was in a privileged position, and his views were adopted and passed on to future generations of scientists in Charles Darwin's *Descent of Man and Selection in Relation to Sex*. Published in 1871, only two years after *Investigations*, *The Descent of Man* pointed to the ways in which "the races of man" are similar and of one species. Linking lung capacity to the cranial capacity measurements of the American ethnologist Samuel Morton, however, Darwin drew on *Investigations* to highlight difference. "When carefully compared and measured, [they] differ much from each other—as in the texture of the hair, the relative proportions of all parts of the body, the capacity of the lungs, the form and capacity of the skull, and even in the convolutions of the brain."[41] He also noted Gould's evidence for "the inferior vitality of mulattoes."[42] Thus, both Gould's empirical data and his theoretical arguments reflected prevailing intellectual currents in America. Importantly, his data on lung capacity helped to shape Darwin's influential theories on the origin of races. In giving an evolutionary cast to lung capacity measurements, Darwin reinforced scientific arguments for a hierarchy of difference.

Medicine, Lungs, and the "Race Problem"

The idea that lungs were key indicators of biological deficiency permeated medical thinking throughout the nineteenth century. During Reconstruction, political commentators invoked the Civil War studies to buttress their beliefs that the emancipated Negro would die out.[43] Joining a long list of differences—such as insanity, promiscuity, and bone development—cataloged by Southern physicians, the lungs, and tuberculosis in particular, stood out as markers portending the future of the black race.[44] In the last half of the century, after the failure of Radical Reconstruction, Northern and Southern intellectuals revitalized extinction theories and continued to marshal notions of deficient lung capacity in social debates. In a long essay titled "The Southern Question," the New Orleans historian Charles Gayaree, for example, suggested that weak lungs might lead to the extinction of blacks:

> Should the black man die out in the end, as he probably will, of
> weak lungs and from the want of congenial air in the more elevated

region to which he has been raised, and to which he cannot be ac-
climated, let it not be recorded that it is due to bad treatment on
our part.[45]

During the 1880s and 1890s, many physicians accepted—and promoted—the notion that reduced lung capacity and predisposition to
respiratory disease marked blacks as inferior in the "struggle for
existence" brought on by emancipation.[46] Invoking statistical studies and postmortem examinations, W. J. Burt, secretary of the Texas
State Medical Association, attributed rising mortality among blacks
from consumption after the Civil War to "two causes—the *less lung
capacity* and the *smaller size of the brain of the negro.*"[47] In a similar
vein, R. M. Cunningham, a physician from the Alabama penitentiary
system, used black prisoners to posit that "normal thoracic movements in ordinary respiration are deficient, and that the thorax is
not capable of as great movement during forced inspiration and expiration." The causes, he argued, are "(a) in less lung capacity; (b) less
muscular development, particularly of the accessory muscles of respiration; and (c) the greater or less encroachment of the abdominal
organs."[48] But such views did not go uncontested. Black physician
M. V. Ball responded that "social conditions," not hereditary or "racial" difference, accounted for high rates of consumption in blacks.[49]

Despite contestation, racialized medical ideas, including those related to lung capacity, were widespread both in the North and the
South. By the end of the century, these ideas had penetrated scientific fields outside of medicine. In an address to the American An-
tiquarian Society in 1895, prominent child psychologist G. Stanley
Hall opined that "the color of the skin and the crookedness of the hair
are only the outward signs of many far deeper differences, including
cranial and thoracic cavity."[50] By the turn of the century, scientists
had implicated virtually every aspect of lung biology—size, weight,
function, susceptibility to disease—in black pathology.

"Race Traits and Tendencies of the American Negro"

The year after Hall's address, Frederick L. Hoffman (1865–1946),
a German-born, self-educated statistician who would become chief
statistician for Prudential Insurance Company, elaborated on the
connection between lung capacity, respiratory disease, and racial
inferiority. His widely reviewed monograph, *Race Traits and Tendencies of the American Negro,* published by the American Economic

Association in 1896, is significant for marshaling the authority of science—specifically the statistical method—to inform debates over the social, political, and economic consequences of emancipation that intensified during Reconstruction and its aftermath.[51] Through Hoffman, Gould's lung capacity measurements on an all-male cohort became a central feature of public discourse about the "race problem," ensuring Hoffman's international reputation for four more decades.

Perhaps because of his association with Frances Morgan Armstrong, manager of Hampton Institute in Virginia, Hoffman took a particular interest in the "race problem" early in his career as an industrial agent in the South.[52] In 1892, while working for the Life Insurance Company of Virginia, Hoffman published "Vital Statistics of the Negro" in *Arena,* a social-reform journal popular with Northern intellectuals. Hoffman's article used mortality data to reinvigorate the long-standing notion that blacks would become extinct under conditions of freedom.[53] This article caught the attention of John F. Dryden, the Yale-educated president of Prudential Insurance and future United States senator from New Jersey.

Differential mortality by race was particularly concerning to Prudential and Metropolitan Life Insurance, the two companies with the largest portfolios in industrial insurance, which catered to the working classes.[54] As many workers turned away from mutual aid societies, industrial insurance became profitable—but only if actuarial risk could be managed in workers who, because of poverty and occupational hazards, bore a high burden of disease. Soon after Dryden assumed the presidency in 1881, Prudential stopped issuing industrial insurance policies to blacks without regard to individual risk. According to historian John S. Haller, insurance companies, including Prudential, based this decision on the statistical evidence of higher mortality of blacks, provided by the Civil War studies, and "attitudes towards the Negro which became 'scientific' as they were mixed in with accumulated statistical materials."[55]

Frederick Hoffman's career brings this intertwining of race and science into sharp relief.[56] Despite a troubled job history, Hoffman's reward for the *Arena* article was a position at Prudential, where he remained for thirty years, influencing—and arguably further racializing—the life insurance enterprise in the United States. At Prudential, Hoffman continued his statistical investigations on the "race problem."[57] Claiming that his status as a German immigrant gave him a more objective view of this uniquely American dilemma,

Hoffman demonstrated his perspectives on the centrality of science to the solution of social problems. "Racial traits and tendencies" are fundamental to the social quandaries of the nation, he wrote. The social situation urgently needed an unbiased "presentation of the facts as they pertain to racial differences," analyzed according to the statistical method. "Race deterioration once in progress is very difficult to check, and races once on the downward grade, thus far at least in human history, have invariably become useless if not dangerous factors in the social as well as political economy of nations."[58] The future of the nation was at stake.

The key elements of Hoffman's argument can be summarized as follows. Blacks were physically superior during slavery because they lived under artificial conditions, protected from the "struggles for existence." Since the 1860s, however, black mortality had increased, owing to consumption, race amalgamation, a "tendency" to migrate to cities—and inferior lung capacity. No amount of philanthropy, education, or benevolent treatment could reverse this decline. The black "race" was doomed to extinction. In making this argument, the skilled statistician did not limit himself to "objective" statistical facts. Rather, Hoffman constructed a complex—and, to many contemporaries, persuasive—argument based on transnational data on racial difference, including government censuses, statistics of the colonial authorities in the West Indies, reports from South Africa, and statistics in the United States. He wove this data together with stories from scientific articles, the popular press, and personal anecdotes. Statistics from the West Indies were of particular import, because emancipation had occurred in the British colonies thirty years earlier than in the United States.[59]

Because the life insurance industry partially funded the United States Sanitary Commission, it is not surprising that Hoffman was acquainted with Gould's anthropometric findings. Indeed, for Hoffman, lower lung capacity was a central marker of racial inferiority. The third chapter of Hoffman's *Race Traits and Tendencies of the American Negro*, titled "Anthropometry," features "the most essential characteristics" to understanding the longevity, social use, and economic efficiency of races: weight, play of the chest, frequency of respiration—and lung capacity.

Combining data from Gould, Baxter, the surgeon general's report, the Freedmen's Bureau, and a study of twenty-four black and white adolescents in a New York reformatory, Hoffman made a rhetorically convoluted—if not tortured and incoherent—argument for degeneration since emancipation. In the process, he reinterpreted or dismissed data that contradicted his thesis. To establish the deterioration of African American "vital power" since emancipation, Hoffman leveraged Baxter's favorable assessment of black soldiers' physical condition in the army surgeons' reports, glossing over Gould's data for inferior lung capacity collected during the same period. In turn, to prove "lower vital power for the negro of the present time than for the negro of about thirty years ago," he highlighted results of a small study at the reformatory in Elmira, New York, which showed 8 percent lower lung capacity in black adolescent inmates.[60] Linking lower lung capacity directly to death rates in blacks, he posited that "the smaller lung capacity of the colored race is in itself proof of an inferior physical organism."[61] For Hoffman, lung capacity measurements taken with a cutting-edge precision instrument offered both an assessment of physiological function and scientific proof for the pervasive belief that "the race" was doomed to extinction, thereby justifying his mean-spirited calls to limit education and philanthropic efforts.

Explanations for racial difference at the turn of the century were simultaneously biological, cultural, and environmental.[62] No one explanation was necessarily less racist than another. Hoffman eschewed any determinist interpretation to explain the origin and persistence of "race traits and tendencies." To build an argument for change in vitality (which for him represented deterioration), Hoffman constructed notions of inheritance that were dynamic, fluid, and rhetorically contradictory—though always rooted in innate difference. Because he saw the physical, moral, and mental deterioration of African Americans as a process that began with emancipation, "race traits and tendencies" had to be changeable. Conversely, because Hoffman blamed "weak constitutions," rather than "conditions of life," for the loss of "vital power," "vitality," "vital resistance," and "vital force," "race traits and tendencies" needed to capture the pathological essence of African Americans. *Race Traits* is thus not only a response to pressing sociopolitical debates over emancipation, race amalgamation and extinction, and empire, but also a key text that invoked science to shape, sustain, and naturalize social debates.

Labor in the South was a pressing and contentious issue during and after Reconstruction. Both Northern capitalists and Southern planters feared that blacks, whose labor they desperately needed, would abandon the cotton fields. Reflecting widespread ambivalence toward free black labor, Hoffman's twisted logic shaped his arguments about lung capacity and black labor. Harking back to Jefferson, he argued that lack of "vital force" made blacks unfit for freedom and unsuitable to urban life and industrial labor. He argued that blacks were biologically and culturally fit only for agrarian labor. Accordingly, blacks should remain on the farms picking "fiber that clothed the masses of a ragged world."[63] Industrial work in factories, cotton and iron mills, or coal mines would, at least theoretically, be reserved for white labor, whether native or immigrant.[64]

While expressing indignation toward the debilitating effects of work on the health of white laborers in the "dusty trades," Hoffman's treatises on occupational disease are silent on the work and health of black workers. When he does address black health, as in the cotton ginning industry, "the susceptibility of the Negro" to consumption is the problem.[65] Thus, using Gould's measurements to mark blacks as biologically deficient, Hoffman marshaled science to restrict African Americans to the land. In Britain, the spirometer was used as a tool to monitor the efficiency of industrial labor; in the United States, it became a tool for marking racial difference and inadequacy for industrial labor.

A prolific writer, Hoffman maintained his interest in the "race problem" for his entire career.[66] In private letters, annual reports, public addresses, and published writings, innate difference between blacks and whites was a persistent theme. In an address to the Association of Tuberculosis Clinics in 1917, Hoffman expressed little uncertainty about the causes of racial differences in lung disease. "Much is said about poverty and its relation to disease, but my own investigations into the underlying condition responsible for an excessive frequency of tuberculosis, with respect to race, are quite convincing that the fundamental basis is heredity, rather than economic conditions."[67] By the Second International Congress on Eugenics in 1921, long after most had abandoned the extinction hypothesis, Hoffman still referred to the lack of "vital power" of people of mixed race and the probability of extinction.[68]

When his predictions of racial extinction were not borne out by the late 1920s, Hoffman's views on the future of blacks shifted slightly. Captivated by the achievements of the United States during its occupation of Haiti, Hoffman envisioned the betterment of the "primitive black race." The "spirit of liberty" exhibited by Haitians was "deserving of praise." Moreover, there was "evidence of the physical regeneration of the Haitian people." He left this "evidence" unstated, a surprising stance for the data-driven statistician. Hoffman's enthusiasm for "a new race of Haitians decidedly more resistant to disease and of a much greater degree of physical efficiency than any previous generation," however, was tentative. It could only be realized under imperialist conditions of white occupation.[69]

Contesting Hoffman

Public and scholarly responses to *Race Traits* were mixed. Judging from the many reviews of the book in popular and scientific journals—such as the *Dial,* the *Nation, Publications of the American Statistical Association, Political Science Quarterly,* and *Science—Race Traits* was a socially important treatise.[70] Most reviewers praised Hoffman's mastery of statistics. Some reviewers uncritically accepted almost all of his findings, including those related to lung capacity measurement.[71] Many who disagreed with him did not question the legitimacy of the statistical analyses.

While taking care to dissociate himself from Hoffman's conclusion that racial traits, not social conditions, caused difference, Gary N. Calkins of Columbia University simply noted the facts of "deterioration and decrease in vital capacity."[72] A skeptical reviewer in the *Nation,* on the other hand, warned that "if the negro in this country does not die out as Mr. Hoffman believes he will, the work as a whole will go its way along with the already almost forgotten articles which, a few years ago, demonstrated to the satisfaction of their authors that the negroes were increasing so rapidly that their ultimate and speedy preponderance in every Southern State was a melancholy certainty."[73] Rudolph Matas, famed New Orleans physician and author of "The Surgical Peculiarities of the Negro," gave Hoffman's monograph unqualified praise in a personal letter, reassuring him that his "views have been largely accepted and favorably discussed by the ablest critics and reviewers." "You are," Matas continued, "everywhere receiving the recognition that is due you for your remarkably conscientious, conclusive and in every sense monumental labor."[74]

As historian Samuel Kelton Roberts observes, the "politics of freedom, color, and labor" shaped medical views on race.[75] Although sometimes constrained by the discourse of black uplift, yet eschewing any notion of innate pathways to racial degeneration, African

American leaders decried Hoffman's racist theories.[76] Kelly Miller and W.E.B. DuBois mounted particularly trenchant critiques of Hoffman. Recognizing that *Race Traits* offered scientific support for racist ideology and harsh public policies aimed at limiting racial equality, both Miller and DuBois developed sharp appraisals of Hoffman's scientific findings, interpretations, and conclusions (Figure 8).

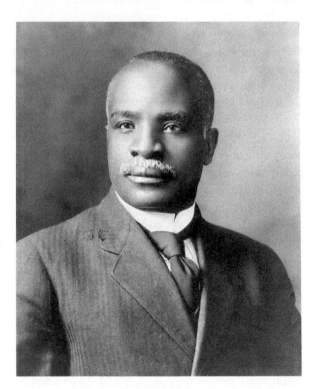

FIGURE 8.
Kelly Miller.
Photograph courtesy of the Moorland-Spingarn Research Center at Howard University.

A prominent Howard University mathematician (and the first black mathematics graduate student in the United States), Kelly Miller (1863–1939) was ideally positioned to engage directly the statistical basis of Hoffman's argument.[77] In "A Review of Hoffman's Race Traits and Tendencies of the American Negro," published in 1897, Miller carefully dissected Hoffman's science and its social implications. While affirming his own belief in "natural laws of population," Miller skillfully deployed many of the same statistics to refute Hoffman's conclusions on population decline. With biting sarcasm, he singled out Hoffman's ill-defined meshwork of innate, environ-mental, and cultural causes, dubbing Hoffman's repeated use of the language of "race traits and tendencies" as nothing more than "a blind force recently discovered and named by him," whose operation could be "suspend[ed] indefinitely or break loose in a day."[78]

Rather than contest the facts of "lung degeneration," Miller at-tributed the high mortality from consumption after emancipation to social conditions under which blacks lived and labored:

> The fact that under the hygienic and dietary regime of slavery, con-sumption was comparatively unknown among Negroes, but that under the altered conditions of emancipation it has developed to a threatening degree, would persuade any except the man with a the-ory, that the cause is due to the radical changes in life which freedom imposed upon the blacks, rather than to some malignant, capricious "race trait" which is not amenable to the law of cause and effect, but which graciously suspended its operations for two hundred years, and has now mysteriously selected the closing decades of the nineteenth century in which to make a trial of its direful power.[79]

Miller went on to question the low vitality of blacks, citing the "un-mistakable evidence of higher vital power among the colored pa-tients" offered by the surgeon-in-chief of the Freedmen's Hospital, Daniel Hale Williams. Dismissing the argument on anthropometry, Miller commented that "the data [on lung capacity and chest expan-sion] are so slender and the arguments are so evidently shaped to a theory, that we are neither enlightened by the one nor convinced by the other."[80] Hoffman's view, based on Gould's data, regarding inferi-ority of mulattoes, he acknowledged, was "almost or quite universal among competent authorities upon this subject." More research was necessary.[81]

Sociologist W. E. B. DuBois (1868–1963) also took on Hoffman's argument about the roots of the "race problem." In "The Study of the Negro Problems," published in 1898, DuBois placed the "problem" in a historical context, arguing that there are many "Negro problems" produced by social conditions, which changed over time. Professing faith in science and professional expertise but frustrated with the uncritical nature of the evidence about African Americans, DuBois historicized race in the United States. For him, "this example of hu-man evolution" required nuanced study that engaged with the his-tory of slavery. Although tinged with racial essentialism, by offering an alternative historical narrative of the life experience of African Americans, DuBois disrupted the notion of white normativity. With *Race Traits* in mind, he questioned how an argument about the physical condition of a race could rest on "the measurement of [lung capacity in] fifteen black boys in a New York Reformatory."[82] Stating resolutely "that there exists to-day no sufficient material of proven reliability, upon which any scientist can base definite and final conclusions as to the present condition and tendencies of the eight million American Negroes," DuBois, like many intellectuals of the day, considered the physical differences between the races striking and worth further investigation.[83]

Historians are rightfully cautious in ascribing intent to historical actors. Hoffman's views, however, can only be understood as racist, even in the context of the times. Ever fearful of the specter of socialism, Hoffman was a political and social conservative, a harsh apologist for vicious racist practices, including lynching.[84] At the same time, he was neither an extremist nor a marginal figure in his celebration of the physical and moral virtues of Anglo-Saxonism. Hoffman was a highly respected statistician whose ideas reflected contemporary views on race and influenced the thought and practices of antiblack propagandists, mainstream scientists, and liberal reformers.[85] In many ways, Hoffman defined the field of insurance medicine. While eschewing Metropolitan Life Insurance Company's more philanthropic reach, he shared with other Progressive-era reformers an enthusiasm for the political, economic, social, and moral principles of American industrial capitalism.[86] He also espoused faith in the expertise of middle-class professionals who were reshaping the culture of knowledge production in the United States.[87]

Hoffman's influence was vast. Through publications, speaking engagements before popular and scientific audiences, extensive foreign travel, and service on the boards of insurance, public health, and statistical societies, as well as his role as government adviser and educator, Hoffman worked indefatigably to shape policies of the state and civil society in the late nineteenth and early twentieth centuries.[88] His reputation continued to grow throughout his career, especially in the field of occupational health. Years later, Alice Hamilton, the highly respected occupational health physician and progressive reformer, referred to him as a "voice from the wilderness" on matters related to occupational health.[89] In her tribute, Hamilton—like other liberal occupational health reformers at the time—ignored that Hoffman spoke only for white workers.

Despite the eloquent critiques of Miller and DuBois, the idea that blacks and whites had different lung capacities became further entrenched in scientific theory and practice. Using innovative technology, Hutchinson had tentatively introduced the idea of hierarchical difference in lung capacity through his limited studies on occupation and gender. Building conceptually and empirically on this work, Gould studied exclusively male military populations to establish the "fact" of hierarchically ordered racial difference. Hoffman popularized this fact, linking lower lung capacity to inherent inferiority and slave labor to race.

Why have the arguments of Gould and Hoffman been so widely accepted? (As noted earlier, Gould continues to be cited to the present day.) This chapter has proposed some possible explanations for Gould's and Hoffman's credibility: their deployment of the statistical method at a moment when statistics was consolidating its legitimacy as a science; the separation of the social from the scientific in matters of health; and a long history of racist ideas about "pulmonary dysfunction." Yet, such explanations are incomplete. Although Miller, the mathematician, and DuBois, the social scientist, also drew on modern statistical methods to mount their critiques, mainstream racial discourses overwhelmed their criticisms of using lung capacity measurements to mark inferiority. How else, then, might we explain the persistence of ideas of innate racial difference in lung capacity?

One possible explanation is the prevalence of tuberculosis among lower classes, especially blacks. Tuberculosis was a leading cause of death in the United States well into the twentieth century, when chemotherapy became widely available. In the profound social dislocation induced by the Civil War, black mortality from tuberculosis soared.[90] Explanations for mortality, as Roberts has shown, drew on and contributed to earlier racial theories about biology and lungs. Yet, black medical opinion and an increasing acceptance of environmentalist theories in public health began shifting the discourse away from racial predisposition to tuberculosis by the 1910s. By the 1930s and 1940s, theories of racial predisposition to tuberculosis declined, at least for the moment.[91] Despite this shift, the notion of racial difference in vital capacity of the lungs, as measured by the spirometer, became more firmly entrenched in biomedicine.

Moving through Social Worlds

Another possible explanation for the persisting racialization of spirometric measurement could be the epistemic authority spirometry gained as it moved among the social worlds of medicine, anthropometry, and life insurance. During the second half of the nineteenth century, discussion continued in medical journals on the technical specifications, safety, reliability, accuracy, expense, ease of construction and use, and diagnostic value of the spirometer.[92] As in Britain, physicians in the United States were intrigued by but ambivalent about precision instrument-aided physical diagnosis.[93] Technologically oriented physicians, however, collaborated with instrument makers and other technical experts to modify the apparatus and promote its use in the clinic.[94] Drawing on eighteen years of experience with the spirometer, Dr. Joseph Jones, president of the Louisiana State Medical Society, promoted a modified device, termed the vacuum pneumatic spirometer. This instrument, which he used for eighteen years, "gives precision to diagnosis, and accuracy to prognosis."[95] By the turn of the century, physicians had considerable experience using the device to evaluate respiratory disease, while affirming the central role of medical judgment in interpreting numerical values produced by the machine.

In the second half of the nineteenth century, American scientists undertook more systematic measurement of human growth, development, "physique," and "bodily constitutions." Rooted in the climatological theories of French natural philosophers, the science of phrenology, technical innovations in statistics, and the ideas of positivist philosophy, the emergence of anthropometry as a scientific discipline coincided with the professionalization of the social sciences and the rise of insurance medicine. Some U.S. physicians, such as Henry P. Bowditch, respected Quetelet's anthropometric studies and had close contacts with European anthropometrists. However, according to James Allen Young, life insurance companies were the first to apply anthropometric measurements to disease prediction and the field of public health. With tuberculosis mortality a major concern, a simple anthropometric tool for screening applicants appealed to life insurance companies. Life insurance companies considered vital capacity a particularly important marker of life expectancy. As was the case for natural philosophers, anthropometrists, however, found the meaning of race to be ambiguous. For some races, anthropometric measures were changeable, whereas for other races, anthropometry defined a fixed essence of hierarchically organized difference.[96]

Screening applicants for life insurance, recruits for the military, candidates for police forces and fire departments, and workers in industrial settings was increasingly important to the burgeoning insurance industry in the nineteenth century. During the 1860s and 1870s, insurance medicine emerged as a distinct medical specialty in the United States. In a poorly regulated, fiercely competitive, corrupt, and rapidly expanding industry, however, the status of the profession was tenuous. The organization of professional societies and journals in the late nineteenth century that carved out a space for the specialty in an increasingly scientifically based medicine partly resolved the status question.[97]

Insurers were desperate to find a simple method—more precise than height and weight—to assess the risk of developing disease. But the most informative instruments to use as adjuncts to medical examinations remained unclear.[98] As a purportedly value-neutral device and despite the formidable challenges presented by its use and interpretation, the spirometer offered hope for the rational administration of life insurance policies. Responding to the high mortality rates from phthisis and the move to professionalize insurance medicine, William Gleitsmann, head physician at the Mountain Sanitarium for Pulmonary Disease in Asheville, North Carolina, promoted a quantitative cutoff in diagnosing incipient phthisis with the spirometer: "According to the unanimous consent of all investigators, the deviation from the normal figure, under ten or fifteen per cent, of the physiological capacity, allows us to assume the probability of an existing, although latent disease, whilst a decrease of twenty per cent gives almost certainty."[99] Based on ten years' experience with the device, Dr. Alexander Rattray in California argued that, while useful in private practice for assessing pulmonary disease, the spirometer held far greater potential in life insurance and screening for the armed forces.[100]

Conclusion

Although not used systematically in private practice or in insurance deliberations, by the mid-nineteenth century the spirometer had acquired credibility as an instrument of precision among forward-thinking scientists. As soon as the technology reached the United

States, Samuel Cartwright built a spirometer and applied it to documenting racial difference. Lung capacity measurements thus acquired a different meaning in the United States than in Britain, where occupation was the dominant analytic frame. Machines were still the "measure of man," but now they were a measure of a profoundly racialized "man." By the beginning of the twentieth century, lung capacity had been deployed in contentious societal debates and authorized by quantitative measures produced with a precision instrument. In doing so, spirometric measurement became a tool to mark blacks as physiologically most suited to agricultural labor. It was white labor that would fuel factories of the northern and southern United States.

Although the idea of racial difference in lung capacity was widespread, racialization of spirometry was not yet cemented in the popular and scientific imagination at the end of the nineteenth century. The idea might have died out (along with drapetomania) had the connections between degeneration, race, disease, and vitality not been taken up by researchers in different social worlds. To gain further insight into the ideological, social, and material processes by which race became attached to spirometry, the next chapter considers anthropometric measurement in nineteenth-century physical culture, where physical educators marshaled spirometry to describe, define, and craft a very Anglo-Saxon form of whiteness.

3

The Professionalization of Physical Culture

Making and Measuring Whiteness

Race is not an attribute that inheres in bodies, but rather attaches itself to bodies through the ideological and material work of things like law, medicine, science, economy, education, literature, social science, public policy, and popular culture.

> LAURA BRIGGS
> "The Race of Hysteria: 'Overcivilization' and the 'Savage' Woman in Late Nineteenth-Century Obstetrics and Gynecology"

At the same time as Civil War physicians and statisticians were inscribing pathology onto the bodies of African Americans, midcentury physical culturalists took up spirometric measurement. Enmeshed in the spirit of religious revivalism, physical culture was a social movement centered on cultivation of the fitness of a white race that was beset with anxieties about mass immigration from Ireland and southern and eastern Europe. According to historian David Roediger, "the state of 'conclusive' whiteness" that played out in various social domains "was approached gradually and messily."[1] What role did anthropometry and the physiological sciences play in ordering this messiness?

For more than half a century, physical culturalists systematically collected data on lung capacity of male and female students, most of them white. In the domain of physical culture—later formalized as

physical education—spirometric measurement focused on the measurement and hierarchical ordering of white bodies. Guiding individual physical training plans and serving the lofty goal of measuring
"the typical man"—of a decidedly Anglo-Saxon variety—anthropometry would be crucial to conferring scientific legitimacy on the field
of physical education. Later in the century, lung capacity measurements would flourish at women's colleges, measuring the "typical"
woman—again understood to be of an Anglo-Saxon sort. The story of
how and why spirometric measurement became part of the project
of whiteness begins at midcentury with the promotion of physical
culture at Amherst College in western Massachusetts.

Physical Culture and Amherst College

In 1854, the board of trustees of Amherst College persuaded William
Augustus Stearns, pastor of the Church of Cambridgeport in eastern
Massachusetts, to become the fourth president of this small rural
college. During his tenure, Stearns would consolidate Amherst's reputation as an educational center for the promotion of Christian pi-
ety, scientific excellence, and Anglo-Saxon manhood.[2] His leadership
saw the establishment of three new academic departments—Biblical
History and Interpretation, Mathematics and Astronomy, and Hygiene and Physical Education—each supported by a new building
dedicated to the discipline.

Established in 1821 as an alternative to Boston's Unitarianism
(especially at Harvard), Amherst College was for the next half century a site of religious orthodoxy, revivalism, and scientific innovation. Among the estimated eight revivals between 1855 and 1870,
the "Great Revival of 1858" had a particularly powerful impact at
Amherst in spiritually aligning the faculty and students. In his *History of Amherst College,* W. S. Tyler quotes Stearns on the significance of this revival for faculty–student relations:

> The year past has been characterized, on the part of the students,
> by general good order, industry, docility, and a manifest disposi-
> tion to do well. . . . The students appear not only more attentive
> to religious meetings, and more generally correct in Christian de-
> portment, but to have much more confidence in the Faculty and a
> greater desire to conform cheerfully to their requirements.[3]

Like other pious reformers, Stearns believed that full development
of mind and body could not be trusted solely to prayer. Christian

duty required care of the body as well as the soul. A systematic training of the minds, bodies, and souls of young men from local farms
and artisan shops shaped his term in office.[4] From the beginning
of his presidency, Stearns expressed concern to the trustees about
"breaking down of the health" of students during their sedentary college years. "No one thing," Stearns told the trustees, "has demanded
more of my anxious attention . . . the waning of the physical energies
in the midway of the College course is almost the rule rather than
the exception among us, and cases of complete breaking down are
painfully numerous." Initially, he proposed a series of lectures on
"the laws of health" to address the problem.[5] By 1859, he argued
that "immediate and efficient action on this subject" was necessary.
In response to his 1859 report, a committee established by the board
of trustees recommended the construction of an indoor gymnasium.
The following year the trustees voted to establish a Department of
Physical Culture at Amherst College. In a surprising move for the
times, the trustees conferred full faculty status on the director.[6]

In his 1860 annual report to the board, Stearns outlined what
would come to be known as "the Amherst Plan." Humane, rather
than militaristic, the Amherst Plan would sustain the "whole body"
in good health through required exercises, cultivation of "regularity, attention, and docility," and, importantly, recreational exercise.
For Stearns, the ideal candidate for the professorship was a physician who was also a gymnast, scientist, and an expert in the art of
elocution. The first professor of hygiene and physical training was
respected physician and gymnast John W. Hooker of New Haven,
who, for reasons of poor health, resigned after only a few months.

Unable to find a candidate with both gymnastic and medical
training, but confident that an appointee could acquire expertise in
gymnastics, Stearns appointed physician Edward Hitchcock Jr. as
professor of hygiene and physical training.[7] This was a momentous
decision. Yale, Harvard, and Amherst had established outdoor gymnasiums in the 1820s, but by the 1830s, only military schools focused
on physical education. (The University of Virginia's program was not
a formal part of the university curriculum, and it ended with the
Civil War.) Although there was renewed interest in physical education in the 1850s, prior to the 1860s there was no systematic program
of instruction in the United States.[8] Until 1879, when Harvard followed suit, Amherst was the only college with a department of physical education. As trustee Nathan Allen later wrote, it was the "first

instance in the whole history of modern education where the claims of the body, its proper development and healthy training, have been placed upon the same platform, and the same importance attached to them as to any other branch of study or mental equipment."[9]

It was not only the health of individual students that motivated Stearns. Amherst's mission was to educate pious young men of hardy New England stock for the ministry. For these students, the transition to sedentary life and intense mental work posed worrisome moral and physical risks. Taming the unruly "animal spirits" and "vices" of this motley student population required a plan to inculcate balance, self-reliance, and patience, rooted in notions of republican fitness for self-government and later Anglo-Saxon superiority.[10] Students themselves were enthusiastic about the program at Amherst. Supporting the mandatory physical exercise requirement, students testified in 1865 that "a strong body is the best bulwark to a sound mind—that strong muscles and well-developed limbs are powerful aids to the brain."[11] The class of 1869 praised Professor Hitchcock's mandatory exercise program for helping them develop "a more manly physique."[12]

Although an unusual step for higher education, Stearns's program illustrates how ideologically aligned Amherst was with the health reform movements sweeping the nation in the first half of the nineteenth century. Beginning in the 1820s, these movements, led by white middle-class Northerners, converged with millenarian movements. Building on the ideas of Enlightenment intellectuals, such as Benjamin Franklin, reformers tempered puritanical beliefs in predestination with the idea of human agency in matters of health, moral development, and responsible citizenship. No longer a matter of fate, health was an individual moral responsibility. In a rapidly changing society, the future of the nation and improvement of the "race" depended on the systematic pursuit of health and fitness. Health, dietary, and exercise reformers—such as Catharine Beecher, Sylvester Graham, Dioclesian (Dio) Lewis—promoted their cause through lectures, books, health guides, popular magazine articles, new associations, and scientific journals.[13]

Thomas Wentworth Higginson, militant abolitionist, former Unitarian minister, and commander of the First South Carolina Volunteers, one of the black regiments in the Civil War, epitomized middle-class anxieties over bodily deficiencies, loss of vigor, and declining fitness produced by social change. Looking to Britain's Charles Kingsley, Thomas Hughes, and other muscular Christians for guidance,

Higginson argued in the *Atlantic Monthly* for the promise of physical culture. The new republic needed men of vitality; "spiritual sanctity" required "physical vigour." At stake was progress of the people:

> To the American people it [bodily vigor] has a stupendous importance, because it is the only attribute of power in which they are losing ground. Guaranty us against physical degeneracy, and we can risk all other perils,—financial crises, Slavery, Romanism, Mormonism, Border Ruffians, and New York assassins; "domestic malice, foreign levy, nothing" can daunt us.[14]

Through the disciplinary functions of physical culture, Americans could assume their rightful place as world leaders. "When we once begin the competition, there seems no reason why any other nation should surpass us."[15] In such a context, lung capacity measurements, enmeshed in a discourse of vigor and fitness, would emerge as a tool for measuring, monitoring, and disciplining the physical power of young American bodies, ensuring their future as leaders in a new world order.

The Early Years of Anthropometry at Amherst College

Physician-scientist Edward Hitchcock pioneered the use of anthropometry to place the field of physical education on a scientific foundation. A deeply religious man, Hitchcock (called "Old Doc" by his students) was classically educated at Amherst College and received a Harvard medical degree in 1853. In many ways, Hitchcock was typical of middle-class Anglo-Saxon health reformers in western Massachusetts, where evangelicalism was particularly strong.[16] Torn between the life of a farmer and the life of the mind, Hitchcock, like his father, suffered from "disordered nerves" and periodic breakdowns from overwork (Figure 9).[17]

Like many American physicians, Hitchcock traveled to Paris and London after graduation from medical school, but his time there was short and not altogether pleasant. Writing of an agonizingly lonely month in Paris in 1860, he expressed admiration for the "beauty and symmetry" of the Grecian statues in the museums.[18] But Hitchcock found himself more comfortable and intellectually engaged in English-speaking, Protestant London, where he read physiology books, attended events at scientific and arts societies, and studied comparative anatomy under prominent anatomist Sir Richard Owen, with whom he maintained a correspondence for many years.[19]

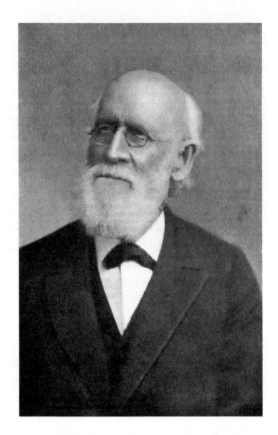

FIGURE 9.
**Dr. Edward Hitchcock,
"affectionately
known to more than a
generation of Amherst
students as 'Old Doc.'"**
Photograph courtesy
of Amherst College
Archives and Special
Collections.

While an instructor in natural sciences and elocution at Williston Seminary in Amherst, Hitchcock coauthored with his father the first of several editions of *Elementary Anatomy and Physiology, for Colleges, Academies, and Other Schools.* Reflecting their simultaneous commitment to science and God, the Hitchcocks devoted an entire chapter to "the religious applications of these sciences," an approach they thought lacking in other texts.[20] Allusions to prominent European scientists—such as physiologist William Carpenter, French comparative anatomist Georges Cuvier, Sir Richard Owen, and Swiss-born naturalist Louis Agassiz—illustrated the broad reach of their scientific knowledge. Notably, they included a long section on lung capacity in this text.

Hitchcock approached his new job as professor of hygiene and physical education as a scientist of faith, quickly establishing a rigorous, yet recreational, program of educating mind and body. Encompassing mandatory exercise, detailed health instruction, and medical care for sick students, Amherst's program conformed closely to Stearns's vision of physical culture.[21] Simultaneous attention to mind, body, and soul, rooted in science and evangelical religion, characterized "the Amherst Plan."

In a move that would profoundly influence the field of physical education, Hitchcock systematically collected anthropometric data on all college students at the beginning and end of each academic year. In the first year of the program—more than a decade before Francis Galton opened his anthropometry laboratory in London— Hitchcock collected data on age, weight, height, girths of the chest, arm, and forearm, and strength on every college student. In the second year, he added lung capacity measurements assessed with the spirometer.[22] In Hitchcock's hand, lung capacity *became* a key anthropometric variable in U.S. physical education, centered on the function and capacity of a vital organ system. Hitchcock's *Second Report to the Trustees of Amherst College* for the 1862–63 academic year contained a table with lung capacity data.[23] Over the next half-century, advertisements for prizes in physical training would feature anthropometric statistics.[24]

The physical space of the gymnasium structured Hitchcock's material practices.[25] Named after its donor, physician and politician Benjamin Barrett, the first gymnasium was a two-story structure of blue-gray granite, the first of several such elegant structures on the campus. The first floor housed gymnastic apparatuses. The second floor featured a bowling alley and anthropometric devices—including spirometers—where results of training programs could be monitored. When Amherst opened the Pratt gymnasium (named after the philanthropic Pratt family) in 1884, it reserved an entire room for taking anthropometric measurements.[26]

By introducing anthropometry to colleges, Hitchcock was charting new territory. In the decade prior to his appointment, there were only two papers on anthropometry published in the United States, one based on records of the surgeon general's Office and two published in the *Charleston Medical Journal and Review*. Elliott and Gould published their army statistics employing spirometry in the 1860s, but not until the 1880s did a significant number of articles (ten) on anthropometry in students appear.[27] According to his biographer Edward Welch, Hitchcock's interest in anthropometry may have stemmed from his admiration for the "natural form" of Greek statues that he scrutinized in Paris.[28] He was familiar with the work of Quetelet, as were many educated men at the time, and he knew of the massive anthropometric study being conducted by the Sanitary Commission.

In the early years of Amherst's program, most anthropometric measurements were simple. The spirometer, on the other hand, was complicated and costly, especially given the college's limited budget. Recall that British physicians complained that the instrument was too difficult to use in their practices. Nor was it widely used in clinical medicine in the United States. Having graduated from medical school in 1853, not long after Hutchinson presented his studies in London, it is unlikely that Hitchcock encountered the instrument in medical school. There is no evidence that he was knowledgeable about life insurance medicine, where there was some enthusiasm for spirometry. Hitchcock most likely learned about the spirometer in physiology texts. From the late 1840s, prominent physiology textbooks in Britain and the United States had discussed the utility of lung capacity to probe respiratory function.

The popularization of a specific exercise spirometer by gymnast, homeopathic physician, and health reformer Dio Lewis may also have persuaded Hitchcock to use the instrument in his gymnasium. In two classic tracts of the health reform movement, *The New Gymnastics for Men, Women, and Children,* published in 1862, and *Weak Lungs and How to Make Them Strong,* published the following year, Lewis highlighted the spirometer as "a direct and effective means of enlarging and strengthening the pulmonary apparatus." For anyone "with weak voice or defective respiration," he advised using it on a regular basis. Cornelius Conway Felton, president of Harvard, testified to the benefits of daily use. The small spirometer "with bronzed case," which he featured on the frontispiece of *Weak Lungs,* was also "a beautiful parlor instrument."[29] Thus distinct types of spirometers— one for exercise (which Hitchcock dubbed the "capacity spirometer"), and one for lung capacity measurement—were popular at the time.

Regardless of how he made his initial decision, by 1866, spirometry was entrenched in Amherst's program, and Hitchcock was corresponding with Gould to acquire the spirometers that the United States Sanitary Commission was distributing to colleges and universities.[30] Despite problems with the spirometer's accuracy, transportation of the delicate instrument to the rural countryside, and the high cost involved, there was great enthusiasm for quantitative measurement of this vital organ system. The spirometer allowed physical educators to quantify the vague concept of physical fitness and to assess the success of their training in building strength and developing a "manly physique." Over the coming century, physical educators continued to refine measures of vitality or fitness, drawing on lung capacity measurement to develop more mathematically complex indices of vitality. By the end of the century, they had measured lung capacity—and other anthropometric variables—on thousands of college students across the nation.

"Without doubt there is an ideal conception—a typical or normal man."

For about twenty years, Hitchcock worked largely in isolation, methodically collecting data on a slowly expanding number of variables (Figure 10). In yearly reports to the trustees, he carefully presented tables with sparse discussion of their meaning. Repeatedly, he emphasized that exercises should be enjoyable for students. Initially, exercises drew on heavy German gymnastics, but influenced by Dio Lewis and the Swedish system, Hitchcock quickly moved to a program of light gymnastics.

In the early years, the daily demands of his job consumed Hitchcock. He conducted numerous physical examinations, taught health

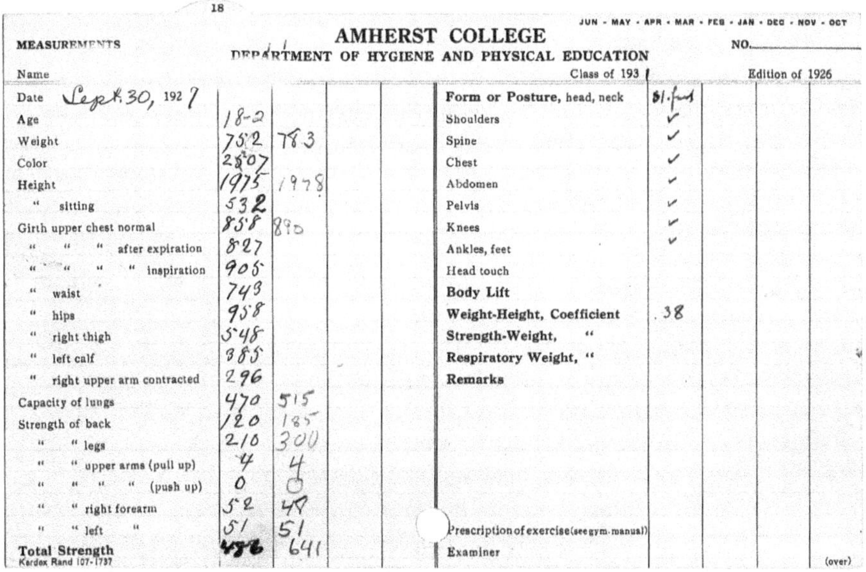

18

MEASUREMENTS

AMHERST COLLEGE

DEPARTMENT OF HYGIENE AND PHYSICAL EDUCATION

JUN · MAY · APR · MAR · FEB · JAN · DEC · NOV · OCT

NO.

Name

Class of 193 1

Edition of 1926

Date Sept. 30, 1927				
Age	18-2			
Weight	75.2	78.3		
Color	28.07			
Height	1975	1978		
" sitting	532			
Girth upper chest normal	85.8	89.0		
" " " after expiration	827			
" " " " inspiration	905			
" waist	743			
" hips	95.8			
" right thigh	5.48			
" left calf	385			
" right upper arm contracted	296			
Capacity of lungs	470	515		
Strength of back	120	185		
" " legs	210	300		
" " upper arms (pull up)	4	4		
" " " " (push up)	0	0		
" " right forearm	52	47		
" " left "	51	51		
Total Strength	436	641		

Form or Posture, head, neck	sl.-fwd			
Shoulders	✓			
Spine	✓			
Chest	✓			
Abdomen	✓			
Pelvis	✓			
Knees	✓			
Ankles, feet	✓			
Head touch				
Body Lift				
Weight-Height, Coefficient	.38			
Strength-Weight, "				
Respiratory Weight, "				
Remarks				
Prescription of exercise (see gym. manual)				
Examiner				

Kardex Rand 107-1737

(over)

FIGURE 10. **Anthropometric health care, 1927.**
Courtesy of Amherst College Archives and Special Collections.

and hygiene, supervised individualized exercise programs, and laboriously collected anthropometric data with little assistance.[31] Hitchcock was so busy with students that statistical analyses of anthropometric observations had to wait for vacations.[32] Not surprisingly, he published very little during this period.[33]

While Hitchcock worked tirelessly to integrate religious ideals into Amherst's scientific training program, American notions of health, fitness, and manhood were becoming more secular. With nearly one-half of northeasterners living in urban areas and working in sedentary occupations, physical culture as a means of improving health became more popular during the 1870s.[34] Increasingly, physical culture converged with an emerging—albeit ambivalent—faith in science, technological innovation, and expert knowledge.[35]

By the mid-1870s, the Amherst Plan began to attract international attention. With more than a decade of data, Hitchcock gave keynote addresses to professional societies and meetings of the Young Men's Christian Association. Hitchcock's 1877 address to the American Public Health Association in Chicago was a largely descriptive account of the "Amherst Plan" and a defense of his nonmilitaristic, recreational approach to physical training at Amherst with little theorization.[36] Four years later, in a report to the board of trustees, Hitchcock elaborated on his rationale for collecting anthropometric data. Developing individualized physical training plans to enhance the physical and mental vigor of young Amherst men was important. But his report revealed a grander vision, one he had quietly pursued for twenty years with religious devotion:

> One of the first duties I felt called upon to perform after your appointment to this Professorship, was to prepare blanks for several anthropometric observations of the students of college. This I did partly to enable the students to learn by yearly comparisons of themselves how they were getting on as regards the physical man. The ulterior object, however, was to help ascertain what are the data or constants of the typical man, and especially the college man. I have conceived no theory on the subject, and have instituted but very few generalizations; but my desire has been to carefully compile and put on record as many of these observations as possible for comparison and verification of statistical work in this same direction by many other persons in America and Europe.[37]

Who was this typical man? "Where is he and how can we find him?" Hitchcock asked gymnasium students at the School for Christian Workers in Springfield, Massachusetts, in 1888. Until the Greeks, he argued, the history of humankind was one of degeneracy. It is the "average person" who "now represents the races on earth." Despite progress in the "most civilized nations," however, danger lurked. For Hitchcock, scientific inquiry embodied the hope of capturing and managing the physical dimensions of this typical man (and later woman):

> By observation and study we can find out the averages of dimension, capacity, endurance, power, and certain kinds of ability, as they appear in our civilized society. . . . We should seek for a moderate and perceptible growth beyond this [the limits and dimensions of the average man], rather than to seize upon a magnificent beau ideal of physical and mental excellence, and feel dissatisfied unless we are closely nearing this acme of our desires.[38]

Ever the scientist, Hitchcock was aware of the methodological complexities posed by interpreting and standardizing anthropometry on growing young men. One must be cautious, he observed, in using the "average" for the type. For reasons of "commonsense" and the "law of beauty," Hitchcock turned to Hutchinson's rule. "The physiological fact," Hitchcock wrote, "has long ago been settled that lung capacity has a fixed ratio to bodily height."[39] Accordingly, Hitchcock determined that height would be the standard to which other anthropometric measurements would be compared. This elegant rule would guide standardization of his voluminous data set.

With only an occasional foray into theoretical speculation, Hitchcock's writings on anthropometry describe in painstaking detail each variable measured. Given his dedication to the project, he must have been stung by the thinly veiled criticism of British anthropometrists Charles Roberts and Francis Galton when they questioned the applicability of his data to "the whole of our race." The British were, however, impressed with the magnitude of his database. In a conciliatory tone, Roberts expressed interest in comparing his study of students in Britain to Hitchcock's work with Amherst students. Americans and the English, he claimed, were more like "cousins than we have long imagined."[40] Galton, although impressed by the supposed homogeneity of the sample, was sharper in his critique, and requested that Hitchcock redo his tables "in the form by which the distribution of any faculty among the individual members of a group is usually expressed." Hitchcock heeded the master's request.[41]

Although Galton and Roberts were convinced of the superiority of British anthropometry, transnational exchanges among Roberts, Galton, and Hitchcock also reflected deep differences in the truth claims of anthropometry. For physical anthropologists in Europe, anthropometric variables revealed a fixed state of bodies, reflective of a "type." For physical educators in the United States, the belief that physical training could improve mind, body, and soul meant that anthropometric traits were necessarily changeable. Motivating the individual to improve, even if an ideal body type could never be attained, informed the entire rationale for physical education.

As a measure of organ function, rather than a fixed state, lung capacity was an especially illuminating anthropometric variable, one that was sensitive to the pressures of modern life, yet could be improved with behavioral changes. According to the Hitchcocks,

> The lungs, if compressed by disease or improper clothing, and even in many cases of so-called perfect health and soundness, can be very much enlarged in their capacity. This can be done by loud reading, or by the simple act of filling the lungs with air to their utmost capacity several times each day, after the manner mentioned under inference 3d. If this healthy habit be kept up for a few years even by some considerable effort, nature will at length take up the habit, and we shall ultimately be found involuntarily filling the lungs with pure air, and thus fix upon ourselves a hygienic habit of great importance in preserving health, and of great value in repelling disease.[42]

However, the dual goals of physical education—training for improvement and uncovering constants—presented certain ambiguities for educators. For all his emphasis on improvement through gymnastic training, Hitchcock's search for "constants of the typical man" cast anthropometric variables as fixed entities.[43] Moreover, not all bodies were included in this social project. By the end of the nineteenth century, physical educators would see some body types as more changeable than others.

Dudley Sargent and "A Manly Education"

Enthusiasm for physical culture after the Civil War led to the construction of gymnasiums in institutional settings and upper-class homes; public gymnastic exhibitions; physical training programs in higher education; competitive athletics; public lecture series; and popular magazines articles.[44] To educate themselves in physiology and health, urban middle- and upper-class white women formed private associations, such as the Ladies Physiological Institute in Boston. The health of women and children became a central concern at the end of the century, producing what historian Martha Verbrugge called a "cult of female invalidism."[45] Invalidism and nervous exhaustion—"neurasthenia"—however, were not restricted to women. These afflictions signaled a crisis of manhood as well as of womanhood. As literary theorist Kim Townsend explains in *Manhood at Harvard: William James and Others,* nervous diseases were commonplace—if not de rigueur—among the male intelligentsia in the last quarter of the nineteenth century.[46]

Although professionally accomplished and much loved by his students, Hitchcock was an unassuming man. He certainly was not a self-promoter. Consequently, Hitchcock and Amherst College have been neglected in the history of anthropometry. In the history of spirometry, in fact, they are completely invisible. More attention is given to Dudley Allen Sargent (1848–1924), the controversial director of physical education at Harvard, who was appointed by President Charles Elliot in 1879.

Born in the small town of Belfast, Maine, in 1848, Sargent was a self-described lover of adventure and "hazard," who came from a working-class family. His education disrupted by the Civil War, Sargent worked as a shipmate, carpenter, and gymnastics performer in a traveling circus before assuming the position of director of the gymnasium at Bowdoin College in 1869. At Bowdoin, he began to theorize his notion of physical culture, combining anthropometric measurements with innovative exercise apparatuses. Initially, he did not include lung capacity measurements.

Like other Americans, Sargent registered the poor quality of recruits during the Civil War and devised a remedy. Like Hitchcock, he opposed military drill in gymnastic programs, arguing for a more holistic program of physical culture to "develop strength of body, dignity of bearing, courtesy of manners and a spirit of obedience, self-possession and honor . . . to enable the student to make the most of himself as a man." What Sargent promised was "a manly education" for the athletic and nonathletic alike.[47] Harmony was everything. Under his direction, Bowdoin was the first college in the United States to require daily gymnastics sessions.

In 1872, Sargent enrolled as an undergraduate at Bowdoin, maintaining his position as director while he pursued his studies. When Bowdoin denied him a full-time position after graduation, he left in 1875 to run Yale's physical education program and study medicine. After obtaining a medical degree, he presented a plan for the development of physical education at Yale, but the administration rejected his plan. Frustrated, he then moved to New York, where, most likely influenced by New York lawyer and physical culture enthusiast William Blaikie, author of the 1879 best seller *How to Get Strong and How to Stay So,* Sargent opened the private Hygienic Institute and School of Physical Culture for those who were "physically weak, or who had run down in the race of human endeavor."[48]

In New York, Sargent began to situate physical culture in the context of preventive medicine. "I felt that I had seen a gleam which I must follow, and that gleam was preventive medicine. . . . I hurled myself at the goblin, disease, from an unconventional angle, with all the sincerity and force that was in me. . . . I wished to fortify well people rather than minister to the wreck of humanity."[49] As an accomplished gymnast, he developed—and promoted—a system of apparatuses to work particular muscles and exercises to develop symmetry in body form and strength. Unlike Hitchcock, Sargent thought exercises should be hard work, not fun.

At the Hygienic Insitute, Sargent developed a comprehensive program of physical examinations and body measurements, including lung capacity, with new apparatus-driven tests, all of which informed individualized exercise plans. He clearly drew on the "Amherst Plan" and the theories of Oxford gymnastic director Archibald MacLaren, among others.[50] Blaikie's popular *How to Get Strong and How to Stay So* featured Sargent's System, bringing his apparatuses with illustrations to a broad audience.[51] For everyone—whether man or woman, sedentary businessman or manual laborer, old or young—simple exercises with dumbbells, clubs, and elegantly designed pulley weights could develop weak arms and flat chests into a robust and vigorous form. A graduate of Harvard College and Law School, Blaikie urged Harvard Corporation to hire the ambitious innovator to direct its gym. In 1879, Sargent became assistant professor of physical training and director of Hemenway Gymnasium, which opened at Harvard a year later. Despite almost constant turmoil, he remained in this position for forty years, until his retirement in 1919.[52]

While Hitchcock labored alone in rural Massachusetts for nearly twenty years, Sargent emerged in a cosmopolitan space at a moment of growing interest in public health and enthusiasm for more secular approaches to physical culture. At Harvard, Sargent fashioned himself as an innovator of exercise equipment, expert teacher-trainer, and ardent popularizer of his methods and theories. In 1887, he established the popular Harvard Summer School of Physical Training to train physical education teachers in gymnastics, anatomy and physiology, principles of education, physical diagnosis, and preventive medicine.[53]

Sargent sought to establish physical education on a scientific foundation, but with a more complex program of physical training techniques, improved anthropometric measures, and physical examination than Hitchcock employed. Featuring new technologies—intricate gymnastic apparatuses, spirometers, dynamometers, and manometers—the technical aspects of gymnastic and anthropometric apparatuses informed this gifted designer's program. Notoriously demanding in his specifications for apparatuses, he worked with talented Boston-based carpenters and mechanics in designing, constructing, and supervising the manufacture of apparatuses, which he distributed widely to educational institutions. Without patent protection, however, the supply houses that developed with the expansion of gymnasium building and anthropometric testing were the ones who profited. Edward Hitchcock's son, director of physical education at Cornell, had already formed the Cornell Gymnasium Outfitting Company, which supplied spirometers and gymnastic apparatuses to the growing market. Running afoul of Harvard's policy proscribing patents by faculty, Sargent was forced to contract with Narragansett Machine Company and Boston mechanic Thomas Upham to make his apparatuses, one of which was a spirometer that Narragansett would manufacture for decades (Figure 11). His entrepreneurial instinct crushed, Sargent remained bitter that others had profited from his inventions.

Harvard's push for competitive athletics irked Sargent. Writing in the popular *Scribner's Magazine,* he critiqued the cost, inefficiency, and antagonistic nature of elite sports. Conventional anthropometry, with its routine collection of simple measurements, fared no better in Sargent's view. Dismissive of Hitchcock's years of toil, he wrote somewhat unfairly, "aside from the investigations of the Provost-Marshal-General's Bureau, of the Sanitary Commission, on recruits during the late war, and of the Anthropometric Committee of the British

Association for the Advancement of Science, but little systematic effort has been made to obtain reliable information by means of physical measurements."[54] For Sargent, muscle development was key to the "power and efficiency of mind and body." Shortly after assuming his position at Harvard, he devised his famous strength tests, which used lifting, hand and chest dynamometers, gymnastic rings, and parallel bars to determine an individual's "physical power, working capacity, and efficiency" and to provide means for remediation. He recorded the anthropometric details on charts for future reference. Like Dio Lewis, Sargent incorporated lung capacity measurement with a spirometer into strength testing.[55]

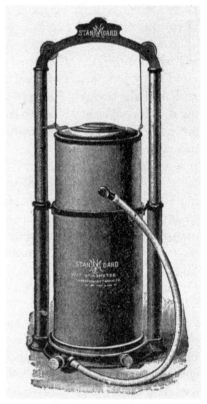

FIGURE 11. **Standard spirometer manufactured by Narraganset Machine Company.** From Jay W. Seaver, *Anthropometry and Physical Examination* (New Haven, Conn.: Dorman Lithographing Co., 1905).

For Sargent, anthropometric measures were changeable. The primary purposes of the anthropometric charts were to motivate students to compare themselves with others and to judge the success of physical training.[56] According to Sargent, strengthening the lungs would improve respiration and increase lung capacity.[57] For students whose "heart is weak, the lung capacity small, the liver sluggish, the circulation feeble, or the nervous system impaired," Sargent had a plan.[58] Bolstered by Harvard's prestige, Sargent's innovative tests moved physical education away from routine collection of anthropometric information, making the measure of manhood a more precise, complex, and dynamic undertaking.

By all accounts an irascible man, Sargent had a contentious relationship with the Harvard's Board of Overseers. Equipping and managing the gymnasium at Harvard was a more complex endeavor than Hitchcock had faced at Amherst almost twenty years earlier. Caught in the battle over athletics, the corporation stripped Sargent of faculty status in 1889. Limited resources left him feeling exhausted and unappreciated, although he never lost enthusiasm for technological innovation.

Professionalization and the Science of Anthropometry

Although tumultuous politically, the 1870s and 1880s were an intellectually invigorating time for physical education—and a critical moment in the history of anthropometry in the United States. Leading medical journals, such as the *Boston Medical and Surgical Journal,* reported favorably on physical culture—particularly Hitchcock's program at Amherst.[59] Many colleges and universities adopted elements of Hitchcock's approach to gymnastics and incorporated anthropometry and lung capacity measurements into their physical education programs. Expansion of higher education after the Civil War and the increasing complexity of industrialization led to a proliferation of experts. With the emergence of professional societies, the social sciences undertook to order expertise.[60]

In 1885, physical educators began to professionalize, forming the Association for the Advancement of Physical Education, renamed the American Association for the Advancement of Physical Education (AAAPE) the following year. The association's *Proceedings* of the annual meetings, published yearly from 1885 to 1895, became the *American Physical Education Review* in 1896. Endorsement of the association by leading medical journals illustrated the medical profession's interest in physical culture.

Professional organization enhanced the public profiles of both Hitchcock and Sargent. Hitchcock was a founding member of the AAAPE and its first president. Sargent would serve as president three times. The National Education Association established a Department of Physical Education in 1894, and the Physical Education Society of the Northeast was organized at Clark University in 1895. Professional meetings and associated publications provided a rich space for theorizing and circulating information related to the profession. Sorting through the place of physical education in the educational system required standardization of testing and measurement, teacher training, curricular development, and assessment of the various systems of gymnastics. Although no simple consensus on the theories, methods, and goals of physical education, and anthropometry was ever achieved, technical innovation with apparatuses and an industry for their manufacture flourished.[61]

Standardizing anthropometric measurements was one of the first objectives of the AAAPE. Along with Sargent and William Anderson, president of the Brooklyn Normal School for Physical Training, Hitchcock served on the Sub-Committee upon the Method of Physical Measurement, which submitted an influential report standardizing measurement to the association in 1886.[62] During this period, Hitchcock began publishing his anthropometric theories and practices in American and British journals, arguing for the "need for anthropometry," to "ascertain the ideal or typical man," and to "give advice as to the physical condition of our young people who are not typical or ideal."[63] He participated in the "battle over the systems" (Swedish, German, Dio Lewis, or Sargent), but with less intensity than other physical educators on the scene. The AAAPE recognized Hitchcock for his contributions to anthropometry at its third annual meeting: "Anthropometry . . . gives a standard and reduces to a positive knowledge what before was merely impressions as we looked a man over. . . . Now we are able to foretell the ultimate result of training with greater accuracy. Anthropometry now seems to be doing more to reduce this work to a positive science than any other single branch of study."[64] According to historian Roberta Park, "without question, anthropometry was the major 'scientific' preoccupation of professional physical education in the late nineteenth century."[65]

Sargent was an influential, though controversial, figure in the AAAPE. As he details in his *Autobiography,* he had many conflicts throughout his career. While these conflicts reflected tensions in the institutional frameworks in which he worked, the context of the times, and his own personality traits, especially as they manifested in entrepreneurialism, many of Sargent's battles represented the pains of professionalization, particularly underlying conflicts over the role of physical educators in higher education. Were physical educators scientists or practitioners?[66] What was the importance of anthropometry to physical education?

Despite growing interest in the scientific basis of physical culture, the identity of the profession remained rooted in service. Considered by many physical educators to be a science, anthropometry also fit comfortably into this service mission. This, as it turned out, was both its strength and its limitation in the field of physical education.[67] The daily labor of this first generation of physical educators was inherently service-oriented, but many of the field's leaders were medical doctors and considered themselves scientists. Both the service dimension of gymnastics and the science of anthropometry, albeit with radically different approaches, engaged Hitchcock and Sargent. Their tireless collection of data solidified the importance of anthropometry to an increasingly scientifically rooted physical education. The broad scope of anthropometric measurement also gave a major impetus to the manufacture of equipment, which included spirometers.

In the late nineteenth century, the experimental laboratory-based sciences gained ground and scientifically oriented proponents of physical education looked to experimental physiology, rather than anthropometry, as the foundation for the discipline. Here spirometric measurement again proves an adaptable scientific object. George Wells Fitz, for example, who directed a short-lived undergraduate program in anatomy, physiology, and physical training at Harvard's Lawrence Scientific School, advocated for a science-based, rather than gymnastics-based, curriculum. By science he meant physiology, not anthropometry. Designed to train directors of gymnasiums and premedical students, Fitz's program centered on a physiology and physical training laboratory, where students studied the mechanistic effects of exercise on muscle contraction, the circulatory system, metabolic activity—and lung capacity. For complex reasons, Fitz's contract was not renewed and he left Harvard, ending a more experimental curriculum.[68] Nonetheless, as a marker of physiological function rather than a fixed anthropometric variable, the experimental study of exercise and lung capacity remained important research topics in physical education into the twentieth century.

Cultivating Whiteness

In the last quarter of the nineteenth century, under the pressure of the explosive growth of urban centers, the beginnings of African American migration from the South, and massive immigration of the "darker races" from southern and eastern Europe, a crisis of Anglo-Saxon manhood emerged.[69] The result would be what Matthew Frye Jacobson and David Roediger argue—though from different perspectives and with slightly different periodization—was a destabilization of the category of "white" or what Nell Painter refers to in her *The History of White People* as the second great enlargement of the white race. The history of physical education provides insight into the role of science in stabilizing or enlarging a unified white race from the messy vestiges of unrestricted immigration before 1924. In this context, anthropometry and lung capacity measurements became racialized in a new way.

Framed in the language of race, civilization, and manhood, and shedding its religious (but not moral) underpinnings, discussions of health and sanitary reform soon transformed into dire predictions of physical, moral, and intellectual deterioration. By the end of the century, discourses of "race suicide," supported by "scientific" evidence, were so commonplace that in 1902 William Hastings, Chief of Anthropometry and Physical Training at the International Young Men's Christian Association Training School in Springfield, Massachusetts, could assert "the persistent decline in the vitality of the racial stock" owing to the "deleterious effect of city life" as fact.[70] While the language of race was fluid at the time, there was little question that the "race" physical educators needed to measure and cultivate was Anglo-Saxon, modeled on middle-class New Englanders.

Dedicated to improvement of an Anglo-Saxon "race," physical education programs in public schools and colleges positioned themselves to arrest this deterioration. The basis of physical training, according to Hastings, "must naturally be physical measurement, diagnosis, and the graphical representation of development upon anthropometric tables."[71] The science of anthropometry offered the promise of precisely quantifying the success of physical education in improving the race. Lung capacity measurements were included in anthropometric measurement in Hastings's training programs. Yet, unlike physical anthropology, where comparative race studies dominated, physical education rarely made direct racial comparisons. Rather, anthropometry in physical education was a project of whiteness, centered on cultivating Anglo-Saxon manhood and womanhood.

Hitchcock did not collect data on ancestry in the first twenty years of the program; therefore, he had no method for tracking race. Even when he and his son added ancestry, they only made limited comparisons between men and women and between Japanese and Amherst students.[72] In 1878, the Japanese government asked Amherst to send someone to Japan to develop a physical education program based on the Amherst Plan. George Leland, a student of Hitchcock's, accepted the invitation. While in Japan, Leland collected anthropometric data on fourteen variables—one of which was lung capacity—on young men and women at a variety of educational institutions, which he then brought back to the United States for analysis. In 1903, Hitchcock and Paul Phillips, his successor at Amherst, prepared a table for the Leland Prize exhibition at Pratt Gymnasium, presenting a comparison of Japanese anthropometry with those of men and women from Amherst, Williston Academy, Smith, and Mount Holyoke. Japanese lung capacity was lower at all ages for men and women. Even with this rich data set, the brief narrative attached to these tables did not seem to attach much significance to the difference between Japanese and Americans. They did not explain the differences or provide causal explanations.[73]

On the other hand, for Hitchcock, lung capacity measurements helped to establish gender difference as truly "fundamental." He noted that races have "their own distinctive characteristics" and that "different classes in the same race are distinguished from each other but not in so marked a degree. . . . In all tests of strength," he wrote in a short pamphlet, "man is naturally the stronger as he is superior in the capacity of lungs."[74] Preparation of young Anglo-Saxon males for their rightful place as world leaders in an increasingly frenetic "Gilded Age" was Hitchcock's primary concern. For this project, he drew on concepts of efficiency and training, rather than race deterioration. Prominent former student and oil executive Charles Pratt credited his physical education under Hitchcock's tutelage for helping him "carry heavy responsibility in business."[75] Quoting President James Garfield, the program for the 1887 Ladd Prize competition touted the benefits of physical training in an imperial world order: "There is no way in which you can get so much out of a man as by training; not in pieces, but the whole of him; and the trained men, other things being equal, are to be the masters of the world."[76]

Although Hitchcock paid little attention to direct racial comparisons, his anthropometric studies served to establish the "average man" as a white Anglo-Saxon one. Although tacit, the racial dimensions of Hitchcock's project are evident in his 1887 *An Anthropometric Manual*, published with Dr. Seelye, featuring twenty-five years of data collection. Here he made clear that the typical man is Anglo-Saxon, well represented by middle-class college students of New England. According to Hitchcock, "it seem[ed] fair to judge that the New England College Student, averaging about 21 years of age, who is neither overworked in body or pampered by luxurious ease or indulgence, would furnish an average, or a mean, that could be used in an Anthropometric study of the Anglo-Saxon race."[77] In calling attention to the "exceptionally homogeneous" material on "students [who] were very largely (90–95 per cent.) native-born Americans," Paul Phillips underscored the significance of Amherst's sample.[78]

Still, white maleness required careful cultivation to reach its full potential. "With a more thorough attention to the physical man," Hitchcock and Seelye wrote, "the many who were defective . . . might be improved and made more efficient men now and hereafter."[79] Instruments for increasing chest size and lung capacity included chest weights, a chest expander, and capacity spirometer.[80] According to Edward Mussey Hartwell, racial improvement through scientific training was an evolutionary imperative. "Muscular exercise," he claimed, "may make a boy into a better man, in many respects than his father was, and enable him to transmit to his progeny a veritable aptitude for better thoughts and actions. Herein lies the power of the race for self-improvement, and the evolution of a higher type of man upon earth."[81]

Sargent, on the other hand, subscribed to a crude notion of progress through evolution, as illustrated in his comments at the 1889 Physical Training Conference in Boston: "Variation in size, form, and feature" marked "progress in civilization." But for Sargent, progress brought deformity. Physical training in "civilized communities" was a matter of great urgency.[82] He limited his theorizing on race, at least in print, to simple assertions of difference: "For every age, each sex and all the different races," there was a "probable standard of height, weight, and chest girth."[83] He singled out the Japanese for their "racial habits." In comparison to an English man and an Irish man, the American man showed superior anthropometric measurements in all categories. Thus, at a historical moment when the United States was embroiled in wrenching debates over immigration, imperialism, and who was white and American, anthropometry offered the possibility of discriminating racial characteristics with precision.

For physical educators, however, the extent to which anthropometric differences among new immigrants were innate or changeable remained unclear. Yale professor Jay Webber Seaver's widely read 1896 monograph *Anthropometry and Physical Examination: A Book for Practical Use in Connection with Gymnastic Work and Physical Education,* published in the same year as Frederick Hoffman's *Race Traits,* interprets racial difference in anthropometric measurements as inherent. For Seaver, the study of body proportions was the study of racial difference: "In studying different races of men, it was found that they had marked peculiarities of physique, as well as marked mental peculiarities and customs." Different races "follow special laws . . . those types having comparatively longer trunks and short limbs possess higher resisting power than the opposite types. We also find that the size of certain physical organs, like the chest has a direct relation to the working power of the individual when considered a machine." Anthropometry provided the opportunity for "graphically representing the racial type."[84]

With such robust data, the next step was to construct standards. That same year, Sargent took his ideas to the esteemed *Boston Medical and Surgical Journal*. According to Sargent, distinct races had distinct normal standards: "The aims of physical training . . . embrace a consideration of the normal proportions of the individual of different races and types in order to determine normal growth and development."[85] Sargent, however, was less certain than Seaver that race difference was fundamental.[86] In an address to the American Association for the Advancement of Science at Yale, Sargent used his formidable database to weigh in on the heated debate over the superiority of the dolichocephalic (Nordic) as compared to the brachycephalic (Alpine) races, famously promoted by Dr. John Beddoe. The story he told revealed an openness to widening the circle of whiteness. The dolichocephalic type of race was stronger and a higher proportion was of American parentage than the sub-dolichocephals, mesocephals (medium), sub-brachycephals, and brachycephals, but he considered the differences for most variables to be small. Even more confusingly, college performance indicated that the brachycephalic type were more intelligent than the dolichocephalic type. Other racial characteristics were evenly distributed. Tentatively concluding that the dolichocephals were probably superior, he nonetheless offered that the racial type most likely to prevail in America was a mixed one—the mesocephalic, "coming to us through a general and more widespread diffusion of races."[87] Out of this complex mixture would emerge an expanded—yet supposedly pure—white race.

Anglo-Saxon Womanhood

Throughout the nineteenth century, women were both the objects of and passionate advocates for health reform. Early health reformers asserted that both girls and boys needed physical education.[88] Writing in the newly established *Journal of Health* in 1829, physicians argued for equal attention to the physical condition of girls.

Strengthening the constitution, preserving the limbs in all their motions, and protecting the system from deleterious influences were essential to the "vigour and usefulness of their future lives."[89] Although these writers thought that exercises should be similar for boys and girls, the types of physical activity appropriate for the sexes would be debated for the rest of the century.[90]

As director of physical training at Harvard, Sargent concentrated on providing the young men of Harvard with a "manly education." His influence on physical education, however, extended far beyond the walls of the Hemenway Gymnasium. Sargent's vision for physical education featured teacher training for both women and men. Excluded from most professions, women were turning to the expanding field of education for employment, teaching in public and private schools, teacher-training institutions called normal schools, or at elite private colleges for women. For the most part, this first generation of college women came from the middle and upper classes, the same classes of women whose childbearing practices—especially in relation to those of eastern and southern European immigrants—triggered such anxiety about the future of the "race."

Soon after his arrival at Harvard, the Society for the Collegiate Instruction of Women (known informally as the Harvard Annex) approached Sargent to develop a program of physical culture for the Society, initiating a relationship that continued until 1892, when the Annex created its own gymnastic space. After that, what was first called the Sanatory Gymnasium and later the Sargent College of Physical Training trained normal school students and private pupils, the majority of them women. In 1887, Sargent established the Harvard Summer School of Physical Training.[91] For more than a half-century, the summer school drew on accomplished scientists from Harvard Medical School and leading gymnasts to train teachers from across the country in the theory and practice of physical training. Designed to equip students with tools for teaching, the Summer School attempted to inculcate "correct habits of living" in the students through their summer experience of a "regular, hygienic life."[92]

Combining mental and physical work, the curriculum of both the Sargent School and the Summer School included lectures on anatomy, physiology, anthropometry, and hygiene; a range of gymnastics exercises from the many competing "systems"; and athletic games, such as boxing, fencing, and wrestling. Although he was ambivalent about women's suffrage, Sargent fought against constrictive clothing and ardently supported coeducational exercise classes. For women, exercises consisted primarily of light gymnastics and dancing. Central to the science-based curriculum was anthropometric theory, instruction in the use of apparatuses, and training in precision measurement.

Women physicians were well represented in physical education.[93] Early graduates of the Sargent College and Harvard Summer School included physicians Delphine Hanna of Oberlin College, Carolyn Ladd and Alice Foster of Bryn Mawr, and Helen Putnam of Vassar, all of whom became intellectual leaders in physical education. These female directors of physical education programs at colleges and universities dutifully collected anthropometric data on lung capacity, along with other anthropometric measures, on all incoming students in much the same way their male colleagues did. In his article "Physical Examinations," Edward Hitchcock Jr. singled out Wellesley's program, directed by Lucille Hill, for its good work in anthropometry—which he considered representative of women's colleges more generally.

Fitness circumscribed a racialized womanhood that would ensure the future of the nation. During a discussion at the Physical Training Conference, Lucille Eaton Hill, director of the gymnasium at Wellesley, affirmed the importance of women's physical training for the nation: "If strong be the frames of the mothers, the sons shall make laws for the people."[94] The vitality of future generations depended on intelligent and vigorous women, for whom childbearing embodied the essence of responsible citizenship. At the same conference, physician to the New York State Reformatory Hamilton D. Wey argued, "physiological laws know neither sex nor conditions, and what is applicable to the male applies more forcibly in the case of the female." By 1902, anxieties over the racial stock, womanhood, and the future of the nation had intensified. For Hastings, physical training for women and girls was an even more pressing matter than it was for boys. Despite adequate opportunity to adopt "hygienic habits . . . the intense strain of study, together with outside interests, is too great a drain upon a delicate, highly organized nervous system."[95] Thus, just as anthropometry and physical training cultivated and monitored white manhood at the end of the century, so too did physical educators deploy anthropometry to cultivate and monitor white womanhood—of a decidedly elite variety. Physical education, Verbrugge writes, was always about difference and its relation to science.[96]

Standardizing Anthropometry

Overlapping theoretically with medicine, basic science, social science, and sport, physical education was a bitterly contested terrain by the end of the nineteenth century. Replaced by a growing interest in hygiene, play, and the more spectacular competitive athletics, anthropometry lost ground as the central scientific practice guiding physical education. Sustained for more than fifty years by cultural enthusiasm for technological innovation, faith in quantification, and an anxiety-ridden quest for fitness, physical educators had tirelessly measured lung capacity on thousands of students.[97] Although this database of anthropometric measurements on mostly white male and female college students was vast, its meaning was unclear.

To bring coherence to this vast enterprise, physical educators published manuals with precise instructions for taking measurement, illustrations of instruments, and sample anthropometric cards to facilitate examinations on masses of students. Experimentally oriented physical educators, however, had concluded that this project yielded little of scientific value.[98] In the first decades of the twentieth century, the situation shifted and research-oriented physical educators again turned to lung capacity measurements as a marker of physical fitness, now using more rigorously scientific, experimental approaches and more precisely defined tests. The result was a flurry of more statistically grounded studies on college students that probed the relationships among lung capacity, height, weight, and surface area; their relevance to early prediction of disease; and their potential connection to other conditions, such as mental retardation.[99]

Problems of individual and technical variability in spirometric measurements bedeviled researchers. Yet, despite technical constraints, researchers forged ahead, linking race to anthropometry and spirometry in ever more explicit ways. As study design and statistical methodologies became more sophisticated, greater care was taken to assure racial homogeneity of samples. Although these early efforts at standardization were uneven, it was "white" lung capacity that would become the standard of "normal"—and it would remain so into the twenty-first century.

The deployment of spirometry in constructing whiteness rested in part on the development of an industry for the manufacture of the instrument. Whether viewed as a home exercise device, a parlor trinket, a medical research tool, or an instrument for routine anthropometry, by the early 1860s, there was sufficient demand for

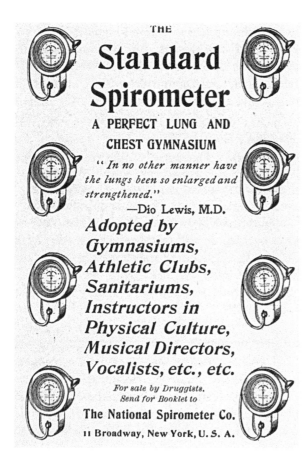

FIGURE 12.
Advertisement in
the *Independent
Magazine*, the
National Spirometer
Co., 1898.

the spirometer to support a burgeoning manufacturing industry. In an exhibit to the Academy of Natural Sciences in 1858, physician S. Weir Mitchell claimed that the manufacturing firm of Messrs. Code, Hopper & Co. of Philadelphia was making "vast numbers" of spirometers, some of which the United States Sanitary Commission used in its studies.[100]

To meet the demand for spirometers by physicians, the AAAPE, the YMCA, most colleges and universities, and many public schools, entrepreneurs founded new manufacturing and supply companies, among them the Harvard Instrument Company, Cornell Outfitting Company, the Narragansett Machine Company, Tiemann Brothers, A. G. Spaulding & Company, and the National Spirometer Company (Figure 12).[101] By the early twentieth century, mechanics had developed extensive technological expertise for modifying, manufacturing, and marketing the spirometer, providing the infrastructure for its uptake in domains other than anthropometry, most significantly that of clinical medicine. Whether the typical, average, or ideal man or woman displayed by the machine was truly "normal" remained uncertain. What was perfectly clear, however, was that whiteness represented the standard of normal.

Conclusion

By the early twentieth century, questions related to ancestry were commonplace in physical education programs, but physical educators mostly assembled databases on white populations. If people from other races managed to get into elite colleges, researchers excluded them from their analyses. In one study, for example, investigators eliminated "students of different racial inheritance, African or Asiatic" for "obvious reasons."[102] Such exclusions, seemingly to enhance the homogeneity of the sample, would become commonplace in the twentieth century. Although not the centerpiece of physical education, anthropometry and lung capacity measurements would remain important measures of fitness. Testing and measuring continued, increasingly cast in a language of efficiency. Bolstered by research across the Atlantic by physician-scientists during the First World War, the statistical analyses of lung capacity measurements would become more complex, increasing their authority as a measure of overall physical fitness.

4

Progress and Race
Vitality in Turn-of-the-Century Britain

Imperialism . . . was the discourse which sought to
bind the myriad realities of the colonial "power" into
a discursive unity. Social Darwinism and other social
evolutionary theories in the later-nineteenth century
underpinned the supremacist rhetoric, but the spectre
of internal degeneration continually haunted it.

> DANIEL PICK
> *Faces of Degeneration*

Innate qualities are needed to prove the justice—
the naturalness and inalterability—of the status quo.

> NELL PAINTER
> *The History of White People*

The masses were restive. The revolutions of 1848 were sweeping the Continent, threatening to spread across the Channel and
disrupt the fragile social order in Britain. In February, Karl Marx
and Friedrich Engels published the *Communist Manifesto*. In April,
Chartists descended on London to demand suffrage for working-
class men. In July, the Young Irelanders took up arms. The moment
felt like a crisis of capital—if not of civilization—and the middle
classes responded with fear, anxiety, and arrogance, urging patience and discipline on the angry crowds. Charles Kingsley—whose
writings were foundational to the social, and religious movement
later called "Muscular Christianity"—was summoned to quiet the

Chartists. Kingsley admonished the impatient masses to "be wise, and then you must be free, for you will be fit to be free."[1]

Although the discourse of fitness had many meanings at midcentury, the concept had long been invoked during war, most especially the Napoleonic Wars. Kingsley's words signified a new moment in England, during which notions of manliness, freedom, fitness, godliness, and knowledge would be deployed to tame and discipline workers in the service of an expanding British empire. Like the Americans, the British became preoccupied with physical culture.

The precise meanings of "fitness," "manliness," and "freedom" and their relation to scientific knowledge were debated in literary journals, scientific treatises, and churches and fought out in the factories, streets, and fields of empire.[2] What were the essential qualities of fitness? Who embodied fitness? And how could it be measured? Initially focused on elite bodies, physical culture would, by the end of the century, become more centered on the bodies of the middle and lower classes. The physical culture movement was important to the development of anthropometry in Britain, but it would have a different emphasis than in the United States. In addition to its role in physical education, lung capacity measurements in Britain gained credibility in the context of the statistical theorizing of Francis Galton and social debates over race deterioration. To stave off or reverse race deterioration, anthropometric projects would be marshaled to measure, mark, and rank bodily efficiency and fitness.

Physical Culture at Midcentury: From Sport and Games to Gymnastics

With the 1859 publication of Darwin's *On the Origin of Species,* social analysts across the political spectrum began to articulate new discourses of fitness, degeneration, and the body, and methods for bodily discipline and control were enmeshed in evolutionary theory.[3] Working-class bodies were a source of both wealth and disorder that could not be easily contained. Physical education in British schools became a culturally acceptable way to promote social stability. In considering physical education as a historically significant "site of production," theorist David Kirk writes that "the themes of egalitarianism and social cohesion, consensus and nationalism were reworked and remade within physical education discourse and re-entered the endless cycle of cultural production to be appropriated by particular conditions and interests."[4] In Britain as in the United States, the tensions of nation-state formation and social class stratification—as well as growing anxieties about labor efficiency—shaped physical culture, the field of physical education that emerged from it, and the technological tools deployed to measure its bodily effects.

Initially, physical culture was most fully developed at British public schools as sport and games, rather than military drill and gymnastics. Sport and games played a key role in the transformation of the public school system during the nineteenth century, producing the famed "cult of athleticism."[5] Adapting to the rising middle class's quest for higher social status, and ideologically informed by the manly ideals of muscular Christianity, public school reform began in the 1840s.[6] Along with courage and self-reliance, for the muscular Christians, sport and games—supplemented later by gymnastics—imbued young men with self-control, patience, and vigor, while also solidifying their class, racial, and gendered identities. Success on the playing fields was linked to success on the battlefields of the British Empire. The constellation of these characteristics—cultivated by sport and games—constituted the nebulous ideal of fitness.

Military concerns profoundly shaped physical education in Britain. No longer the sole province of gentlemen, the military professionalized in the early nineteenth century, integrating physical exercise along with sport and games into its training regimes. New military academies became a testing ground for the theories and practices of physical culture. During the Napoleonic Wars, the army framed its concern with the health of recruits in an ambiguous language of "fitness," but an organized approach to cultivating fitness only emerged when P. H. Clias, an officer in the Swiss army, came to Britain in 1822 to organize gymnastics at military academies.[7] By the 1820s, gymnastics had been established in military schools and colleges as a means to cultivate physical fitness. By the end of the 1850s, efforts were under way to implement a program of physical training for all ranks of the army.[8] After the Crimean War (1853–56), sport and games were extended to the lower ranks. After the Caldwell reforms of the 1870s, and another spate of military reforms in the 1900s, systematic physical training and sport had become firmly established in the British army.

For reasons related to the educational system, military engagements, the muscular Christianity movement, and the proclivities of educators, anthropometric measurement was initially taken up at midcentury by elite public schools, universities, and the military where gymnastics was finding its place. The humiliations of the Crimean War, a new phase in imperial expansion, and a spirit of liberal reform provided the context for the development of more systematic approaches to cultivating the bodies and minds of the upper classes.[9] The first public school gymnasium opened at Uppinham in 1859, the same year that the Oxford gymnasium opened under the direction of pioneering gymnast Archibald MacLaren.[10]

The Theories and Practices of Archibald MacLaren

Anthropometric measurements—including those involving the spirometer—did not assume the same significance as scientifically informed, objective markers of physical fitness in physical education in Britain as they did in the United States. Yet, as a physiological marker of labor value, lung capacity figured in the theories of physical culture elaborated by Scottish gymnastics pioneer Archibald MacLaren, a seminal figure in British physical education. Working at Oxford, an institution influenced by the manly ideals of muscular Christianity, MacLaren used anthropometry in a limited way to develop his ideas and to promote his system of gymnastics for military, university, and public school physical education programs. MacLaren's concern was physical culture both as a state of being and as a physiological state, assessed through an incremental program of exercise, rather than precise physical measurement.

Born around 1820 in Alloa, Scotland, MacLaren studied medicine in Paris, while also pursuing fencing and gymnastics. Returning to Oxford, he opened a fencing school and gymnasium in the mid-1850s, at a moment when liberal reform was reshaping this medieval university.[11] In 1858, he directed the building of the University Gymnasium at Oxford, a space where young intellectuals could cultivate body and mind (Figure 13). According to historian J.W. MacKail, undergraduates at Exeter College were sharply divided between those who engaged in classical study and those who "rowed, hunted, ate and drank largely, and often sank at Oxford into a coarseness of manners and morals distasteful and distressing."[12] MacLaren's gym and home in Summertown provided a stimulating haven from a boring routine of lectures for a small group of disillusioned intellectuals around the artists William Morris and Edward Burne-Jones. Voracious readers, this group at Oxford engaged the works of Ruskin, Wilberforce, and Shakespeare, along with the iconic muscular Christian Charles Kingsley.[13]

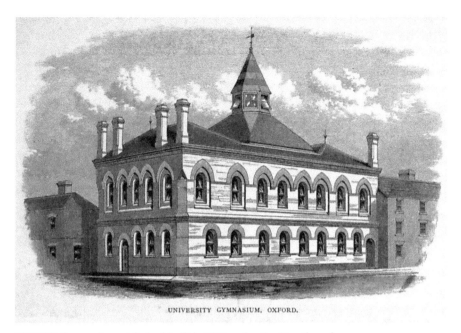

UNIVERSITY GYMNASIUM, OXFORD.

FIGURE 13. **Gymnasium at Oxford built in 1858 under the direction of Archibald MacLaren.** From Archibald MacLaren, *A System of Physical Education: Theoretical and Practical*, (Oxford: Clarendon Press, 1869).

At the gymnasium, MacLaren approached physical culture from a holistic perspective, which for him meant gymnastic training based on the physiology of bodily labor "in all its physical essentials."[14] MacLaren's approach to gymnastics was a synthetic one, which incorporated elements of different systems to develop a coherent program of exercises that would enhance the physique of the "whole man." Rather than measurement, gymnastics with new apparatuses were used to monitor and improve the young male bodies under his charge.[15] For MacLaren, recreational gymnastics (sport and games) had its place, but only as a supplement to a scientific program of apparatus-assisted exercise.

In 1860, MacLaren's career shifted when the army invited him to develop a system of physical training. Shaken by the Crimean War and the Indian Mutiny, the War Office decided that the physical deterioration of army recruits, as well as the stresses of difficult military campaigns in extreme weather, required a dedicated program in physical fitness training. MacLaren's first book, *A Military System of Gymnastic Exercises for the Use of Instructors,* published in 1862, was an instructional manual outlining the contours of the program, which brought him fame. This progressive program of exercises both contributed to physical culture and, more practically, enhanced the "professional duties [of the soldier] by systematically teaching him how to overcome their principle obstacles, difficulties, and dangers."[16] In 1862, the War Office ordered the construction of gymnasiums in every garrison. Subsequently, military and civilian gymnasiums throughout the empire adopted MacLaren's program of exercise.[17]

In later writings, MacLaren made sweeping claims for exercise. Exercise, he argued, was the primary mechanism of achieving the exalted state of physical culture. It was "the agent for renewal of that which is continuously lost—vital power."[18] As he outlines in 1869, in the influential book *A System of Physical Education: Theoretical and Practical,* "it is to Exercise almost exclusively that we must look as the means of actual physical culture during the greater part of the period of growth and development."[19] Ever the synthesizer and aware that he was at a world-class center for sport and games, MacLaren's second book, *Training in Theory and Practice,* applied his theories to rowing, then the most popular sport at Oxford, and gave recommendations for diet, sleep, clothing, and hygiene for athletes.[20]

Like other physical culturists on both sides of the Atlantic, MacLaren was concerned with the demands that constant study made on the fragile young men with whom he worked. His writings articulated contemporary anxieties about modern civilized life, business, mental work, and the demands of empire on male English bodies. Importantly, his system offered a means of control. While he foresaw broad applications for his system, "embryo soldiers, lawyers and doctors which were a product of the elite public schools" preoccupied him. For MacLaren, the public school was the "centre and source of its [England's] vitality and power."[21] To support his claims, he drew on the notion of vital capacity, though it is not clear that he considered it a measureable entity. Nonetheless, linking vital capacity to labor, he claimed that the systematic pursuit of exercise would develop "the condition of the body, and that amount of *vital capacity,* which shall enable each man in his place to pursue his calling, and work on in his working life with the greatest amount of comfort to himself and usefulness to his fellow men."[22] Almost immediately, his theories went transnational, influencing the American Blaikie, who popularized the system and its apparatuses, which—as we have already seen—profoundly shaped Dudley Sargent's program at Harvard.

MacLaren's experience with the army informed physical training programs in the military for years to come. It also shaped the theoretical and practical development of his system of gymnastics at Oxford that placed less emphasis on measurement than on systematic exercise. Initially "discomfited at the appearance of this detachment" of army recruits and their lack of fitness, he nonetheless recognized the opportunity for testing his system on "the weak and the strong, the short and the tall, the robust and the delicate."[23] Although his use of anthropometric measurements was limited, he did measure chest circumference. And physical educators widely acknowledged MacLaren as a pioneer in anthropometry. For MacLaren, anthropometric measurement was not an end in itself. Rather, anthropometry provided insight into the physiology of growth and development and monitored the impact of his system of exercises on individual bodies.[24] Periodic measurements—supplemented with other technologies, such as photography—provided evidence for his system's effectiveness.[25]

In the appendices to *A System of Physical Education*, MacLaren published tables with height, weight, forearm, upper arm, and chest measurements to characterize the effects of his system on two cohorts: university men and army NCOs attending his course. Colonel Hammersley continued periodic measurements on military men when he was director of gymnastics in the army.[26] Although MacLaren's anthropometry was rudimentary, British educators, such as the muscular Christian H. H. Almond, founder of a private school near Edinburgh, looked to him as they incorporated gymnastics, including anthropometric measurement, into health education programs to prepare their charges for the "struggles of life."[27] Ultimately, though, MacLaren's association with the military was difficult to shake, and it led to the downfall of his system in Britain.[28]

Despite MacLaren's attention to chest measurements as a marker of physical power and his understanding of vital capacity as shaping a man's place in the world, he relied on technically simple chest measurements—rather than the spirometer—to measure lung capacity. Spirometric measurement was not an important scientific tool in the hands of this renowned physical educator. Not until the 1880s, when Francis Galton used anthropometry to amass large databases of physical measurements for testing his statistical theories, would lung capacity measurements become a part of the anthropometry programs of British public schools and universities.

Francis Galton's Anthropometric Laboratories

Quetelet conducted his early anthropometry studies with simple tools, allowing anthropometric theories and practices to move easily across borders and to acquire increasingly practical applications in rapidly industrializing societies. In Britain as in the United States, lung capacity measurements would be enmeshed in discourses of labor. Physical educators used anthropometry to monitor individual performance in the gym. Francis Galton (1822–1911), on the other hand, drew on anthropometry for the lofty scientific goal of developing statistical theory and methods to help frame a broad social agenda of race improvement.

Galton is well known for his association with eugenics, a social movement of the professional classes dedicated to the improvement of "the race." In fact, he coined the term "eugenics" in 1883, a year before establishing the anthropometric laboratory in Kensington. Less well known is that Galton measured "breathing capacity" with a spirometer in his anthropometric laboratories. The horror of eugenics as it played out in Nazi Germany—and less prominently in the U.S. sterilization campaigns—has led to a cultural amnesia about how influential Galton's scientific and social ideas were in the late nineteenth and early twentieth centuries. Consequently, Galton's work on lung capacity has been overlooked in most scholarly analyses of eugenics.

Explorer, geographer, ethnologist, geneticist, and statistician, Galton was born into a wealthy Quaker family in 1822, near Sparkbrook, Birmingham. He studied medicine at King's College and math at Cambridge, where, like many of his social class, he suffered the first of several nervous breakdowns. After his father's death, the unsettled Galton traveled to Africa for several years, returning to London in 1852. Working independently of academic institutions and often with few staff, Galton was nonetheless a well-connected and respected figure among Britain's intelligentsia. Half-cousin of Charles Darwin, grandson of Erasmus Darwin, and descendant of members of the Lunar Society, Galton's scientific pedigree was impeccable. His African travels—and his geographic publications based on these travels—established him as a credible scientist. In 1854, he received the gold medal of the Geographical Society, and he was elected a Fellow of the Royal Geographical Society in 1856. Both honors recognized his research in southern Africa. He served as honorary secretary of the Royal Geographical Society from 1857 to 1863. Although he never left Europe again, his experiences in Africa shaped his scientific pursuits, including his understandings of "race."[29]

The breadth of Galton's interests was staggering. In addition to his involvement in geographic societies, he played important roles in a broad range of scientific organizations. From 1863 to 1867, he was the general secretary of the British Association for the Advancement of Science and president of the Anthropological Section from 1886 to 1889. In 1890, he was awarded the Royal Society's gold medal for his anthropometric research. University College, London named its Eugenics Laboratory—established in 1907—for him, and knighthood followed two years later.[30]

A creative innovator, Galton was fascinated by instrumentation. While a student at Cambridge, he began designing machines, an interest he continued during his travels in Africa. Galton's *Hints to Travelers,* published by the Geographical Society, contains a wealth of instrumentation. He made highly regarded contributions to standardization projects for apparatuses as a member of the managing committee of Kew Observatory. He was intimately involved in the design of many of the apparatuses used in his anthropometric work. In the 1880s, Galton initiated collaborations with his relative Horace Darwin, son of Charles Darwin, a talented engineer and cofounder of the Cambridge Scientific Instrument Company, to develop anthropometric instruments. One instrument that piqued his interest—and that of the Cambridge Scientific Instrument Company—was the spirometer, which measured what he referred to as "breathing capacity."

Until his death at age eighty-nine in 1911, Galton continued to develop his theories of inheritance and to use them to influence social debates. His legendary contributions to statistical theory and methods include correlation, regression, and pedigree analysis, many of which were developed with anthropometric data he collected himself.[31] Although a "gentleman amateur," Galton was also influential in the professionalization of anthropology, particularly physical anthropology.[32] Writing in his three-volume biography of Galton, Karl Pearson, Galton's most prominent disciple, claims that recognition of anthropology as a science rested in part on his mentor's methods: "Anthropology was considered as a field to be left for a recreation ground almost entirely to men busy in other matters, for it had developed no academic discipline of its own, until Galton's methods gave it the status and dignity of a real science."[33]

Profoundly influenced by Darwin's *On the Origin of Species,* Galton published *Hereditary Genius* in 1869, outlining his developing theories of inheritance based on a literature review of English men of "high ability." In contrast to Quetelet's interest in the average man, Galton focused on the exceptional. He considered the average man to be mediocre, and his methodologies and theories stressed human variation. Developing statistical methods to quantify the exceptional, Galton believed that, through scientific measurement of physical characteristics, he could predict intellect—and the future of the nation. At this point, though, his theories lacked empirical proof. Proof would require collecting data on "every measurable faculty of body or mind."[34] For this, Galton turned to anthropometry, and proposed that the Anthropological Institute establish anthropometric laboratories in schools and, eventually, at universities and factories. With a few simple measurements, he believed he could assess whether the nation was progressing, deteriorating, or remaining the same, and he could compare Britain to other nations. Which measurements would be the most informative had yet to be determined.

Only a few schools, however, established anthropometric laboratories and collected data.[35] After Cambridge appointed Galton as Rede Lecturer in 1885, he presented the university with a set of anthropometric instruments and persuaded it to create a laboratory.[36] Not until 1908 did Oxford University follow suit. Although mass anthropometry in schools was not adopted in the nineteenth century, Galton remained indefatigable, promoting his theories and methods in scientific journals, literary magazine, books, and popular periodicals.[37] He argued endlessly that the systematic collection of life histories—including anthropometric measurement, photographs, and medical information—would show that inherent capacity, rather than education, circumstances, or free will, drove the physical and psychological evolution of individuals and the race.

Galton's appeal coincided with the empirical turn in anthropology, and his efforts were partially successful by 1875, when the British Association for the Advancement of Science established an Anthropometric Committee with William Farr as chair.[38] Charged with conducting the first systematic study of the "height, weights, &c, of human beings in the British Empire, and the publication of photographs of the typical races of the empire," the committee functioned until 1883.[39] Among the nine measurements selected—along with documentation of birthplace, residence, and "race"—was "breathing capacity." From the beginning, however, the spirometer posed technical problems for users. The measurements taken by London surgical instrument maker Mr. Coxeter were inaccurate in large men. Ultimately, the results were so uneven that the Anthropometric Committee had to jettison breathing capacity measurements in its final report.[40]

The Anthropometric Laboratory at South Kensington

The Anthropometric Committee's data was insufficient to answer Galton's pressing questions regarding the condition and future of the race. He was not, however, to be deterred. The following year, he opened an anthropometry laboratory at the International Health Exhibition in South Kensington (Figure 14).[41] With an impressive array of new and refined anthropometric instruments—including the spirometer—Galton designed the Anthropometric Laboratory to demonstrate to the public "the simplicity of the instruments and methods by which the chief physical characteristics may be measured and recorded." Through scientific measurement, the efficiency and progress of both the individual and the nation could be assessed—and, importantly, comparisons made.[42] "Anthropometric records," he told the public, would enable us "to compare schools, occupations, residences, races &c."[43]

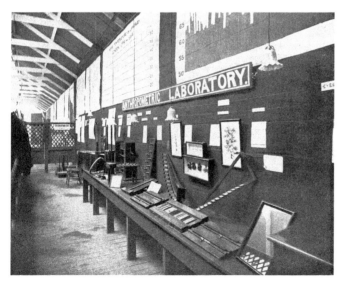

FIGURE 14.
Francis Galton's first anthropometric laboratory at the International Health Exhibition, South Kensington, 1884–85. From Karl Pearson, *The Life, Letters and Labours of Francis Galton*, vol. 2, *Researches of Middle Life* (New York: Cambridge University Press, 1924). Copyright 2011 Cambridge University Press.

In a space measuring thirty-six by six feet, with walls decorated
with charts and pedigrees, and instruments neatly displayed on a
long table, there was one station for each measurement. Open lat-
ticework along one side of the gallery allowed the curious public to
view the laboratory and its instruments, (hopefully) consent to be
measured, and learn about the relationship of statistical measures
of mind and body to social progress. Attendees could purchase a
pamphlet explaining the measurements for threepence. The laboratory, Galton advertised, would measure one's "height, weight, span,
breathing power, strength of pull and squeeze, quickness of blow,
hearing, seeing, colour-sense, and other personal data," all of which
would be recorded on a card for personal use. Galton would keep
another (anonymous) copy from which he compiled a large data set
(Figure 15). During the exhibition, Galton measured approximately
ninety persons a day, or a staggering total of 9,337 males and females from five to eighty years of age, in seventeen different ways.
After the exhibition closed in 1885, he continued his "hobby," securing space in the Science Galleries of the South Kensington Museum,
where he remained for six years, collecting life histories on an additional 3,678 people and conducting more detailed studies of various body parts—including breathing capacity—and extending his
observations to fingerprints.[44] In later years, fewer people visited the
laboratory, and Galton shifted from anthropometry to the anthropological value of fingerprints.[45]

The Anthropometric Laboratory proved successful for a time,
both nationally and internationally. Galton published two papers
from the laboratory in the *Journal of the Anthropological Institute
of Great Britain and Ireland*. The first described the operation of
the laboratory, and the second showcased Galton's laborious work
making tables and analyzing data.[46] As he received many requests
for instruments from "foreign countries," Galton appealed for standardization of instrumentation, something he appreciated from his
experience at Kew Observatory. Noting the extensive anthropometric work being carried out in American colleges, he renewed his call
for a school of anthropometry in Britain.[47]

Technological innovation undergirded Galton's theories and practices. Proud of his flair for design, he continuously modified and developed new anthropometric instruments. With the exception of the
spirometer (made by Hawksley of London), the weighing machine,
and instruments for testing muscular strength, Galton designed

MR. FRANCIS GALTON'S ANTHROPOMETRIC LABORATORY

The Laboratory communicates with the " Western Gallery " in which the Scientific Collections of the South Kensington Museum are contained. The Western Gallery runs parallel to Queen's Gate, and is entered from the new Imperial Institute Road. Admission is free.

Date of Measurement. Day. Month. Year.			Initials.	Day.	Birthday. Month.	Year.	Eye Color.	Sex.	Single, Married, or Widowed ?	Page of Register.
8 4 93			J E	14	11	72	Grey	m	S	4669

Head length, maximum.	Head breadth maximum.	Height standing, see heels of shoes.	Span of arms from opposite finger tips in front of chest.	Weight in ordinary clothing.	Strength of grasp. Right hand. / Left hand.		Breath capacity.	Interval perceived across nape.	Color Sense.	Keenness of Eyesight. Diamond Numerals. read at inches. Right eye. / Left eye.	Smallest Snellen's type read at 6 metres. Right Eye. / Left Eye.
Inch. Tenths.	Inch. Tenths.	Inch. Tenths.	Inch. Tenths.	lbs.	lbs.	lbs.	Cubic inches.	mm. ? Normal.		No.	No.
7.69	6.05	67.5	72.9	161	112 / 108		230	8	?/8	25 25 / 5	5

Height sitting above seat of chair.	Length from elbow to finger tip. Left arm / Right arm		Length of middle finger of left hand.	Keenness of hearing.	Highest audible note. (by whistle)	Reaction time, in handredths of a second.	Greatest speed of blow with fist.	Norm.—Snellen's types are legible by normal eyes at as many metres distance as the numbers they severally bear. Left Thumb. / Right Thumb.	
Inch. Tenths.	In. tenths.	In. tenths.	In. tenths.	? Normal.	Vibrations per second.	To Sight / To Sound	Feet per sec.		
35.5	18 6	18.7 4 6		Yes	19,000	19	13 broken		

One page of the Register is assigned to each person, in which his measurements at successive periods are entered in successive lines. A copy of these made at any specified date may be obtained on application by the person measured, or by his or her representative, at the cost of sixpence and postage.

FIGURE 15. **Card for recording anthropometric data on volunteers at the Anthropometric Laboratory, 1893.** From University College London, Special Collections, Francis Galton Papers.

most of the measuring instruments used in the Anthropological Laboratory. A year before the exhibit opened, Galton asked friends and colleagues for a list of instruments for outfitting an anthropometry laboratory.[48] Simplicity of design and ease of use were critical features for mass anthropometry. Instruments had to be inexpensive and easily transported. Galton often displayed instruments at his lectures.[49] By 1887, his work with the Cambridge Scientific Instrument Company led to the marketing of numerous instruments for measurement of human physical characteristics.[50] Cambridge Scientific continued to market anthropometric instruments, including the spirometer, during the twentieth century.

Although the sample size was impressive, Galton was well aware that exhibit attendees were a heterogeneous population, not a random sample. In his view, however, precision of measurement trumped the limits of sampling. Galton collected his data with careful attention to detail. He used the data on static variables—such as height—as evidence for his theories of human variation and heredity, correlation, the novel concept of the percentile, and the law of error, all of which would contribute to a system of comparing and ranking differences in people.

As he ventured into comparative studies, gender difference stood out for Galton, as it did for Hitchcock. To Galton, the superiority of men was scientifically incontrovertible. He commented glibly that, although "very powerful women exist, but happily perhaps for the repose of the other sex, such gifted women are rare, [as] men generally surpassed women in almost every anthropometric variable."[51] Acknowledging—though ultimately dismissing—"irregularities" in the data, Galton concluded that breathing capacity increased with age to the middle years, declining thereafter. Only after age twenty did a marked difference in male and female breathing capacity appear. For the most part, however, Galton did not conduct extensive comparative study of males and females. His theories would be gendered male.

Unlike social Darwinist Herbert Spencer, who believed physical power was depleted in men of high intellect, Galton found no essential conflict between intellectual and physical abilities.[52] To understand better the physical and intellectual potential of the English male elite (which he could not do with the limited sample of Kensington Laboratory volunteers), Galton turned to Cambridge University's Anthropometric Laboratory, where he could obtain a more homogeneous sample of public school boys from the "upper professional classes." This sample allowed Galton to test rigorously his theories of heredity, intellect, and physical characteristics, using the new statistical tool of correlation, and then promote his findings in prestigious scientific journals.

To complete these studies, Galton invited the esteemed logician John Venn to analyze measurements from 1,450 young Cambridge men and to compare them to those taken from public participants in the Health Exhibition. In each of five measures (height, pull, squeeze, weight, and breathing capacity), the Cambridge men surpassed the heterogeneous Kensington sample, even after taking age differences into account. These results confirmed the "high physical characteristics of the English upper class."[53] Venn was particularly impressed by the "largely superior breath capacity [in Cambridge men]," whether "inherited or acquired by the practice of continued out-door exercise from childhood."[54]

Classifying their intellect by "level of distinction" as a purportedly objective measure of intellect ("first-class man in any Tripos examination" or scholar; remaining "honour men"; or "poll-men"), Venn concluded that "there does not seem to be the slightest difference between one class of our students and another: that is, they are equally tall, they possess the same weight, the same muscular strength of hand, and the same breathing capacity,—this last characteristic probably carrying a good deal along with it."[55] By studying various parameters of physical fitness, including breathing capacity, in university men of the English upper classes, Galton confirmed what he had long believed: superior physique and intellect were tightly correlated. Breathing capacity was a key marker of this group's superiority. In an interview with the London newspaper the *Pall Mall Gazette,* Galton summarized his position, claiming that university athletes "belong to quite another race to those measured in my laboratory in the Health Exhibition. Their breathing capacity and strength are of a far higher order."[56]

Why Measure? Bodily Efficiency and Breathing Capacity

Galton's passionate—if not obsessive—commitment to the practical application of his theories informed the statistical methodologies he developed to test these theories. For Galton, anthropometry was a rational ordering project, one made scientifically and socially credible through theorizing and empirical study. He also deeply believed in the social importance of his project. Armed with a vast amount of data from the anthropometric laboratories of South Kensington, Cambridge, Eton, and Marlborough, Galton began a public relations campaign in 1889 to convince scientists, politicians, and the public of the benefits of measurement, marking, and ranking for the efficient ordering of society. In an article printed in the February 1890 issue of *Lippincott's Magazine* and reprinted the same year in *Anthropometric Laboratory: Notes and Memoirs,* Galton posed a series of questions: "Why should you, the reader, put yourself to the trouble of being measured, weighed, and otherwise tested? Why should I, the writer, and why should others, take the trouble of persuading you to go through the process? Are the objects to be gained sufficient to deserve this fuss?"[57] His publications and public addresses in the coming years repeatedly returned to these questions.

In this period, civil-service candidates in Britain were selected based on their performance on a literary examination. In privileging the upper classes, not known for their hard work, Galton considered the exam inadequate to assess the complex labor needs of Britain's empire. One of the most notable features of Galton's public-relations campaign for the history of spirometric measurement was his articulation of the concept of "bodily efficiency" as a more objective and rational marker for the civil service than the literary examination. He argued that "bodily efficiency," comprised of a series of physical tests—breathing capacity, strength, keenness of eyesight, height, weight, and arm span—promised to erase examiners' "uncertainty of judgment."[58]

In written communication to the 1889 meeting of the British Association for the Advancement of Science, Galton described the importance of bodily efficiency for government posts. Drawing on Venn's analysis, he critiqued the literary examination as an effective measure of prowess. Ever concerned with men of exceptional ability, whom he considered most likely to succeed in the competitions of life, Galton's goal was not to eliminate the literary examination or individual physicians' judgment. Rather, he advocated tests of bodily efficiency to "save from failure a few very vigorous candidates for the Army, Navy, and Indian Civil Service and certain other Government posts in which high bodily powers are of service."[59]

Hierarchical ordering was embedded in Galton's conception of bodily efficiency. Writing that same year in the prestigious journal *Nature,* for example, he rationalized the superiority of relative over absolute ranking, a method for correlating faculties such as breathing capacity with other variables, the statistical place of the probability integer for analysis, and specific techniques for applying these principles in practice.[60] In Galton's mind, relative rank, as opposed to absolute rank, was critical to individual, national, and race improvement. "Relative rank," he wrote, "has an importance of its own, because the conditions of life are those of continual competition, in which the man who is relatively strong will always achieve success, while the relatively weak will fail. . . . The strongest even by a trifle will win the prize."[61] Not only could bodily efficiency be ranked, it could also track maintenance of rank over time, diagnosing defects in efficiency at early stages. For reasons never fully explained, Galton considered breathing capacity and strength measurements to be particularly informative indicators of bodily efficiency:

> The best general test of bodily efficiency is the breathing capacity, taken not by itself, but with reference either to the stature or the weight. Lungs that are amply large enough for a small man would be wholly inefficient for a large one, as the tables of averages and of "rank" show very distinctly. . . . The possession of a considerable amount of breathing capacity and of muscular strength is an important element of success in an active life, and the rank that a youth holds among his fellows . . . is a valuable guide to

the selection of the occupation for which he is naturally fitted, whether it should be an active or a sedentary one. As life proceeds, the strength declines somewhat, and the breathing capacity is materially reduced.[62]

In lectures and publications, Galton demonstrated the power of the statistical principle of correlation by illustrating ranking cards of bodily efficiency. The principle of correlation allowed certain variables, such as lung capacity, to be understood in relation to other variables, such as height and weight. Thus, in highlighting breathing capacity, a dynamic variable, which could easily be tracked over the life course, Galton drew on Hutchinson's hierarchical ordering of lung capacity measurements to address questions of labor. Unlike Hutchinson, Galton did not limit himself to evaluating candidates for the police and armed forces. Instead, he appealed more broadly to "employers of labour" to use breathing capacity in competitive examinations.

The civil service met Galton's ideas with skepticism. In 1878, the War Office and Civil Service Commissions established a joint committee to investigate the addition of a physical examination to the literary examination.[63] Amid concerns about cost, difficulty, and strain, however, they abandoned the recommendations for the next decade. By the late 1880s, circumstances had changed. With growing interest in scientifically informed efficiency in administrative matters, a marker of physical efficiency made political and scientific sense and Galton gained support for his initiative. In their 1889 report, the Civil Service commissioners acknowledged the ease with which physical examinations could be conducted, an admission that likely encouraged Galton to promote his test again.[64] The British Association for the Advancement of Science (BAAS) backed a pilot study of Galton's system of marking physical efficiency, and submitted a memorandum to the War Office, H. M. Civil Service commissioners, the Admiralty, and the Secretary of State for India urging further investigation.[65] But, what appeared so obvious to the rational Galton was not so to the War Office, which affirmed its satisfaction with the current system of literary exam and the overall physique of its recruits. His efforts were again unsuccessful and the debate over civil-service examinations would continue.

Why was Galton so consumed with this campaign to reform examinations for the civil service? Reflecting and informing prevailing notions of efficiency in 1889 and 1890, he presented reform as self-evident. Any objections to the improved physical exam were "preposterous." According to Galton, even slave owners resorted to "minute inspection" to rank their human property.[66] At this time, however, Galton generally avoided broad statements regarding his social agenda. By the turn of the century, as debates over the physical deterioration of the race and the "quest for national efficiency" intensified, he became less cautious in his political prescriptions.[67] A short but telling article published in the *Daily Chronicle* in 1903— soon after the humiliating South African (Anglo-Boer) War—illustrated the connections among Galton's preoccupations with civil-service examinations, physique, race, and national deterioration.

For Galton, race improvement was the critical issue. At stake were the deleterious effects of "town life and sanitary conditions" on the working classes, determining the "prospects for the British race," and taking measures—perhaps "drastic" ones—to improve it. Was Britain "equal to its Imperial responsibilities? . . . How far is it feasible to make it more capable of the high destinies that are within its reach if it possesses the will and power to pursue them?" While concerned with the differential fertility of "the exceptional," in matters of race improvement, Galton could not ignore the largest producers of wealth—a group he had previously referred to as the "passables." Colonial expansion depended on a healthy, efficient, and disciplined civil service, which was partly comprised of lower-middle-class Britons of a "coarser fibre than the Latins," whose "manners [were] vulgar and noisy," and whose physiques were overstated. Only through the careful scientific study of the limits of nurture would "material improvement in our British breed" be accomplished.[68] Studies of the male elite would no longer suffice for the British imperial project.

Galton knew of the extensive anthropometric work being done in American colleges and used it to call for anthropometry in British schools, a cause he pursued zealously in the last years of his life.[69] Hitchcock sent him a number of pamphlets and anthropometric tables from Amherst, Wellesley, and Oberlin.[70] In the last of three public lectures on heredity and nurture at the South Kensington Museum, Galton specifically referred to the work on physical culture at Amherst and Harvard Colleges (Figure 16).[71] A demonstration of anthropometric apparatuses accompanied each lecture. In the 1884 Rede Lecture at Cambridge, Galton commented wistfully that "America, in some of her colleges, has instituted a system of physical measurements, and is turning them to good account, going further

LECTURES ON HEREDITY AND NURTURE, S. KENS. MUSEUM,

November 26, December 3, December 10, 1887,

ON BEHALF OF THE ANTHROPOLOGICAL INSTITUTE,

By FRANCIS GALTON, F.R.S., *President.*

PROGRAMME OF LECTURE III.

The study of different conditions of life on large groups of men. Increase of the white races in modern times. Diversities in marriage, birth, and death-rates, and their effects in varying the proportions among men of different races. Also, in causing the breed of a nation to improve or degenerate. Unforeseen and wide consequences of apparently small reforms. The large infant mortality in the lower classes is followed by few of the beneficial results of natural selection. Want of statistical imagination and our consequent carelessness as to undoubted social duties. Modern instances of stringent State interference when its utility has become appreciated. Avowed cultivation of the physique of men. Professorships of physical culture at Amherst and Harvard Colleges, in America. Effects of gymnastics on national health in Germany and elsewhere. School hygiene and medical inspection. Civilised men are a costly stock to rear. Need for further social inquiries, and remarks on conducting them.

Retrospect of the three lectures. Briefly expressed, their object has been to discuss the influences that tend to " Eugenism."

Demonstrations—(1) **Testing the color-sense by the instrument devised by Capt. W. de W. Abney, F.R.S., and General Festing, F.R.S.; (2) other Anthropometric Apparatus.**

FIGURE 16. **Notice on lecture by Galton where he indicates the work at Amherst College and Harvard University, 1887.**
From University College London, Special Collections, Francis Galton Papers.

in this direction than the public opinion in this country is probably prepared for."[72] Jay Seaver, secretary of the American Association for the Advancement of Physical Education (AAAPE), invited Galton to speak at the AAAPE's sixth annual meeting in 1890 on "the physical side of heredity."[73] In his address, he called on the Americans to join the British in developing anthropometric tests for physical efficiency—a suggestion that was greeted with enthusiasm by army physician Lieutenant Colonel Charles R. Greenleaf. Still, Galton had limited respect for the work of American physical educators. Their atheoretical "accumulation of neatly tabulated figures, carefully added and averaged, quite irrespectively of any use to which those figures can be applied," exasperated him.[74]

In Galton's hands, constructing a marking system for open competitive examinations became an explicit project of ordering difference hierarchically. Galton frequently referred to U.S. Army statistics compiled by Baxter and Gould in his writings. Despite promoting the use of breathing capacity for ranking labor, however, he never published any breathing capacity rankings by race. Although focused on the races of the British Isles, the "dark- and yellow-skinned savages" of Britain's far-flung empire were always lurking in the background, threatening to overrun British civil servants. Like many of his scientific peers, Galton's deployment of race was fluid and adaptable, moving seamlessly between internal and external enemies.[75] For Galton, race meant several things: a sharply class-differentiated human race, a way to discriminate between peoples of the British Isles, a method to construct a notion of "Englishness," and a marker of civilized and savage societies. Each of these uses was embedded in his concept of race improvement, as materialized in his detailed system of measuring and ranking bodies.[76]

In a context of widely shared enthusiasm for hereditary explanations for physical features, anthropometry became a respected science, and lung capacity measurements were established as part of the anthropometric armamentarium in Britain. By the end of the nineteenth century, physiologists, anthropometrists, instrument makers, and engineers had constructed a technical infrastructure for continued innovation with the spirometer and the statistical technologies with which it was intertwined. In other words, lung capacity had become an anthropometric variable of some predictive value, linked scientifically to concepts of fitness and efficiency, its full social implications to be shaped and reshaped by its travels through new socioscientific domains. Wartime anxieties about the fitness of recruits would continue in the twentieth century, providing a stimulus for further innovation with spirometric measurement. In the process, the sociocultural, political, and scientific meanings of this scientific object would expand.

Fitness, Degeneration, and National Efficiency

In his concern for the future of the race, Francis Galton was a man of his times. In the late Victorian and Edwardian periods, anxieties about race degeneration reached a fever pitch. Lagging industrial productivity, military weakness, working-class revolt, and national rivalries for trade and imperial dominance combined to cast narratives of degeneration in increasingly pessimistic terms. Unbridled working-class sexuality—especially that of the "residuum"—that lurked in overcrowded urban spaces filled the ruling classes with fear and loathing. The lower classes appeared to procreate at higher rates than the educated classes, producing mentally and physically inferior offspring. For social analysts, the course of biological evolution was in jeopardy. Despite factory and sanitary reform measures, the physical and economic conditions of the working classes worsened and a general angst about classical laissez-faire liberalism, democracy, and the notion of progress settled on Britain.

In his study of European discourses of degeneration, cultural historian Daniel Pick captures the mutually reinforcing relationship between racial and class identities at the time. The essence of "Englishness" was at stake:

> The notion of degeneration was used at once to signify the urgency of intervention and, still more alarmingly, the potential impossibility of constituting the nation from society in its entirety. "Englishness" had to be defined in a double movement of inclusion and exclusion, ideological assimilation and expulsion. In the light of changing political circumstances, for instance the increasingly wide electoral constituency, the criteria for social "fitness" changed. It was not a question of rejecting the whole urban working class as a "rabble", nor of accepting it wholesale, but of constructing cross-class ideologies of patriotism shored up against the combined internal and external threat of degeneration.[77]

The meanings of physical and social fitness, how they related to degeneration, and how they should be cultivated all remained fluid.

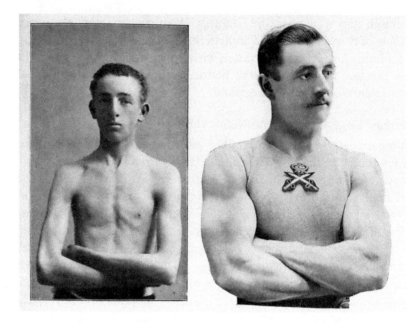

FIGURE 17. **Photographs of young men before and after scientific physical training, 1920s.** The original caption read: "The first photo shows the physical condition of the youth of the nation as revealed by the war. The second shows what can be achieved by scientific methods of physical education and culture, and how imperative such methods are to safeguard us against physical deterioration and disease in the future." From Wellcome Library, London.

Over the course of the century, two models of fitness would replace the ideal of the military man: the athlete, embodied in the public school boy, as discussed earlier, and the professional fitness entrepreneur, embodied in the German immigrant Eugen Sandow. As historian Michael Anton Budd explains in *The Sculpture Machine,* by the 1870s fitness regimes and sport were institutionalized in an increasingly receptive consumer society. It was Sandow who popularized fitness, transforming it into a public spectacle and a lucrative commodity (Figure 17).[78] Intrigued by these displays, Galton the scientist attended Sandow's competitions. The sociocultural and scientific project of individual bodily reform thus coexisted uneasily with broad-based social-reform movements, including sanitary reform, eugenics, and ideologies of national efficiency.

Medical journals and the popular press took note. According to an 1888 article in the *Lancet,* "degeneration . . . is undoubtedly at work among town-bred populations."[79] In 1892, the *Times* reported on a survey of the physical condition of the Army Corps. Of concern was that "their vital capacity is in the majority of cases below Hutchinson's standard of health." Among the suggested steps for improvement were "to use the spirometer once a week," and to measure vital capacity periodically.[80] The times were ripe for scientific interventions.

At the turn of the century, a politically complicated, scientifically oriented elite ushered in a "cult of the expert." United by a commitment to "national efficiency," best understood, according to historian George Searle, as "a convenient label under which a complex of beliefs, assumptions and demands could be grouped," they attempted to rationalize government, the military, education, public health, and empire according to scientific principles.[81] One of the many social reforms supported by "national efficiency" proponents was eugenics.

There has been much scholarly debate over the actual influence of eugenics on public policy. Although contested in its purest form, eugenical thinking was pervasive among segments of the British intelligentsia, shaping literary, scientific, medical, journalistic, and public policy discourse in complex—and often contradictory—ways.[82] Rather than a coherent program, what emerged in late Victorian Britain was a set of interlocking social concerns about the body, the nation, the race, and degeneration, framed in discourses of fitness, and authorized by the theories of evolution, heredity, and scientific management, to which shifting politics were attached.[83]

Although social commentators at the time disagreed about the exact nature of the problem, anxieties about fit male bodies grew as Britain engaged in numerous colonial wars in Africa, Asia, and the West Indies. Whether cast as national decline, race degeneracy, or physical deterioration (deterioration, unlike degeneration, was considered amenable to intervention), concern about the national physique deepened among the British middle classes—imperialist and anti-imperialist alike—in the aftermath of the South African War, a brutal and dehumanizing conflict that spanned 1899 to 1902. In alarmist language, the popular press reported on the high rates of rejection (between 40 and 60 percent) of young British volunteers from urban slums. Again, anthropometric variables loomed large as indicators of fitness for war. "Under chest measurement" of these young working-class men was evidence of a threatening social problem.[84]

What was to be done about the rapidly degenerating masses? Was "the vital capacity of our race deteriorating?" queried one writer to the *Times*.[85] For George Shee, military statistics demonstrated that declining physical fitness in Britain as compared to Germany and France threatened British imperial power. His solution—universal naval and military training—would "arrest the physical deterioration of our population and enable us to maintain that vigour and strength without which we cannot hope to maintain our commercial supremacy among the energetic and virile nations which are now competing with us in the markets of the world."[86] On the other hand, such dire pronouncements conflicted with notions of the inevitability of progress, and statisticians, public health officials, and medical professionals from the Royal College of Physicians and Surgeons viewed the evidence of declining physique among the working classes with skepticism.[87]

In Scotland, the Unionist government appointed a Royal Commission on Physical Training in 1902. In England, the government appointed an Inter-departmental Committee in 1903. Charged with investigating "the deterioration of certain classes of the population as shown by the large percentage of rejections for physical causes of recruits for the Army and by other evidence," the Inter-departmental Committee was composed of representatives from the board of education, reformatory and industrial schools, the military, and the General Registrar's Office.[88] It called sixty-eight witnesses from England, Scotland, and Ireland, most of them male experts and many of them medical professionals, to testify. In the future, medical expertise would be marshaled to find solutions to the problem of fitness.

Cognizant of the poor quality of evidence for deterioration (e.g., lack of anthropometric data on homogeneous comparison groups; shifting criteria for rejection in the military; lack of compulsory military service; and the problem of categorizing the laboring classes), the committee assumed the lower classes, especially "the residuum" or casual laborers, to be unfit. Consequently, it focused its attention on elucidating causes and offering solutions.[89] Sweeping in scope, the strongly worded report was reassuring, if not optimistic. To eugenicists' consternation, the committee determined that the primary causes of unfitness were environmental, not hereditary, and therefore amenable to reform measures, albeit highly coercive and invasive ones for the poor. Success was a matter of political will. According to Dr. Eichholz, a witness whose statement featured prominently in the final report, "there is, accordingly, every reason to anticipate RAPID amelioration of physique so soon as improvement occurs in external conditions."[90]

Historians have analyzed the importance of this report in refuting hereditary explanations for bodily fitness and the extent to which it actually influenced popular and scientific views of race degeneracy.[91] Of note is the centrality of anthropometry to the committee's analysis and recommendations. Agnostic on whether the physique of potential recruits represented the working classes as a whole, the committee and its witnesses agreed that more data was required as a "means by which those interested in the subject may at any moment satisfy themselves of the progress of the nation."[92] In making this point, the committee turned to what was now a credible scientific tool, the anthropometric survey, so avidly promoted by Galton for more than a quarter century. On the basis of testimony by D. J. Cunningham, professor of anatomy at the University of Edinburgh, the Inter-departmental Committee recommended the organization of a permanent anthropometric survey, which would target young people in schools and factories and eventually the population at large.[93]

While environmentalist notions of inheritance inform Cunningham's testimony to the Inter-departmental Committee of Cunningham, they coexist uneasily with an emphasis on biologically fixed and measurable standards of bodies and peoples:

> In spite of the marked variations which are seen in the physique of the different classes of the people of Great Britain, anthropologists believe, with good reason, that *there is a mean physical standard, which is the inheritance of the people as a whole, and that no matter how far certain sections of the people may deviate from this by deterioration . . . the tendency of the race as a whole will always be to maintain the inherited mean. . . .* To restore, therefore, the classes in which this inferiority exists to the mean standard of national physique, all that is required is to improve the conditions of living, and in one or two generations all the ground that has been lost will be recovered.[94]

To measure the physical state of the people and monitor their improvement, Cunningham proposed the establishment of a Central Anthropometric Bureau in London. Although he did not mention the spirometer, second among eight simple measurements to be collected systematically was chest measurement at inspiration and expiration, a common proxy for spirometric measurement.[95] Ultimately, the committee, supported by the College of Physicians, decided that the resources to establish such a complex enterprise as a British Anthropometric Survey were lacking. As a viable alternative, it

proposed the collection of anthropometric data on all children entering primary schools and factories. At some later date, the committee
noted, the survey could be expanded to include workers at a variety
of governmental institutions.[96] Thus, with chest measurements firmly established as "a critical test of physique," the report catapulted
anthropometry to center stage in the administration of British primary schools. The recommendations of the committee became the
foundation of the British welfare state.[97]

As anxieties about degeneration sharpened at the turn of the century and enthusiasm for "national efficiency" gathered steam, Galton's calls for a national anthropometric survey had slowly gained
acceptance. For Galton, statistical analyses of anthropometry measurements were a means to "discover the efficiency of the nation as
a whole, and in its various parts, and the direction in which it is
changing, whether for the better or worse."[98] In 1908, Oxford opened
the Anthropometric Laboratory under the direction of the biome-
trician and eugenicist Edgar Shuster. Its first report, read to the
British Association for the Advancement of Science and published
in *Biometrika,* featured lung capacity measurements, using a spirometer modeled after Galton's at the International Health Exhibit.

Conclusion

Sometimes considered hereditary and sometimes considered changeable, by the beginning of the twentieth century chest and spirometric measurements were accepted as scientifically valid measures of
fitness, vitality, and progress of "the race." While public-health epidemiologists and eugenic biometricians continued to debate nature
versus nurture, violent human conflict again ushered in a period of
anxiety over the physical fitness of recruits.[99] In the early years of
the Great War, fit young men rushed to enlist, and quotas were easily filled. As the war dragged on and Britain's youth were slaugh-
tered, an increasingly dissatisfied public demanded explanations for
the appalling loss of life. As the next chapter illustrates, spirometry
provided a way to assuage these social anxieties over the fitness of
recruits. War would provide a space for technological innovation.

5

Globalizing Spirometry
The "Racial Factor" in Scientific Medicine

Processes of standardization . . . do not themselves
follow a standardized, uniform path. The large
number of elements involved, and the concurrent
presence of multiple actors attempting to pull
the developments in different directions, ensure
that the trajectory of development is jagged and
unpredictable. . . . Different standards bring along
different worlds.

STEFAN TIMMERMANS AND MARC BERG
The Gold Standard

Hutchinson's elegant machine and the "rule" around which
he organized the meaning of vital capacity measurements captivated research-oriented scientists throughout the nineteenth century. Indeed, his attempt to standardize vital capacity stood the test
of time. The transnational infrastructure for manufacture and refinement of the spirometer that emerged in the second half of the
nineteenth century is a testament to his achievements.

Yet uptake of the device was mostly restricted to physiology or anthropometry research laboratories and physical education programs.
Its use among nineteenth-century clinicians was limited. Physicians
were not actively opposed to the spirometer; they simply did not find
the device relevant to the clinic.

Enthusiasm for the spirometer would shift dramatically in the
early twentieth century. As part of the rise of laboratory-based med-

109

icine and public health, American physicians began to reexamine the spirometer's potential as a diagnostic tool. At the same time, physician-scientists in Britain were using the spirometer as a screening tool for the air force and as a marker of individual and national fitness. In such varied contexts, standardization of the apparatus and the entity it described emerged as a pressing theoretical and practical problem.

A new breed of scientifically oriented physicians in the United States began to shift their focus from the bedside to the laboratory, increasing the use of tests, implementing technologies of hospital management, and transforming medical education.[1] Central to changes in medicine were the integration of basic sciences into clinical training and the move to hospitals as sites of innovation, where, as historian Joel Howell writes, "people worked out new ideas that were later applied more widely."[2]

Public health was also professionalizing at this time. With funding from the Rockefeller Foundation, laboratory-oriented schools, such as the Johns Hopkins School of Hygiene and Public Health, were established to train researchers and practitioners in the science of public health.[3] Thus, in the early twentieth century, a broad-based, transnational project of laboratory-based clinical and public health research began to flourish, reinvigorating research on vital capacity and intensifying efforts to standardize the methods, machinery, and interpretation of measurements.

Renewed interest in spirometric measurement was not an inevitable consequence of the move from symptom-based medical practice to laboratory-assisted diagnosis. Medical devices appeared and quickly disappeared from the medical marketplace. The spirometer stood out to researchers for a variety of reasons. It produced numerical values that could be analyzed, categorized, and graphed; it measured the dynamic state of physiological function and allowed for precise monitoring over time; and it lent itself to innovation to accommodate changing applications. Finally, part of the spirometer's appeal undoubtedly stemmed from its ability to make the cultural notion of "efficiency" scientific.

For the spirometer to realize its potential in the clinic or as a marker of fitness and efficiency, reliable standards of "normal" had to be developed. Transnational experts scrutinized the many factors that might influence the assessment of lung function—the technicalities of the instrument, operator methods, patient behavior, physical activity, statistical methodology, and anthropometric variables. Despite such careful analysis, lung capacity, the entity being measured, proved more resistant to standardization than anticipated.

In his analysis of the history of race and normal values in clinical pathology laboratories in the early decades of the twentieth century, historian Christopher Crenner astutely observes that "judgments about normality entailed judgments about human difference; and among the many categories of difference, none in the day entailed greater risks or harm than race."[4] Comparative studies of vital capacity in racial groups were integral to standardization, and race quickly became embedded in the technology as a key variable—similar to age, height, and weight. By 1930, physician-scientists in Europe, the United States, China, and India had established the scientific "fact" that vital capacity was lower in "nonwhite," "non-European," or "non-Western" populations than in those considered "white." In so doing, they naturalized a hierarchy of difference, establishing "white" norms as the standard to which all other groups would be compared.

Early Standardization Projects

Born to an elite Boston family, Francis Weld Peabody (1881–1927) was emblematic of a new generation of physician-scientists who helped to establish the clinical utility of spirometric measurement in the United States. Despite a career cut short by his untimely death, Peabody played an important role in the transnational spread of the technology when he disseminated the virtues of spirometry to China in a 1921 lecture at the Peking Union Medical School dedication ceremonies. Shortly thereafter, comparative racial studies would begin in China.

Clinical training was in transition with the emergence of new technologies of hospital administration based on models of scientific management that shaped the relationship among physicians, patients, and machines. The professional identities of this new generation of clinicians were tied to hospital laboratories. According to Howell, "laboratory tests and x-ray images were thought to provide physicians with useful data . . . data they believed to be valuable, in large part, because that data was seen to be objective and scientific. Patients, too, had come to share their physicians' faith in objective, scientific medicine."[5]

With the widespread adoption of technology, vague notions of efficiency, vitality, and fitness, so pervasive in the first decades of the twentieth century, became measurable, acquiring the authority of

scientific fact.[6] Consistent with the privileging of expertise characteristic of the Progressive Era, the laboratory became a source of expert knowledge that marginalized the knowledge and experiences of
laypeople and community physicians.[7] As a member of this new generation, Peabody saw himself as an experimental clinical researcher
applying basic principles of physiology to disease. Rooted in the expertise he acquired in U.S. and European research laboratories, he
conducted physiological studies of lung capacity in animals and hu-
mans. While known as "a caring physician" to medical students, the
instruments of the laboratory animated Peabody's practice.[8]

Peabody's career followed the trajectory of many elite young physicians educated in the early twentieth century. Graduating from
Harvard Medical School in 1907, just prior to publication of the
Flexner Report, a course in clinical investigation with Johns Hopkins
University–educated Dr. Joseph Pratt piqued Peabody's interest in
research. With generous family financial support, Peabody pursued
a one-year internship in medicine at Massachusetts General Hospital, followed by in-depth training in pathology, physiology, and organic chemistry at Johns Hopkins, the newly established hospital
of the Rockefeller Institute for Medical Research in New York, and
German laboratories. Recruited back to Boston in 1912, he became,
in the words of his biographer, "a pioneer member of a small group
initiating a novel role for the physician—the full-time academic physician concentrating on research and teaching, with private practice
only a minor activity."[9]

Before becoming the first resident physician at Peter Bent
Brigham Hospital, Peabody made another trip to Europe in 1912,
visiting laboratories, hospitals, and clinics. In addition to revisiting
German laboratories, he spent several weeks in Copenhagen, in the
laboratory of famed physiologist August Krogh, winner of the 1920
Nobel Prize in Physiology and Medicine. There, Peabody studied
respiratory function and likely became acquainted with spirometers
built by Krogh. Peabody and other researchers at the Rockefeller
hospital later employed Krogh's spirometer in studies of vital capacity in the United States.

Building on the work of an earlier generation of German investigators, Peabody experimented with a variety of American and
European spirometers for more than a decade. Initially focused on
the instrument's clinical applications, he soon became interested in
developing standards of normal. Beginning in 1916, Peabody and

John Wentworth analyzed the relationship between vital capacity and dyspnea (difficulty breathing) in cardiac disease. "As an objective method which will give even approximately exact evidence with regard to dyspnea," vital capacity measurements, they argued, could circumvent both clinician observation and patient experience.[10] In a lecture to the prestigious Harvey Society of New York, Peabody singled out "the application of the methods and instruments of the physiological laboratory to the study of patients in the wards" as revolutionizing clinical research.[11]

For Galton, the study of individual variability in relation to the "exceptional" was the stuff of statistical theory; for clinicians, this variability represented a serious challenge to the clinical utility of technology. Variability—and the uncertainty it generated—had to be "tamed."[12] To categorize a patient's lung capacity as normal or abnormal and to tailor treatment accordingly, clinicians needed a definition of normal. But determining a precise cutoff for a continuous variable was—and remains—problematic. The challenge of expressing a patient's lung capacity as a percentage of normal drove the early resurgence of interest in standardization of lung capacity measurements, which was part of a flurry of interest in normal values in clinical pathology.[13]

In the clinic, a working standard had to be practical, simple, and precise, even at the risk of erasing biological complexity. Vital capacity measurement varied greatly in individuals of the same age or height. Peabody and Wentworth realized that the many factors that might modify lung capacity made a fixed standard challenging. "The vital capacity varies normally . . . with many conditions. . . . Age, sex, height, weight, the size and flexibility of the thorax and physical training may each and all influence it." Although there was no uncomplicated solution to variability, the principle of simplicity won out. "In the present clinical study," they wrote, it was necessary "to have as simple a method of standardizing results as possible and, after attempting in various ways, it was found that a classification based on sex and height was practical and sufficiently accurate."[14]

While consistent with Hutchinson's elegant "rule," standardizing by height (and sex) did not eliminate ambiguity. Peabody and Wentworth noted that there still "may . . . be quite a variation in the actual vital capacity of normal persons of approximately the same height."[15] Moreover, patient cooperation could influence measurements: "Weakness of the will or failure to cooperate and give the maximum expiration" risked rendering "observations on the vital capacity worthless and misleading."[16] Despite these serious limitations, they set 90 percent as the lower limit of normal (that is a 10 percent cutoff for pathology), thus establishing a standard around which future adjustments would be made.

Although Peabody and Wentworth are credited as the first investigators to improve significantly on Hutchinson's standards, the problems of variability and standardization also captured the attention of scientists at newly established research institutions in the United States. Drawing on German and Scandinavian research on lung capacity, Christen Lundsgaard and Donald Van Slyke of the hospital of the Rockefeller Institute for Medical Research introduced new definitions of residual air, complementary air, and middle capacity into the literature. Dimensions of the chest, they optimistically suggested, might provide a more accurate method of standardization than height.[17]

Several years later, Harvard Medical School professor Howard West boldly proclaimed that Hutchinson's rule did not hold up. Citing previous work of British physician-scientist Georges Dreyer, West proposed that body surface area rather than height correlated most closely with vital capacity. Yet his comments did not unequivocally endorse using body surface to standardize vital capacity. Reflecting on the broad diversity of factors influencing lung function, he observed:

> Since the earlier studies on this subject, it has been recognized that healthy individuals vary considerably in the volume of air which they can expire after a full inspiration. Age, sex, height, weight, the size and flexibility of the chest, muscular strength and physical training are factors which may singly or jointly affect the vital capacity. As an example, trained soldiers, and especially athletes, tend to show higher vital capacity readings than clerks of the same age, height and weight. The probability, therefore, of finding a single standard for all classes of individuals that does not involve numerous measurements and complicated formulas, and that is at the same time not subject to rather wide variations is, to say the least, remote.[18]

West's emphasis on the impossibility of a single standard "for all classes of individuals" is noteworthy. Perhaps classifying people into distinct groups would bring order—as it had for Hutchinson and Gould. According to West, future research should focus on "the more important groups representative of the habits of life of the present day."[19] But what were the most important groups? And how should spirometry be managed until all the variables were understood? Despite their limitations, researchers from the United States to China adopted West's simple formulas based on body surface area, erasing the messy array of factors that influenced lung function, factors over which West himself had agonized. A complex scientific problem became a narrow technical quest to devise a rational system for classification, whether utilizing anthropometric variables, stage of disease, occupation, or—as we shall see—race. Consequently, three interlocking projects emerged—standardization, classification, and establishing norms—that would profoundly influence future research on lung capacity measurements.

Meanwhile, at the University of Minnesota, clinician-scientist J.A. Myers was building an impressive academic medical career. Myers's research applied vital capacity to the diagnosis and monitoring of tuberculosis. Like previous researchers, Myers thought lung capacity tests might elucidate underlying pathologies in the heart and lungs. For Myers, spirometry complemented visual imaging with X-rays, another relatively new technology. The spirometer was especially valuable in monitoring the course of disease because it "measures the ability and power of the lungs to function, while the X-ray records the nature and extent of the disease. Therefore, each has a different part to play. Neither one is infallible, but both are very valuable."[20]

Myers was a prolific researcher, publishing more than twenty articles in only a few years. At first glance, the array of factors affecting vital capacity seemed an insurmountable obstacle to its clinical application. One potential solution involved establishing a baseline in each individual before the onset of disease. "There is no small individual variation in vital capacity," he observed. "It depends upon many factors, such as physical development, occupation, nationality and age. Therefore, lung capacity readings in any given case are of greater significance when the individual's normal has previously been established by actual observations, at a time when that individual was in good health."[21]

In 1925, Myers published a handbook that would become the standard reference guide for clinicians and researchers the world over. With its simply organized tables, a comprehensive history of lung capacity measurements, and extensive bibliography (with more than two hundred listings), a busy physician could simply plug his patient into ready-made tables.[22] No complicated mathematical calculations were necessary. Although certainly convenient, the tables ignored the chaos of variability, making it more difficult to critique the new standards.

Reflecting a growing cultural enthusiasm for record keeping and a fascination with medical technology, the handbook made grand claims for the spirometer in the clinic, public health, and preventive medicine:

> Many persons would become familiar with their actual vital lung capacities if spirometers were made available as weighing scales are. To install accurate spirometers and tables with normal vital capacities and weights in many places where they would be available to the public, would be an excellent public health measure. . . . The taking of one's vital capacity and its comparison with the theoretic normal is so fascinating as to insure extensive use of spirometers if they were made available to the public. Moreover the readings obtained from scales, and spirometers are so concrete as to be convincing to the ordinary citizen. I am convinced that such a method would result in bringing many who suffer from heart or lung disease for definite diagnosis and treatment long before they would, otherwise, present themselves. Thus many more persons would arrive while in the curable stages of disease.[23]

Myers's vision of mass spirometry was never realized. What did survive, however, was his codification of a 15 percent cutoff for normal (slightly different from Peabody), the principle of practicality in standardizing spirometry, and a handbook with reference values embraced the world over—values that incorporated distinctions among racial groups.

War, the Spirometer, and the Exact Sciences

In the United States, the potential clinical applications, particularly for diagnosing heart disease and tuberculosis, motivated standardization of vital capacity measurements and innovation with the spirometer. In Britain, however, it was the First World War that generated renewed interest in tests of physical fitness and fostered technological innovation.

Medical practitioners had long declared recruits fit for service. For the expendable men of the regular army, a cursory examination sufficed. The bodies of the elite Royal Air Force (RAF), however, required careful attention. World War I was the first war in which airpower played such a strategic role, but the initial loss of life among RAF men was staggering. Perhaps more rigorous selection criteria would ameliorate the problem. On both sides of the Atlantic, military researchers worked to develop objective tests to measure all aspects of bodily efficiency for pilots—the simpler the test, the better. Under the influence of Lieutenant Colonel Georges Dreyer, one of the most promising tests—that of vital capacity—became a screening tool for the RAF.

Georges Dreyer (1873–1934) was born to Danish parents in Shanghai, where his father, Captain Georg Hannibal Napoleon Dreyer of the Royal Danish Navy, was a diplomatic adviser to the Great Northern Cable Company (Figure 18). Like others in his family, Dreyer had planned a career in the Danish navy, but poor health led him to pursue a medical degree. In 1900, he graduated from the University of Copenhagen School of Medicine, after which he pursued postgraduate training in mathematics, physics, and chemistry. Having demonstrated talent in research and "passionate precision of technique" in pathology during his schooling, Dreyer was appointed chair of pathology at Oxford University in 1907, a post he retained until his death from heart failure.[24]

Inspired by Louis Pasteur and Paul Ehrlich, Dreyer is best known for his "devotion to quantitative methods and close application of mathematics" as applied to biological problems.[25] His list of scientific accomplishments includes conducting experimental research in bacteriology and mechanisms of immunity, standardizing reagents for serological diagnosis and treatment of disease, developing a vaccine for typhoid and paratyphoid fevers, and measuring blood volume. After controversy broke out over his mathematics, however, he dropped his investigations of vital capacity and focused on experimental bacteriology for the rest of his career.

According to Dreyer, "the question of the Vital Capacity of man was brought into prominence during the War in connection with the problem of high flying."[26] High flying had numerous physiological effects tied to oxygen deprivation.[27] During the Great War, Dreyer served in the British Expeditionary Forces in France as a lieutenant colonel in the Royal Army Medical Corps. First studying methods for diagnosing enteric fever, a major cause of death, he later worked with the RAF and pursued problems related to high-altitude flying. His most important contributions included developing an apparatus to deliver a precise concentration of oxygen to pilots and creating a method for detecting hypoxia. Partly triggered by a report attributing a high percentage of pilot deaths to "physical unfitness, recklessness or carelessness," toward the end of the war Dreyer studied vital capacity measurements and their relationships to anthropometric variables, measuring and ranking physical fitness with mathematical exactitude.[28]

Like American researchers studying lung capacity, Dreyer was committed to a medicine based on scientific principles. Standardization of vital capacity measurements was integral to this vision. During the war, he traveled to the United States to obtain respiratory apparatuses previously supplied by Germany. His Harvey Lecture in New York City on October 18, 1919, emphasized the need for biological standards. It was now necessary, he claimed, to "accomplish for scientific medicine what has already been done in the

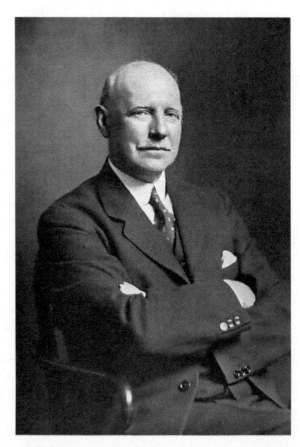

FIGURE 18.
Georges Dreyer.
From Wellcome
Library, London.

field of physics."[29] Following the Harvey Lecture, Dreyer continued to publicize his research in the United States when he traveled to Cleveland, Ohio, to deliver a lecture on the topic "Vital Capacity and Physical Fitness" at Western Reserve University.

In the same period, Dreyer was invited, along with E. W. Ainley Walker, to contribute a chapter, provocatively titled "Iatro-Mathematics: A Plea for a More General Appreciation of the Value of Applied Mathematics and Exact Quantitative Methods in Biological Science," to a Festschrift honoring physician Sir William Osler, formerly of Johns Hopkins and then Regis Chair of Medicine at Oxford. Embracing scientific medicine, Dreyer and Walker explained the importance of quantitative methods to the biological sciences.[30] Dreyer would pursue his study of vital capacity firmly rooted in mathematics.

Ranking Vital Capacity Measurements

The vital capacity cutoff for the RAF during the war was based on an absolute volume of air, not standardized in any way. To the precision-driven Dreyer, who assisted in the assessment of the candidates, this cutoff—which failed to take into account the height, weight, chest size, or body surface of the men—was arbitrary. He wanted to pursue the study of vital capacity after the war.

Dreyer was a member of the Anthropometric Committee of the Medical Research Committee (MRC, later Medical Research Council) and his interests in mathematical description of anthropometric variables intersected with the MRC's desire for a comprehensive anthropometry survey of the population. In 1919 Dreyer submitted a summary of his previous work on vital capacity and a critique of Hutchinson's rule to the MRC and requested funds for additional studies. Specifically, he planned to investigate in more depth his mathematical formulas describing the "true relationship" between vital capacity and other body measurements, especially body surface and stem height (trunk length) as compared to full height. In his analysis of Hutchinson's data, he focused on the hierarchical ordering of occupation, with Hutchinson's Chatham recruits representing "the *best class*" with 100 percent fitness. In the present day, Dreyer argued, "the active athletic class of gentlemen heads the groups of my own observations."[31] In June 1919, he received approval from the MRC to hire physiologist F. W. Hobson to set up the necessary collaborations and secure the required apparatuses.[32]

Dreyer's goals and broad vision for vital capacity measurements are captured in the 1919 leaflet his assistant Hobson (with Dreyer) prepared for the trained observers who would be measuring subjects. He was emphatic about the significance of Dreyer's findings. "The terms 'good physique' and 'physical fitness', two terms which have hitherto had but a vague and indefinite significance," now had "definite values." Focused on the various classes of society, the document asserted: "As might have been expected, different elements of the population have different standards of physical development and physical fitness, dependent upon their conditions of life and the character of their occupations. . . . Adequate and sufficiently extensive observations have only been made upon the gentlemen class of to-day as represented by the Oxford undergraduate, and observations must now be made upon other classes of the population in order that standards may be fixed for each class."[33] (They later modified the leaflet to remove reference to class, which had offended some observers.)

In reality, the entire project was challenging. Dreyer was an experimental pathologist, not a clinical researcher or a physical anthropologist, and organizing a study with a large number of human subjects from different areas of life was logistically demanding. Nervous and insecure throughout the project, Hobson seriously underestimated the problems involved in securing apparatuses, including spirometers, and gaining access to different groups. There were numerous delays in delivery of apparatuses because of labor strife and difficulties with a manufacturer, Boulitte of Paris. Even with collaborators, the logistics of assembling populations of schoolchildren, university students, air force trainees, policemen, firemen, and factory workers were frustrating. To expand his analysis of occupation, Dreyer hoped to gain access to the trade unions, although this proved to be difficult. Moving apparatuses to different sites only added to Hobson and Dreyer's worries.[34]

Dreyer and Hobson persevered, and by 1921 they had collected a massive amount of data on schoolchildren and published several articles in the *Lancet*.[35] Bringing his expertise in blood volumes and aorta and trachea sizes to bear on lung capacity, Dreyer argued that vital capacity had a constant relationship to body surface area. Labeling spirometric measurement an "index of fitness," Dreyer, for the first time, used Hutchinson's same occupations, now for the explicit purpose of making comparisons between males and females and adults and adolescents and ranking the different trades and occupations. Dreyer compared his sample of sixteen fit young men to Hutchinson's original data, ranking the various occupations in relation to Hutchinson's Chatham recruits.

Dreyer's investigations culminated in a transnational collaboration, *The Assessment of Physical Fitness by Correlation of Vital Capacity and Certain Measurements of the Body,* which appeared in 1921. Written with American G. F. Henson and reviewed widely in both Britain and the United States, this compilation of tables and instructions for taking measurements with little text made sweeping claims for the value of vital capacity assessments in measuring physical fitness, assessing the health of "the nation," and distinguishing normal and abnormal bodies. Dedicated to Hutchinson, the monograph aimed "to supply medical men and others directly interested in the subject with a method, new only in the details of its application, whereby physical fitness can be assessed on the basis of a few simple, physical measurements."[36] For these researchers, "War has . . . thoroughly awakened public interest in the importance of physical fitness, not only to the individual but also to the nation."[37] Vital capacity measurements, they hoped, would "remedy the evils of under-development, and . . . promote the cultivation of health and good physique" (Figure 19).[38] Dreyer and Henderson do not mention race in their discussion. Reflecting anxieties about the poor quality of draft recruits during the war, however, American physician Charles H. Mayo, founding member of the Mayo Clinic, frames his "Foreword" in the eugenical language of "race betterment." According to Mayo, "Dr. Georges Dreyer has shown that the estimation of vital capacity is more than a mere test."[39]

"The Dreyer Controversy"

With the publication of his monograph, Dreyer became embroiled in controversy over mathematical formulas. Major Greenwood, a medical officer at the Ministry of Health, began to question "the Dreyer Method" and its claims for assessing fitness. Others, such as A. V. Hill of Manchester University, expressed similar doubts.[40] Karl Pearson wrote a confidential and sharp letter in 1922 to Walter Fletcher, castigating Dreyer's method.[41] The Anthropometric Standards Committee brought in statistical experts to analyze Dreyer's data.

Although Dreyer had many supporters in public health and on

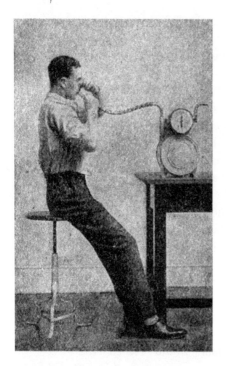

FIGURE 19. **Using the spirometer, "Testing the vital capacity."** From Georges Dreyer, *The Assessment of Physical Fitness by Correlation of Vital Capacity and Certain Measurements of the Body* (New York: Paul B. Hoeber, 1921).

the MRC, the critique of his crude mathematical methods went public when Lucy Cripps, Major Greenwood, and Ethel Newbold presented at the London meeting of the Society of Biometricians and Mathematical Statisticians in October 1922. *Biometrika,* the journal established by Francis Galton in 1901, published their paper the following March, refuting Dreyer's conclusions and confirming Hutchinson's. Like Dreyer, Cripps, Greenwood, and Newbold believed in the reality of vital capacity as an object for scientific investigation. At issue was "the simple biometric question" of the mathematical relationship between vital capacity and various body measurements. Were "the formulae used for the tables or similar formulae," they queried, "better descriptions of a sample population than those based upon elementary biometric considerations?"[42]

In August, former collaborator Alfred Mumford and MRC statistician Matthew Young published a gentler critique of Dreyer's formulas in *Biometrika,* using data from the anthropometric screening of 1,100 boys, "selected by innate powers," at the Manchester Grammar School. They also included data from the police force, Westminster School, and L. C. C. School. Manchester Grammar School had collected physical measurements since 1881, but only in 1921 did it add vital capacity as a marker of vigor. Calculating standard deviations, coefficients of variation, multiple regression formulas, and power formulas, Mumford and Young confirmed the linear relationship between height and vital capacity established by Hutchinson seven decades earlier—but with a caveat. This relationship, they wrote, "cannot be expected to hold from case to case with unfailing accuracy on the average; it was only intended to be applicable to typical cases or to cases on the average."[43] In what would prove to be a fatal flaw, Dreyer's small sample size failed to capture the range of variability.[44]

Despite devastating critiques, popular enthusiasm for Dreyer's method remained high. The *Times of London* featured their results and those of the School Medical Department of Nottingham. According to a school officer in Nottingham, "in no case has Professor Dreyer's method let us down."[45] Four years later, the high master of Manchester Grammar School pointed to the school's long experience of collecting measurements on vital capacity. Boys who "had gained high distinction in the sixth form" had "a large vital capacity." Improving vital capacity made the boy "a more efficient intellectual machine."[46]

The biometrics debate over Dreyer's methods had little impact on practitioners' interest in measuring vital capacity. In 1922, tuberculosis specialist Charles Cameron published his study of patients at a Glasgow sanatorium according to "Dreyer's standards."[47] Attempting to correlate vital capacity with clinical stage of disease, Cameron concluded that the spirometer was useful for diagnosing and monitoring disease and assessing treatment. "The test is a simple one, and appreciation of the various previously detailed causes of decrease is quickly gained," but only as a supplement to the clinical examination.[48] And the test is not a marker of fitness to work. Cameron's paper was reviewed shortly after publication in the United States with interest but skepticism.[49]

The statistical controversy had minimal impact on American researchers. Still, reaction to Dreyer's work in the United States was mixed. For Louis I. Dublin, statistician at Metropolitan Life Insurance Company, Dreyer's conclusions faltered on grounds of accuracy, application, and—most importantly—significance in measuring that elusive entity "physical fitness." Ignoring the statistical dispute, Dublin argued that Dreyer's research opened up a new area of investigation, but in the short term "the use of this rather expensive instrument must be limited to laboratories."[50] Eugenicist Eugene Lyman Fisk of the Life Extension Institute differed from Dublin. In a review of Dreyer's book, Fisk argued that, in thousands of examinations at the Institute, vital capacity measurements were found to be "very useful in distinguishing between substandard types and light weights of sound constitution."[51] Like Dublin, Fisk ignored the mathematics of the dispute. In his handbook, Myers indicates an awareness of the differences between Greenwood and Dreyer, but he, too, avoids substantive discussion of the controversy. According to Myers, it was Peabody and Wentworth who introduced the notion of surface area in relation to vital capacity; West and other American researchers confirmed this view. (Although Dreyer never cites American researchers, his American travels suggest that he was aware of their findings.) Despite devastating critiques in Britain, Dreyer would be cited by researchers into the twentieth century.[52]

Spirometry in South Africa

Dreyer trained many young men at Oxford, including Eustace H. Cluver, who became one of South Africa's most distinguished public-health researchers and administrators. Awarded a Rhodes scholarship, Cluver conducted physiology research at Oxford and received a medical degree in 1918. After returning to South Africa, he eventually became known for his career as director of the South African Medical Institute, dean of the Faculty of Medicine at the University of Witwatersrand, and Secretary for Health. Less well known is Cluver's early interest in vital capacity measurements, which he pursued at the University of Witwatersrand.[53]

In 1921 and 1922, the Smuts government deployed bomber aircraft to crush the Rand Rebellion, an uprising of white mine workers opposed to eliminating the color bar. The mission was contentious, marked by "strain" on the pilots. Interested in medical problems of the air force, Cluver collaborated with the newly organized South African Air Force to create better tests to assess the physical fitness of its pilots.[54] Among the many tests Cluver developed to assess pilot adaptability to high-altitude flying was vital capacity. Although he considered vital capacity as standardized by Dreyer to be "of considerable scientific value," he underscored the importance of the respiratory rate and the ventilation rate, both determined by breathing into the spirometer. In 1923, Cluver devised a scorecard incorporating eight different tests for assessing physical fitness. Consistent with the guidelines of the *Medical and Surgical Aspects of Aviation,* the minimal vital capacity for the air force was set at 3,000 cc.[55]

Over the next decades, Cluver would attach new meanings to vital capacity measurements. With racial segregation hardening and black South Africans increasingly marginalized, the social and political consequences of the perceived deterioration of "white" bodies captured the attention of the U.S. Carnegie Corporation in the 1920s.[56] A concern from the beginning of the twentieth century,

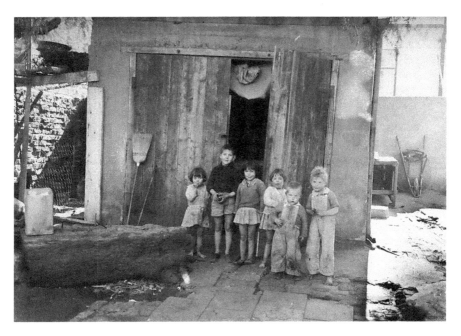

FIGURE 20. **Poor white children living in a garage in South Africa, 1944.**
Reproduced with permission of Museum Africa.

anxieties about "poor whites" reached a fever pitch in South Africa during the Great Depression of the 1930s. Intent on constructing a comprehensive scientific assessment of the well-being of South Africa's poor whites, the Carnegie Corporation funded the Commission of Inquiry into the Poor White Problem, an ambitious interdisciplinary initiative. Informed by experiences in the American South, South African and American experts began their fieldwork, traveling to remote areas in search of poor whites to interview (Figure 20). What they found, according to Columbia University–trained South African educator Ernest Gideon Malherbe, was a "poor black problem" as well as a poor white problem.[57] It was, however, the state of white bodies, so vastly outnumbered by "natives," that required immediate attention. Was "the existence of the evil," queried the *Cape Times,* the result of competition with nonwhites?[58] The survival of the "race" was at stake. Significantly, official unemployment figures did not include black South Africans.

As a member of the health section of the Commission of Inquiry, Cluver introduced physical tests, including vital capacity, which he had developed working with the air force. Later he published numerous papers analyzing vital capacity in poor whites. Cluver's goal in studying poor whites was to use physical tests to improve the national physique and productivity. Although technically complicated tests like vital capacity were soon abandoned, Cluver constructed a "Nutrition Index" based on bodily measurements, such as weight, trunk length, and chest circumference—the familiar substitute for vital capacity.

Applying the index to the study of eight hundred children from the Transvaal, Cluver concluded, "physical unfitness was primarily due to ill-feeding, and was therefore remediable."[59] The state began additional testing on poor white children, with a focus on improving the physique of the Special Service Batallion of the South African Army. Cluver's conclusion was unambiguous: "the physical inferiority of the section of the community loosely referred to as poor whites is attributable to environmental rather than hereditary factors."[60] With proper training, poor whites could become good citizens. Still concerned with the country's young white bodies years later, Cluver continued to study physical efficiency as director of the South African Institute for Medical Research, publishing frequently in the 1940s with Ernst Jokl, head of the Department of Physical Education at Witwatersrand Technical College.[61]

Physical efficiency—also referred to as "physical working power" —was comprised of skill, endurance, and strength, each measured separately. Fitness for labor was a matter of national defense. "It is insufficiently realized," they wrote, "that the standard of physical efficiency dictates largely the rate of industrial and agricultural production, that it is one of the primary determinants of military preparedness, that it has a bearing on the health of the nation and it influences the rate of progress of physical education."[62] As part of a larger project of "intelligent planning," physical tests could assess physical efficiency with precision; functional tests, such as vital capacity, quantified "organic" efficiency.[63]

According to Jokl and Cluver, the growth of physical efficiency was surprisingly similar among racial groups, strong evidence "for the basic equality of man."[64] The "Bantu" were educable, "another deposit of gold in South Africa."[65] As Cluver would argue in addresses to the South African Association for the Advancement of Science during the Second World War, experimental study of physical fitness indicated that improved nutrition and programs of physical training would enhance the working capacity of the population —white, black, and Indian—whose labor was necessary to produce wealth and win the war. But there were limitations to equality. The Bantu were "physically educable," but physical training had better results for the "socially superior type of youth" than the "less plastic human material."[66] "Intelligent plans," with state compulsion, if necessary, were required to "lead the powerful stream of labour into well defined channels of production."[67] In *Training and Efficiency: An Experiment in Physical and Economic Rehabilitation,* Cluver, Jokl, and collaborators analyzed the effects of training on poor white recruits.[68] Among the many tests performed was vital capacity. The book's "vital discovery," concluded the *Johannesburg Sunday Times,* was "that the poor-white is biologically sound and can be turned into a valuable citizen."[69] Left unstated was the status of the South African black majority.

Whether using sophisticated technology or crude measures, Cluver, like his mentor Dreyer, connected physical fitness, efficiency, and whiteness to the future of this African nation-state. South Africa researchers would not conduct systematic studies of racial differences in vital capacity until the 1960s. But the use of this device to probe the science of difference in South Africa was established in this period.

A Racial Factor

Stamped with the imprimatur of "science," nineteenth-century research on lung capacity in physical education and anthropometry laid the foundation for the scientific framing of racial difference in lung capacity in the twentieth century. As laboratory-based scientists marshaled "the increasing armamentarium of instruments of precision in clinical medicine," race became embedded in the larger project of standardizing lung assessment technology—and the many uncertainties associated with vital capacity measurements became increasingly invisible. As Stefan Timmermans and Marc Berg argue, standardization elides careful explanation in favor of "predictability, accountability, and objectivity."[70] This erasure of "careful explanation" would prove consequential for future understandings of variability in lung function measurements.

As mentioned earlier, from the time of slavery American physicians played a key role in producing a science of racial difference in respiratory disease.[71] It remained for laboratory-based scientists to provide more precise and objective evidence. During the 1920s, there was a brief—though epistemologically significant—flurry of interest among biomedical, public health, and physical education researchers in analyzing lung capacity through the lens of race. By the end of the decade, race became a credible causal "factor"—like age, sex, weight, or height—to explain variability in lung capacity. Over the course of the decade, eight papers—six of which were published in the *Journal of the American Medical Association* and the *Archives of Internal Medicine*—compared blacks, Chinese, and Indians to groups referred to as white, Western, or Occidental. That the research and instrumentation were transnational only served to entrench an explanatory framework centered on innate racial difference in lung capacity. A close examination of a few of these seminal studies will illustrate the process by which lung capacity in "whites" or Westerners became the standard of normal and innate racial difference became a scientific fact.

Comparisons between blacks and whites were a prominent feature of the American literature. Working in the tradition of Dreyer, Peabody, West, Van Slyke, and Lundsgaard, May Wilson and Dayton Edwards, two physician-scientists at Cornell University, studied standardization of lung capacity in children in the early 1920s. By this time, precision instruments were becoming more common in hospital settings.[72] To the constellation of well-studied factors of age, sex, height, and occupation, Wilson and Edwards added nutrition, development, activity, social status, environment, and—most notably—race. Using a spirometer made according to Peabody's specifications—with the addition of a self-recording dial—they constructed a normal standard, corrected for body surface area, from measurements taken in three groups of children. Differentiated by ethnicity and social class, the groups were defined as (1) those "representative of the average New York City public school child from homes of moderate income, chiefly of Irish and American nativity," (2) those from "poor Italian and Irish homes, representative of the dispensary type of child in New York City," and (3) private schoolchildren of unspecified ethnicity "residing in the best section of the city and suburbs." Almost as an afterthought, they included a fourth sample (without any socioeconomic descriptors) of "38 average normal colored children."[73] When constructing the normal standard, they excluded "colored" children. It was a range of socioeconomically differentiated ethnicities collapsed into a single "white" category that became the standard of normal. (While the category constructed through this scientific sleight of hand was clearly white, this first publication did not use the term. All future references to this paper used the term "white.") Unifying various ethnicities, whiteness became normal, "colored" aberrant.

The selection of groups and the interpretation of results reflected early-twentieth-century concerns with the social disruption of eastern and southern European immigration and the migration north of African Americans. According to investigators, race and sex—but not socioeconomic—differences stood out. Girls had lower lung capacity than boys. Normal values in "colored" children were "strikingly below that obtained for any of the other groups." Because poor white children, who were quite active, had higher averages than the middle- or upper-income children, "poverty, environment and social statues, with the ensuing advantages and disadvantages, do not seem to influence the lung capacity of children growing up in these respective environments." Lower vital capacity in "the colored race" was due, they concluded, to "a possible racial factor."[74] Moreover, there was no question that lower capacity signaled pathology. According to Wilson and Edwards, vital capacity reduced by more than 15 percent of normal required medical intervention.

By excluding social factors and eliminating "colored" children, this first analysis of racial difference since Gould's Civil War studies projected the material existence of a factor inherent to blacks. (Investigators did not invoke racial factors in relation to whites.) Consequently, an explanatory framework of innate racial difference took hold, which would prove hard to dislodge.[75] Subsequent studies in the 1920s and 1930s built on this framework. Although interpretations would vary, the notion of innate difference in lung capacity continues to inform the interpretation of these measurements to the present day.

Two philanthropic efforts of the Rockefeller Foundation, one focused on medical education in China and another on hookworm among poor whites and blacks in the southern United States, would help solidify the notion of racial difference as an unassailable scientific fact. Committed to introducing Western scientific medicine to China and developing a plan for assisting its medical schools and hospitals, Peabody joined the Rockefeller Foundation's First Medical Commission in 1914.[76] Over a period of four months, the commission visited hospitals and medical schools throughout China. Finding poorly trained staff, bleak facilities, and inadequate equipment for clinical diagnosis, the commission recommended that the foundation expand its support for medical education, hospitals, and medical research. In 1915, the foundation purchased the Union Medical School of Peking from a consortium of missionaries, establishing it as an elite site of Western medicine in China.[77]

Retaining its Christian character and directed and staffed by Western (British, Canadian, but mostly American) medical men who contributed knowledge, equipment, and laboratory techniques, Peking Union Medical College (PUMC) was, to the foundation, an exemplar of Western scientific medicine—a "Johns Hopkins implanted in China."[78] Indeed, PUMC attracted many accomplished physicians from top academic medical centers in the United States as permanent staff and visiting faculty. Among them was Peabody, who returned to China as a visiting professor for three months in 1921. His visit coincided with lavish dedication ceremonies in September, where he joined an international cast of dignitaries to deliver a lecture on the topic "The Clinical Importance of the Vital Capacity of the Lungs."[79] In making his case for the use of vital capacity measurement in clinical medicine and as a measure of physical fitness, Peabody singled out the "quantifying function" of spirometry, a function he thought was enhanced by "graphic expression."[80]

Among the dozens of medical missionaries in the audience at Peabody's lecture was the young American John H. Foster, a physician in the Department of Medicine at Hunan-Yale College of Medicine in southern China.[81] We do not know whether Peabody and Foster discussed the topic, but within two years of attending the dedication, Foster published the first systematic study of vital capacity among the "Eastern races" with his Chinese collaborator P. L. Hsieh.[82]

The son of missionaries, Foster was born in China. After attending college and medical school in the United States, he returned to China in 1919 to work at the Yale-in-China Medical School. By this time, the spirometer had reached the East. Using a water spirometer replicated by a local brass smith from one manufactured by the Narragansett Machine Company and owned by the Chinese chapter of the YMCA, Foster and Hsieh published the first "normal" standards on a Chinese sample, organized by occupational group—soldiers, policemen, workmen, coolies, and so on—and compared them to Western (referred to as foreign or Occidental) norms. Compared to West's standard, 80 percent of the men and 85 percent of the women were below 90 percent of normal.[83]

When measurements revealed that "the vital capacity of the Chinese fell considerably below the standards adopted for Americans," they realized the need to determine normal standards for Chinese "and incidentally, to study the effect of various occupations on the vital capacity." The study design, the questions asked, the references cited, and interpretation of results all reveal the influence of Wilson and Edwards. Noting the difference in "negro children," they invoke the involvement of "a racial factor" to explain lower vital capacity in Chinese relative to "foreigners" whose "measurements were taken under the same conditions." While structuring their research in terms of an East/West binary, they nonetheless recognized the heterogeneity among Chinese, commenting that central Chinese standards would not necessarily apply "to the different races of the Chinese."[84]

Published in the prestigious *Archives of Internal Medicine,* Foster and Hsieh's research soon reached international audiences. Myers featured their work in his handbook, claiming that "various races of people would probably be found to show differences in normal vital capacities."[85] As illustrated by citation patterns, explanations for racial difference in these early-twentieth-century papers shaped future research.[86] Over the next decade, researchers worldwide would study the problem of racial difference in lung capacity. The most immediate task they considered was the seemingly simple—but in practice daunting—development of normal standards for people of all races, ages, and occupations. In framing the scientific problem as a matter of standardization, careful explanations for any observed differences were ignored.

Layered onto the compelling narrative of innate difference in vital capacity were studies from the southern United States and India. With improved study design, more complex statistical methodologies, and new transnational populations, explanations for difference began to harden around a "racial factor." Again, the Rockefeller Foundation would play a crucial role.

According to one popular account, while touring the southern United States, John D. Rockefeller was moved by the "pitiable conditions of a half million hookworm victims." As a result, he selflessly established the Rockefeller Sanitary Commission for the Eradication of Hookworm in 1909.[87] In contrast to the popular account, the genesis of this campaign was more complex, building on earlier

Rockefeller initiatives and the microbiological findings of Charles Wardell Stiles, the cantankerous parasitologist at the U.S. Public Health Service, who had long advocated for a campaign against hookworm. In fact, it was a journalist's sensationalist account of a lecture by Stiles that excited popular opinion in 1902, when he dubbed hookworm the "germ of laziness."[88]

In 1910, cooperating with state and local health departments—organizationally fragile, legally constrained, and severely underfunded though they were—the Sanitary Commission began an intensive, but brief, campaign against this widespread parasitic disease of poverty in the South.[89] For the commission, the five-year campaign, focused on educational programs in country schools, sanitary privies, treatment, and self-help initiatives, captured its vision of public-health education and disease prevention. Attuned to southern racial sensibilities, health advocates avoided addressing the extreme poverty of black and white sharecroppers and disease in the context of segregation.

This nutrient-depleting worm had economic implications. Inducing severe anemia and lethargy, hookworm sapped the "vitality of our population" and reduced "physical efficiency."[90] Indeed, as argued by the esteemed public-health researcher Wilson G. Smillie and his collaborator Donald L. Augustine, "in the economic control of hookworm disease, the essential factor is not the presence of hookworm infestation in an individual or in a community, but its existence in sufficiently severe form to be of economic importance."[91] Indeed, a major concern for philanthropists and businessmen alike was the effect of hookworm on the shortage of white labor for the mills and mines of the South.

Stiles, now chief of the Division of Zoology at the United States Public Health and Marine-Hospital Service, echoed the views of many when he concluded in his 1908 address to the Alabama Medical Society: "what is our country doing in order to better the conditions of the impoverished rural white people of the South?" Rather than a foreign invader from southern Europe, blame was placed at the feet of the southern black, a "frequent soil polluter . . . and greater factor in the spread of the disease to others." Acknowledging his scant experience working with southern blacks, Stiles nonetheless claimed that the Negro was relatively immune from hookworm infection, resulting from centuries of adaptation in Africa.[92]

In 1917, Smillie began working with the International Health

Board of the Rockefeller Foundation (the successor of the Sanitary Commission). A young trainee in scientific medicine, and later a leading figure in U.S. public health, Smillie established the Hookworm Research Laboratory in Andalusia, southern Alabama, to study soil infestation and the physiological effects of infection. By some accounts, hookworm infection approached 98 to 99 percent in this rural region.[93] Because of its cardiac and circulatory effects, researchers hypothesized that hookworm infection might reduce vital capacity. According to the prevailing scientific view, hookworm affected children more profoundly, and the intensity of infection was highest in rural white children.[94]

In part because of the commission's educational campaign in public schools, by the mid-1920s vital capacity measurements were routinely conducted on schoolchildren in Covington County.[95] As an "index of physical fitness," vital capacity, it was hoped, "might serve as a more accurate index of the injury done to a growing child by hookworms than the measurements of height, stem length, or even hemoglobin." This hope was not to be realized. Instead, these studies found that "negro children . . . had a markedly lower vital capacity than the white children."[96] According to investigators, this "incidental" finding might help explain the susceptibility of Negroes to respiratory disease.

In a study published later that year, Smillie and Augustine confirmed that vital capacity was lower in blacks than in whites.[97] While acknowledging "the sharp social barrier that separated the negroes from the whites" in the South, they nonetheless ignored the health consequences of Jim Crow and asserted comparability of living conditions, nutritional status, and hygiene of poor white and black children in Alabama.[98] They concluded that the "marked difference in vital capacity between the white and negro children . . . was so striking and so constant that it occurred to us that it might be a racial characteristic."[99]

Perhaps Smillie and Augustine were not completely convinced that the euphemistically termed "social barriers" in a violently segregated South were insignificant. They wanted to confirm their findings. To do so, they turned to another source of labor in the South—black and white male contract laborers in an Alabama state prison camp, where the men were all loggers. Ignoring the differential assignments of the worst jobs to black contract laborers, they again claimed comparability: "the men were well housed, well fed and had excellent medical care. They were required to work hard, and most of them were in splendid physical condition." Given that "negroes and whites worked side by side, their food was the same, and all conditions of living may be considered as comparable," socioeconomic conditions could not explain the difference. Rather, it must reflect the operation of some racial essence.[100] Consistent with the explanations proposed in previous studies, Smillie and Augustine continued: "as these negroes whom we studied were all apparently normal, we believe that low vital capacity is a racial characteristic, and that vital capacity standards which may be applied to white people cannot be directly applied to the negro race."[101] With vital capacity in blacks more than 15 percent below that of whites, difference was unmistakably intertwined with pathology. The idea of a racial factor, pathologically expressed in African Americans, was gathering scientific credibility.

Again drawing on children, Frank L. Roberts and James A. Crabtree, state field directors of the State Department of Public Health in Tennessee, undertook a study of racial difference in vital capacity. With access to a large sample of black and white children, they could bring more sophisticated statistical methods—such as probable error of the mean, probable error of difference, and standard deviation—to bear on the analysis of vital capacity measurements. Writing that "the negro child forms an integral part of our population and must be considered in any health program," they turned to the anthropometric variable stem length promoted by Smillie and Augustine as an explanation for observed difference.[102]

By the end of the 1920s, the spirometer and the paradigm of innate racial difference had traveled to India. Influenced by the international literature, including the studies of Dreyer and Peabody, S. L. Bhatia, professor of physiology and dean of Grant Medical College, Bombay, presented his work on lung capacity in Indians in a paper before the Indian Science Congress in January 1929. Bhatia was struck by the marked difference in Indians compared to Westerners. He commented that "no matter what standard is taken into consideration, one fact is perfectly obvious, namely, that the vital capacity of the lungs of this group of 100 Indians is much smaller than the normal standards given for Western people."[103] Western standards were defined as the American standards from Myers's handbook and the Association of Life Assurance Medical Directors and Actuarial Society of America. Consistent with previous work, Bhatia's explanation was simple—"a racial factor." For Bhatia, vital capacity held great promise for diagnosis of many clinical conditions, as well as for physical fitness, and he called for "further investigation." Researchers in India continued to study the problem throughout the twentieth century.

While the empirical evidence for innate difference was building in the 1920s, an alternative view on the causes of racial difference in vital capacity measurements in Chinese and Westerners emerged in the work of American Charles McCloy, a missionary and physical educator working in China. Arriving in China in 1913, McCloy worked with the YMCA until 1921, after which he assumed the directorship of National Southeastern University in Nanjing. He published extensively in Chinese and founded the *Physical Education Quarterly* in 1922. Deeply committed to a scientifically rooted physical education, McCloy emphasized careful measurement and thorough statistical analysis. With the spirometer having made its way to China and in wide use in American physical education, McCloy was drawn to vital capacity measurements as a marker of physical fitness.

McCloy used a machine manufactured by Narragansett Machine Company to compare Chinese students with previously developed American standards. Introducing multiple regressions, McCloy concluded that "there is little difference between American and Chinese data" when controlled for surface area.[104] Of particular note is the environmentalist explanations put forth by McCloy. He believed neither vital capacity nor body surface area was a fixed "racial factor." Both were responsive to environmental conditions. Like Foster and Hsieh, he resisted the tendency to homogenize a group as varied as the Chinese. "The possibility of regional variations should be kept in mind," he concluded. "It may prove that there is a larger variability in nationals of one country, caused by climate, activity and bodily build than is found between nations or races."[105]

Drawing on the literature of physical education rather than medicine, McCloy, like others before him, used laboratory tools to promote the idea that fitness could be both measured and improved through physical training. His interpretations were consistent with views at a very specific and short-lived moment in China, when, as Andrew Morris claims, athletics occupied a new intercultural zone, where both imperialist and nationalist narratives of sameness and difference were fluid.[106] By the mid-1920s, a strident nationalism began to replace this intercultural zone.[107] In the United States, McCloy's research did not fit into prevailing paradigms. Although he reached a broad audience through the *Archives of Internal Medicine,* the impact of his environmentalist views on lung function researchers was minimal. McCloy's paper would be cited infrequently outside the field of physical education, and it ultimately disappeared from the biomedical literature, leaving innate, biological difference as the default explanation.[108]

Conclusion

As Timmermans and Berg argue, "efficiency through standardization became a national preoccupation in the prewar United States."[109] Like the factories of industrial America, the social worlds of medicine and public health were ideal sites to enact this preoccupation. Precise standardization of lung capacity, however, proved elusive. There were too many factors to account for. Most of the standards implemented in early-twentieth-century medicine were quickly abandoned.

At the beginning of the 1920s, research on vital capacity was centered in Western Europe and North America. Bolstered by American imperial interests in the form of Rockefeller philanthropy, by the end of the decade, vital capacity measurements were conducted in China, India, the Philippines, and South Africa. With the global spread of spirometry in medicine and public health came a sharpening of ideas of racial difference. The notion of an innate "racial factor" would linger in the literature, reducing the issue of racial difference in lung capacity to a technical one, but informing future research. Findings from physical education could have troubled narratives of innate difference, but they failed to do so. The notion of innate racial factors made too much cultural sense.

Although efforts to standardize vital capacity measurements were unsuccessful, by the end of the decade, the notion that whites had higher lung capacity than other racial or ethnic groups had an unmistakably scientific foundation. The idea was rapidly assimilated into medical handbooks and textbooks published in the United States. Not until the 1960s did significant interest in the racial dimensions of the technology reemerge. Debates over statistical methodologies and standardization continued, with the basic framing of how race fit into modern standardization projects only rarely disrupted. Before examining the consequences of this racial framework for the contemporary thinking on vital capacity, let us first explore the racialization of vital capacity measurements in yet another social world—that of work-related respiratory disease in Britain and South Africa after World War II.

6

Adjudicating Disability in the Industrial Worker

Orthodox medical knowledge tended to minimize risks and promote the view that hazardous products and toxins could be controlled by science and technological fixes.

ARTHUR McIVOR AND RONNIE JOHNSTON
Miner's Lung: A History of Dust Disease in British Coal Mining

J. A. Myers, respiratory specialist at the Mayo Clinic, began advocating for spirometry in preemployment examinations in the 1920s. With workers pitted against industrial employers and company physicians, workers' compensation—still in its infancy in the United States—was already a polarized terrain. Like other medical experts, Myers viewed spirometric measurement as a tool to manage malingering.[1] Although a promising innovation, with weak trade unions and a politically muddled patchwork of state-based approaches to compensation, the spirometer would not be used systematically in industrial medicine until much later in the century.[2]

The situation differed in Britain. In the aftermath of the technologically "modern" Second World War, bitter societal debates over workers' compensation converged with scientific research agendas to stimulate major innovations in the technology for measuring lung function and fitness to work. Production demands, mechanization, power drills, poor ventilation, and brutally exploitative labor practices left growing numbers of coal miners disabled from respiratory diseases. Demands for compensation grew. With mistrust rampant, the spirometer, a medical device that could mediate opposing interests, appealed to workers, capital, and the state alike. Yet, adapting the spirometer to assessing disability was not a simple matter. Developing a system for compensating disease and adjudicating disability were slow, uneven, and politically fraught processes, shaped by regional, national, and transnational contexts.

In 1945, the British Medical Research Council (MRC) established the Pneumoconiosis Research Unit (PRU) near the coalfields of South Wales to address work-related disease in miners. Initially dedicated to the study of the newly scheduled coal workers' pneumoconiosis (CWP), the South Wales PRU later became a rich site for innovation with the spirometer.[3] An impressive interdisciplinary team of researchers refined clinical diagnosis, standardized X-rays, conducted field surveys, designed and built elaborate laboratory equipment, developed experimental animal models to study disease—and forged new theoretical ground on lung function and disability assessment.

PRU researchers published hundreds of papers on industrial medicine, population-based epidemiology, and respiratory physiology that catalyzed international interest in the mechanics of lung function.[4] They experimented with the machine, attempting to define "normal" and rationalize variability. Eventually they turned to the study of groups, choosing to compare lung function in racial, ethnic, and national groups to people referred to as whites/European/ Western.

From the South Wales PRU came a seemingly simple technical solution to the problem of group difference. Rather than exploring the causes of observed differences, researchers devised a "correction factor" for lung function in people labeled "black." The standard of "normal" was that of "white" lung function. With computerization, correction factors would be built into the software of the instruments. Yet, for all its simplicity and apparent objectivity, the dynamic nature of lung function—and the dynamic nature of groups—limited the utility of this technical fix.

Respiratory Disease and the Dilemma of Disability

By the early nineteenth century, South Wales was a major coal-producing region in Britain (Figure 21). As coal mining expanded to deeper and larger pits and thinner seams and as production demands intensified, mine work became more hazardous. By the mid-1830s, it was clear that miners were suffering from a chronic and apparently disabling respiratory disease, variably referred to as miners' asthma, black spit, melanosis (black deposits), anthracosis, silico-anthracosis, and later, coal workers' pneumoconiosis. The daily risk of death or crippling injury from "accidents" resulting from roof falls, deadly fumes, fire, and gas explosions in the collieries, however, overshadowed the magnitude of disease.[5]

As historians Arthur McIvor and Ronnie Johnston have written, understandings of the health effects of coal dust developed fitfully. In a process they aptly call "discovery and denial," some aspects of disease would be illuminated while others were obscured.[6] Writing in the mid-twentieth century, Scottish industrial physician Andrew Meiklejohn organized the unevenness of development of medical knowledge into three periods, which still help to elucidate the complex recognition of CWP.[7] According to Meiklejohn, the first phase of medical studies, around 1800–1875, reflected the emerging dominance of pathological anatomy in the understanding of disease.[8] During this period, British physicians published microscopic

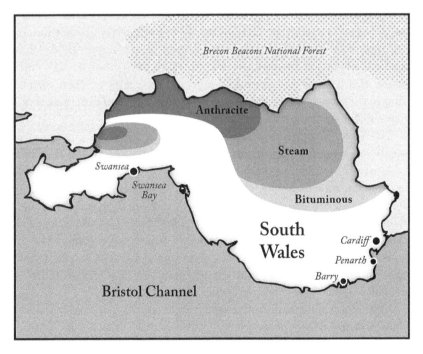

FIGURE 21. **Map of South Wales showing coal deposits.**

descriptions of coal miners' lungs. Although some physicians, such as pathologist and social reformer Rudolf Virchow, denied the existence of coal-induced disease, a consensus was emerging that respiratory disease occurred in coal miners.[9]

This medical consensus was fragile, however, as it was riddled with uncertainties about causal processes. Scientific questions focused on classifying lesions and associating particular agents with specific lesions. Coal miners were, after all, exposed to a variety of dusts, fumes, and soot underground. How could coal dust be distinguished from other hazards? How did coal miners' disease differ from tubercular phthisis, a widespread ailment at the time? Why were some individuals affected and not others? The problem of assessing disabled bodies was not even considered an important scientific question at midcentury. Despite the availability of the spirometer and Hutchinson's use of occupational categories, studies of the effects of work-related disease on lung function had not yet been systematically pursued.

Because of improvements in ventilation, shorter working hours, and the establishment of bathhouses at pit heads—along with a certain amount of wishful thinking—by the late nineteenth century, experts began to report the disappearance of pulmonary disease among coal miners.[10] During Meiklejohn's second phase, about 1875–1920, medical attention focused on free silica in rock dust as the main cause of a fibrotic respiratory disease in coal miners, then termed silicosis. The very existence of disease resulting from coal dust was a matter of dispute in this period (Figure 22).[11]

The 1906 Workmen's Compensation Act ushered in a new era in social relations among physicians, workers, industry, and the British state, in which the problem of disability loomed large. Yet this legislation was a deeply problematic compromise that left many work-related diseases uncompensated.[12] Indeed, compensable conditions in the 1906 act were limited to a few diseases—anthrax, lead poisoning, mercury, phosphorus, arsenic, and anklysostomiasis—for which disability assessment was clear-cut. Additions to the schedule of disease were made cautiously, often the result of contentious battles waged by workers and their allies.

Influenced by international research on silica—especially studies from South Africa—pressure built to schedule silicosis in Britain. For Meiklejohn, the third phase of medical knowledge began in the 1920s, when coal miners who worked seams embedded in silica-

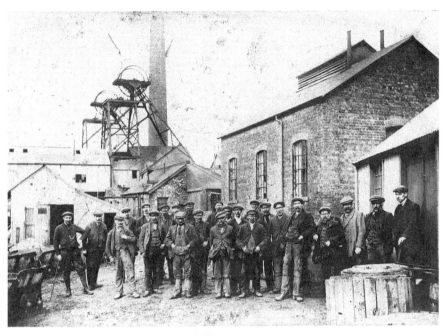

FIGURE 22. **Coal miners at Seven Sisters Colliery, 1911.**
Reproduced with permission of South Wales Coalfield Collection,
Swansea University.

containing hard rock were brought into the compensation system.
But, under the Various Industries (Silicosis) Scheme of 1928, only
cases of death or total disability were compensated.[13] The majority of
miners remained excluded from compensation.

In extending compensation to partial disability, the Various Industries Scheme of 1931 covered more workers. At the same time,
the Scheme introduced new medicolegal challenges in assessing partial disability, setting the stage for the introduction of spirometry
as an objective marker of disability to industrial medicine. Under
the Various Industries (Silicosis) Amendment Scheme of 1934, compensation for silicosis (or silicosis accompanied by tuberculosis) was
extended to all underground coal miners—but only if the nodular
features of silica dust were detected on microscopy and X-ray.[14] Disease without visible nodular silicosis or tuberculosis—"X-ray negative disease"—remained undiagnosed and uncompensated.

Despite a growing consensus that coal dust alone did not cause
disease, respiratory disease had not disappeared among colliers by
the 1930s. With the increased use of machine cutters, conveyors,
air drills, and other mechanized equipment, more men were falling

ill. The rate of workmen's compensation certifications—and rejections—escalated. In 1935, 50 percent of claims were rejected. As the worldwide Depression deepened, the high rate of bankruptcies and resultant unemployment in the coal industry intensified workers' dissatisfaction with the compensation system.[15]

Adjudicating disability—that is, assessing loss of function—was not a simple matter. Even as compensation expanded, new sociomedical and technical questions related to disability emerged. What was the relationship between gross, microscopic, and physiological lung damage? What changes constituted disability? Could one have disease without disability? Although not displaying nodular changes of classical silicosis, the lungs of miners whose claims were rejected were not normal. They often exhibited a distinctive pattern of delicate fibrous shadowing called "reticulation." Whether reticulation was an early stage of disease and whether it was functionally disabling became a matter of intense debate. Physicians, many of whom espoused the values of free enterprise, were increasingly central to mediating this contentious terrain. The profession took its responsibility seriously—researching, describing, and categorizing microscopic lesions. Current technology was not adequate to determine loss of function. For miners, the government, industrialists, and physicians, the spirometer soon emerged as a precision tool that purportedly could assess function.

The Medical Research Council Takes Notice

In the volatile interwar period, disability assessments based on physician interpretation of clinical symptoms of dyspnea on exertion (breathlessness) and radiologically visible tissue damage were highly problematic.[16] Physicians were puzzled by the lack of correlation between the degree of tissue damage and the severity of breathlessness. As radiography became increasingly available, experts focused on technical issues related to imaging, resolution, and reproducibility. But observable changes were difficult to interpret in the absence of agreed-upon standards of normality. The landscape of disease and disability—caught between uncertain diagnoses, the subjective experience of workers, and the subjective interpretations of physicians—continued to be contested.

Eighty-five percent of certifications in Britain occurred in South Wales; the highest rates were in the western anthracite fields. As workers' discontent mounted, and scientific evidence for a "new" chronic respiratory disease in coal miners accumulated, the South Wales Miners' Federation (referred to as the Fed) pressured the government to authorize research on diseases caused by coal dust. Fully aware that money could never compensate for the "loss of health and life that disease entail," the militant Fed focused its attention on prevention as well as compensation.[17] The Home Office and Mines Department responded, directing the MRC to investigate whether coal dust caused a distinct and disabling disease or whether pulmonary disease in coal miners was a form of silicosis. In 1936, physician Philip D'Arcy Hart, staff researcher at the MRC, Edward Aslett, a chest physician from the Welsh National Memorial Association, and a team of interdisciplinary researchers set off for the coalfields of South Wales.[18]

Using portable X-rays, "simple respiratory disability tests" (an exercise test), clinical examinations, and detailed work histories, D'Arcy Hart and Aslett's team conducted the first large-scale survey of an industrial disease. With the cooperation of the Fed, they surveyed miners and examined coal trimmers who were not exposed to silica-containing rock dust.[19] "The remarkable memories of the miners" provided critical information on exposures and disease progression. Respect for miners' knowledge was crucial to the success of the study. (As recounted at a Wellcome Witness Seminar on Pneumoconiosis, D'Arcy Hart and Aslett's respect for miners was deep. For example, they defied the MRC's directive that researchers travel first class to avoid talking with miners.)[20]

In three special reports—detailing clinical, pathological, environmental, and experimental investigations published between 1942 and 1945—D'Arcy Hart, Aslett, and collaborators obtained compelling scientific evidence for something workers and local doctors had long known: coal miners developed disabling respiratory disease that progressed according to length of exposure to coal dust. Crucially, this disease was radiologically and pathologically distinct from that produced by silica or asbestos. Confirming earlier work with coal trimmers and coal screeners, the researchers demonstrated that coal trimmers had lesions pathologically identical to coal face workers and distinct from classical silicosis.[21] Moreover, it appeared to be the same disease the world over.

Among the MRC's most important findings was that early disease—characterized by the X-ray shadowing called "reticulation"—was associated with disability in older miners.[22] The revised 1943 Workmen's Compensation scheme included coal dust–induced respiratory disease and the early stages of "reticulation."[23] While an important step, D'Arcy Hart and Aslett's report also generated new scientific uncertainties through which future research and legislation were filtered.[24]

The recognition of CWP created a crisis of staggering dimensions. Under the act, certifications skyrocketed. In 1945, five thousand men were certified in South Wales alone. By 1948, more than one-tenth of the workforce in South Wales—40 percent of whom were unemployed—were on the disabled register. The Ministry of Fuel and Power that administered the claims and the miners' union that monitored them were both overwhelmed.[25] The "present Pneumoconiosis Scheme," according to H. J. Finch, compensation secretary for the South Wales Area of the National Union of Mineworkers (NUM), "was breaking down."[26] New ways had to be found to contain the crisis. All involved parties invested in scientific research to resolve the crisis.

The PRU in South Wales

The PRU's vision was scientifically exciting. For a generation of medical researchers returning from war and committed to rebuilding Britain, the opportunity to ameliorate a disabling disease was inspiring. A rising star in clinical medicine, Charles Fletcher was, by all accounts, an unusual but excellent choice to head a research unit in South Wales, far removed from cosmopolitan London. He was, according to Sir Christopher Booth, "really a man with quite extraordinarily the wrong qualifications to go to talk to coal miners in south Wales."[27] Son of Sir Walter Morley Fletcher, first secretary of the Medical Research Council (MRC), Charles Fletcher was educated at Trinity College, Cambridge. With additional clinical training at St. Bartholomew's Hospital and research experience at Oxford, a prestigious academic career awaited him. At the suggestion of Richard Schilling, then secretary to the MRC's Industrial Health Research Board, Sir Edward Mellanby, secretary of the MRC, approached Fletcher in 1945. Hoping for a professorial appointment and knowing little about chest disease, Fletcher was torn. But having been excluded from war service because of diabetes, he agreed to direct the unit "because I thought that this was a way that I could serve the country."[28]

Tackling the pneumoconiosis problem required experts and infrastructure. Fletcher settled on Llandough Hospital, five miles outside of Cardiff in Penarth, as the site for his research unit. The unit contained eight side wards that served as laboratories and workshops for equipment and a twenty-bed ward for treatment, rehabilitation, and clinical research. Fletcher recognized that they would soon outgrow the space and immediately began planning for the construction of a new building with laboratories, workshops, radiographic facilities, and clinical departments. The opening event attracted regional and national dignitaries (Figure 23).[29]

Although recruitment to remote South Wales was difficult, Fletcher hired a talented staff of thirty-four, who were interdisciplinary in their expertise and worked well together. By 1951, the staff had grown to seventy.[30] In a vibrant and collaborative "research climate . . . which resulted in day-to-day discussion of ideas and interests in an enthusiastic forum," the unit quickly became recognized as an international authority on industrial disease—and on the technical approaches to identify and measure its disabling effects.[31]

THE MEDICAL RESEARCH COUNCIL

request the pleasure of the company of

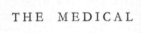

at the opening of the new laboratories of the

Pneumoconiosis Research Unit
at
LLANDOUGH HOSPITAL, Near CARDIFF
by
THE RT. HON. HERBERT MORRISON, *M.P.*
(The Lord President of the Council)
at 2.45 p.m. on SATURDAY, 28th OCTOBER, 1950

Following the ceremony, tea will be provided in the Hospital by kind invitation of the Board of Governors of the United Cardiff Hospitals

R.S.V.P. *to*
The Director, Pneumoconiosis Research Unit,
Llandough Hospital, Near Cardiff.

FIGURE 23. **Invitation to opening of new laboratories at the PRU, 1950.** Courtesy of Cardiff University Library, Cochrane Archive, University Hospital Llandough.

Among the many researchers at the PRU, those most pertinent to the history of research on lung function and disability include Alice Stewart, John C. Gilson, Philip Hugh-Jones, Basel Martin Wright, Archie Cochrane, and John Cotes. All were research-oriented physicians, but their interests varied. Stewart, the lone female scientist, helped Fletcher set up the unit in 1945, after which she moved to the John Ryle's Institute of Social Medicine at Oxford.[32] Having analyzed vital capacity measurements for his MD thesis, chest physician Philip Hugh-Jones joined the staff when Mellanby sent him there after the war. Hugh-Jones worked at the unit until he left to teach medicine at the newly established University of the West Indies before returning to London.

John C. Gilson, a key figure in lung function testing, joined the unit in 1946 as deputy director. He became interested in respiratory physiology while studying with pioneering occupational physician Donald Hunter. Gilson worked in the Physiology Laboratory in the Royal Air Force at Farnsborough during the war. Like Georges Dreyer during the First World War, Gilson's scientific, technical, and engineering skills—honed during wartime—were essential to his work on the physiology of lung function and its application to disability determinations. Hugh-Jones and Gilson collaborated to develop new measures of lung function. Fletcher recruited the pathologist Basel Martin Wright to the PRU in 1949. A self-defined "gadgeteer," Wright spent most of his time developing medical devices. (He is most famous for inventing the peak flow meter.) Archie Cochrane, perhaps the most renowned of the medical staff at the PRU, designed the now famous Rhondda Fach epidemiologic studies of pneumoconiosis in the valleys of South Wales. Cochrane joined the unit in 1948 after meeting with Fletcher in London. He later referred to the job as "almost hand tailored to my dreams and abilities."[33] At the unit, Cochrane developed the theories and methods of population-based research, achieving a high response rate in his surveys.[34]

After seven years leading the PRU, Fletcher left South Wales, returning to clinical medicine at Hammersmith Hospital in London. The more technocratic Gilson succeeded him as director in 1952. Ably guiding the unit for the next twenty-four years, Gilson moved the unit's work in a biomedical direction, one oriented to basic physiology of disease. John Cotes, a later recruit of Gilson's from the Institute of Aviation Medicine, worked at the PRU from the early 1950s until 1979, when he left for the Department of Occupational Health and Hygiene at Newcastle upon Tyne's medical school. An accomplished respiratory physiologist, Cotes was the first staff member systematically to probe racial and ethnic differences in lung function.

The early cohort at the PRU was part of a generation of scientists for whom the brutalities of war, socialist ideals, and a postwar faith in science altered their lives, careers, and worldviews. Many were born before or during the Great War, Cochrane served in the Spanish Civil War, and most served during World War II. Cochrane also was a prisoner during World War II. Several conducted physiological research during the war and became accomplished instrument makers under conditions of austerity. Economically and socially privileged, most were products of public schools and elite universities. Some—though not all—were at least loosely committed to a vision of social medicine. United by a fascination with precision measurement, whether of instrumentation, X-rays, or statistical analysis, this group created an intellectually vibrant research environment dedicated to solving the scientific and social problems of CWP. Especially in its early years, the unit was noted for its commitment to the miners. For the most part, the PRU staff was enthusiastic about the National Health Service and the nationalization of the coal industry. The unit's international reputation in pathology, physiology, dust physics, epidemiology, and statistics of industrial disease would be unrivaled for decades.

A kind man, Fletcher's personality and social commitments (he joined the Socialist Medical Association during medical school) contributed to the respectful working relationship he established with miners and their union. For a brief moment under his leadership, a holistic social medicine approach—though still physician-centered—shaped by the dilemmas of compensation and unemployment, informed the unit's understanding of CWP in South Wales. Fletcher avidly promoted technoscientific research to improve X-ray classification, develop instruments for dust sampling, and measure various parameters of lung function; yet, in his early writings and speeches, scientific and social concerns were intertwined. Fletcher's two Goulstonian Lectures at the Royal College of Physicians, for example, convey remarkable sensitivity to the suffering of miners. He had harsh words for physicians. "It must be admitted," he wrote, "that medical men by their ill-informed complacency have a heavy load of responsibility to bear for the present high incidence of pneumoconiosis among coal-miners."[35] Together with Hugh-Jones, he authored a monograph for the MRC in 1951, *The Social Consequences of Pneumoconiosis among Coal Miners in South Wales,* detailing the hardships that disability and unemployment brought to miners and their communities.

From the beginning, PRU staff members used the spirometer in their studies. Alice Stewart, working with the Social Survey, conducted the first major survey coming out of the unit. Her sociomedical survey examined disability and mortality in men who had been suspended from industry with both early- and late-stage pneumoconiosis. Foreshadowing future collaborations with the Fed, the staff found the miners "keen to cooperate," and achieved a stunning 91 percent participation rate.[36] This was likely the first large survey of the pathogenesis of disease in which vital capacity measurements, using "a simple spirometer," were part of miners' clinical examinations. Although the analysis of vital capacity measurements was limited, Stewart and her colleagues made a cursory attempt to link disease to pulmonary disability. An astonishing two-thirds of men with mild disease and almost all the men with gross disease showed abnormal vital capacity.

Stewart's findings on CWP did not fit into the conceptual framework the unit was developing and her contributions were largely ignored. In particular, Stewart (like D'Arcy Hart) did not subscribe to the sharp distinctions between simple and complicated pneumoconiosis that would define PRU thinking on disease progression. Many years later, Fletcher wrote, "it became clear (but not to Alice!) that there were two distinct types of disease."[37] The independent-minded Stewart left the PRU soon after completing her survey to join John Ryle's Institute of Social Medicine.[38] Cochrane, who grasped South Wales's potential for studying defined populations, continued the survey work, achieving the spectacular response rates for which he is widely praised.

Researchers at the unit worked hard. By any account, their productivity was striking. By the end of 1949, the unit staff had published fifteen research papers, an amazing achievement given the complete lack of a scientific infrastructure before Fletcher's arrival four years earlier.[39] Critical to the success of the PRU—and what distinguished South Wales from the coal-mining regions in Scotland and northern Britain—was the Fed. Sociologist Michael Bloor has insightfully analyzed the Fed's "instrumental" use of expertise in their relations with medical researchers.[40] Articles in the *Miner,* the official publication of the South Wales miners, for example, engaged technical debates over rates of pneumoconiosis, methods of dust suppression, and workers' compensation. Drawing on deep knowledge of mining operations, one writer linked the high rates in anthracite mines to ventilation: "The Geographic position of the Anthracite accounts for the fact that faults . . . are more frequent in that area . . . more hard headings are driven, resulting in a more frequent use of auxiliary fans as the means of ventilation."[41] Miners approved of the research on lung function under way at Llandough Hospital, commenting that "it is important to develop methods of testing the functioning of the lungs, in order to clarify this position [X-ray evidence]."[42] The PRU submitted yearly reports to the NUM, detailing the progress of the unit, including the development of tests to measure breathing problems. The work was frequently the subject of hopeful commentary in the NUM's annual reports of the South Wales area.[43]

Fletcher apparently got along well with the communist Arthur Horner, president of the Fed. (The Fed reorganized as the National Union of Mineworkers in 1945 but would continue to be referred to as the Fed.) (Figure 24) He participated in conferences with unionists and taught at their Week's Summer Schools for Compensation Secretaries.[44] Although not without tension, the agendas of the PRU and the Fed converged for a time (Figure 25). Indeed, much of the most important work in the unit could not have been done without the knowledge, resources, and political clout of the Fed. During this postwar period, the Fed already had a long history with compensation claims. It was acutely aware of the limits of the schedule, the complexity of scientific evidence, and epistemological confusion around CWP. In the early years, some of the PRU staff recognized that workers' knowledge was essential to the high-quality science they produced.[45] Over the next decade, however, the problem of pneumoconiosis would be turned over to specialists.

Apportioning Disability

The Labor Party won a landslide victory in 1945, initiating a period of social reform and state planning amid the continuation of wartime austerity, which informed the vision of the PRU.[46] In 1946, Parliament passed two relevant pieces of legislation: the National Insurance (Industrial Injuries) Act (NIIA), which established a no-fault

FIGURE 24. **MRC poster announcing survey, circa 1950.**
Courtesy of Cardiff University Library, Cochrane Archive,
University Hospital Llandough.

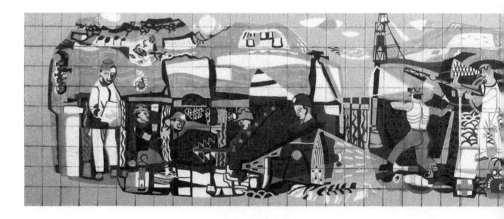

insurance scheme and the Coal Industry Nationalisation Act, which nationalized the industy.[47] Rather than the hated private owners, the National Coal Board would now run the industry. Coal miners invested tremendous hope in these reforms.

Several provisions of the NIIA are relevant to the story of the spirometer. First, as was the case with workers' compensation, the new scheme only covered diseases specifically related to occupation (although the legislation did allow for "special exposure"). Bronchitis and emphysema—diseases that occurred in nonindustrial populations—remained uncompensated. Second, the new scheme included "dust reticulation," the early stage of disease described by D'Arcy Hart and Aslett. At issue was the relationship between dust reticulation and loss of respiratory function. Third, workers were compensated for loss of faculty, not of earnings, introducing new challenges to measuring function. Fourth, the act abolished compulsory suspension from the industry, allowing "certified" workers—those determined to have evidence of dust reticulation—to continue working under "approved conditions." Facing a severe labor shortage in an industry critical to the recovering postwar economy, the government could not allow the departure of large numbers of miners with early disease.

According to Fletcher, this legislation was implemented hastily and without sufficient input from "medical men." Passage of the acts instigated debates about the definition of disease, the assessment

FIGURE 25. **Mural presented to the PRU by the National Union of Mineworkers, 1959.** Courtesy of Cardiff University Library, Cochrane Archive, University Hospital Llandough.

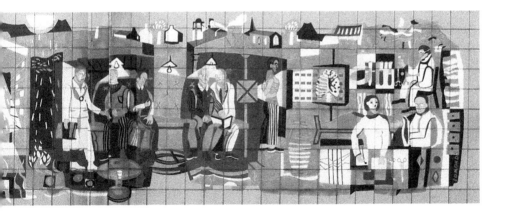

of disability, and "letters of advice" for men regarding work under "approved conditions." ("Approved conditions" referred to conditions that purportedly did not lead to disease progression.)[48] The PRU and miners considered the standard for approved conditions to be arbitrary, and the wording of these letters led to sharp exchanges between the PRU staff and the Pneumoconiosis Medical Panels who distributed letters of advice to miners regarding workplace hazards. Additionally, the panels assigned a precise percentage to a worker's disability and determined the portion of disablement due to work conditions. These were almost impossible tasks.[49]

One major problem was the absence of a direct correlation between tissue damage detectable on X-ray and breathlessness, the most established clinical symptom of disability. Men could be disabled without any visible X-ray changes. Conversely, men could have X-ray changes without any apparent symptoms. The lack of correlation stemmed, in part, from the contested and dynamic parameters of this newly scheduled disease.

By 1947, research at the unit crystallized around the "two-disease" hypothesis of CWP. Promoted at conferences, in lectures to scientists and miners, and in scientific journals, PRU staff argued that CWP presented as two distinct diseases: "simple" pneumoconiosis, which they considered relatively benign, and "progressive massive fibrosis," which they recognized as severely disabling. Progressive massive fibrosis involved tuberculosis infection and was often called "infective pneumoconiosis." They termed the combination of both types "complicated pneumoconiosis."

Fletcher and his PRU colleagues were confident that radiographic imaging could help precisely classify and monitor CWP. Publishing his first exposition of the theory in 1949, Fletcher and colleagues subdivided each form of CWP into four categories defined in the case of simple CWP by the profusion (density of the distribution) of small opacities and in case of complicated CWP by the aggregate size of the opacities larger than one centimeter. For simple CWP they labeled the categories 1, 2, 3, and 4, and for complicated CWP they labeled them A, B, C, and D.[50] Whether these neat categories would actually ensure the miners' safety, however, was unclear. Fletcher told the 1947 Pneumoconiosis Conference that "many of the men in the early stages of reticulation could return to employment underground provided their health was closely watched."[51] Yet, he also acknowledged that the "quantitative aspect of diagnosis is an artificial one resulting from the requirements of compensation legislation."[52] Fletcher's ordering project made X-ray diagnosis of CWP more reproducible. But it also narrowed the definition of disease, leaving many workers at risk.[53] Indeed, certainty was illusory.[54] Despite these ambiguities, the International Labor Organization (ILO) adopted the PRU's classification in 1950 with few modifications.

Treating the two-disease hypothesis as scientific fact, PRU researchers turned their attention to the thorny issue of disability, first drawing on symptom-based questionnaires and later on the spirometer. At what stage of disease did disability occur? Could disability be quantified precisely? Fletcher attempted to quantify breathlessness by devising a graded scale tailored to workers' "habits and activities." Grade 4 disease, for example, would establish whether "the patient [was] unable to walk more than about 100 yards on the level without a rest." Importantly, according to Fletcher, "there is also general agreement between the answers to these questions and an objective measure of dyspnoea."[55] Indeed, Gilson suggested that "objective physiological measurements of function should provide a more satisfactory index of the presence and degree of emphysema."[56]

The PRU questionnaire formed the basis of the standardized MRC questionnaire on respiratory symptoms. Although touted as a technique to "avoid bias," the subjective element to the questionnaire troubled its users.[57] The PRU began experimenting with measures that would eliminate subjective clinical judgments and patients' reports.[58] Concerns about malingering, which permeated the administration of workers' compensation systems worldwide, were not dominant at the PRU when Fletcher was director. They nonetheless hovered over concepts of disease—and the development, interpretation, and application of new technologies, including the spirometer, for disability assessment.

Lung Function Research at the PRU

Beyond the problems of unemployment and disease diagnosis, disability assessments raised a fundamental epistemological question: whose knowledge would prevail in assessing disability—that of workers or of medical experts? The scaled assessment of disability required by the NIIA cried out for an "objective" tool that both the workers and the Coal Board could trust. As an instrument already linked to problems of vitality, efficiency, and fitness to work and fight, the spirometer was ideally positioned to mediate the polarization between workers and the state. Refinement of apparatuses to measure lung function would be undertaken by the unit's medical physiologists, notably Gilson, Hugh-Jones, and the talented instrument makers Wright, Margery McDermott, and Terry McDermott.

The contribution of the PRU's population-based research to chronic disease epidemiology's development as a scientific discipline is well known. Little attention, however, has been paid to the unit's pathbreaking work on the physiology of work-related disease. PRU staff members conducted elegant and technically complex physiological research that both elucidated the mechanics of the lung and established the growing role of research in adjudicating social problems.[59]

Soon after joining the PRU, Gilson and his collaborators set up physiological laboratories and began studying lung function tests. As discussed earlier, numerous tests of lung function were available at the time, but their use as markers of disease and disability had never been investigated systematically. Not all lung function tests, for example, correlated with breathlessness. Because respiratory equipment was not commercially available, PRU staff made the equipment themselves.[60] In a stunningly short period—even by today's standards—staff built or adapted apparatuses, recruited and tested subjects, reviewed the literature, designed and conducted complex experiments, and analyzed and published their findings. Gilson brought some equipment from the RAF and also made his own. Soon after moving to Llandough Hospital, "the side rooms of Ward W3 were . . . overflowing with respiratory apparatus, much of it made by Gilson." Former PRU staff member John Cotes credits Gilson and the McDermotts with building the first UK spirometer for measuring forced expiratory volume, a measure of lung function used in the PRU's industrial surveys.[61]

Like Fletcher, Gilson believed that medical experts should address the new regulations for certification. Writing to E. A. Shearing of the Ministry of Fuel and Power in 1948, Gilson asserted that "ill-advised haste" to certify men with any abnormality on X-ray without significant disability had created a crisis. He called for a conference *with medical men* to prepare a workable scheme. Prioritizing expert over workers' knowledge, he argued that "*after* a scheme has been prepared by the two medical personnel based on our knowledge of the disease, the scheme should be discussed with the administrators including, of course, the National Union of Mineworkers."[62]

Approving the PRU's research, the NUM endorsed "the various improved types of test of breathing function" and hoped that further research would "throw considerable light on the reasons underlying the breathlessness of men with pneumoconiosis."[63]

After surveying the worldwide literature, Gilson and colleagues identified four measures—functional residual air, vital capacity, voluntary maximum breathing capacity (MBC), and radiological chest volume—for additional investigation.[64] Affirming the two-disease hypothesis and Fletcher's grading system of breathlessness, Gilson and Hugh-Jones concluded that the dyspnoeic index (a combination of an exercise test and MBC test) corresponded most closely to radiographic abnormality.[65] In measuring the rate and depth of breathing, the MBC included a timed element, a major advantage over vital capacity in providing insight into lung physiology. Although the measurements were detailed and precise, the study's sample size of seventeen was small. Moreover, measurement of MBC required a skilled operator and was difficult for miners with breathing difficulties. Large-scale surveys outside the laboratory would require new equipment and testing methods that were simple, repeatable, discriminating, and valid.

The unit's basic physiology work was elevated when the more clinically oriented Fletcher returned to London, and Gilson became director. The Ministry of Health took over routine treatment, and the Coal Board assumed responsibility for most survey work on CWP. The study of respiratory function and disability, however, remained in the unit. Over the next decade, Gilson and his "gadget-minded" team of instrument designers created new and simpler instruments. They brought more complex statistics to the analysis. With Owen Wade, they explored the detailed mechanisms of impaired lung function in coal miners by measuring the movement of the chest wall and diaphragm as the disease progressed. They developed new techniques for studying gas transfer. They experimented with closed- and open-circuited spirometers, the placement of valves, electronic timers, timing cycles, calibrating devices, and recording drums. Hugh-Jones devised a simple exercise test, less onerous for the patient. Basel Wright, the pathologist whose "real love was gadgeteering," developed a device called the peak flow meter. Colin McKerrow, one of the technical staff, used rubber bags to build a simple, accurate, and easily assembled instrument for measuring MBC.[66]

In 1955, Gilson and Hugh-Jones published a major MRC (Green)

Report on lung physiology and CWP. *Lung Function in Coalworkers' Pneumoconiosis,* a 266-page volume, was the most comprehensive report on lung function to date. It would remain the authoritative text for decades. Reviewing the methodological limitations of the growing literature on lung function and disability, Gilson and Hugh-Jones examined many tests of lung function, discussed the relevance of their work both to understanding the mechanics of the lung and to compensation and introduced a sophisticated factor analysis of the interrelationship among the different tests of lung function. As with the unit's epidemiological work, technoscientific and social questions were interwoven throughout the text.

In a unit established to address the practical problem of pneumoconiosis, physiological experiments were meaningful only when they provided insight into disability assessment and disease prevention. A "man's complaint" was the single best measure of disability, but it was "subjective." Gilson and Hugh-Jones believed that the dyspnoeic index was closely related to radiological grade and was therefore the "best objective measure" of disability.

Despite their purported objectivity, lung function tests introduced new uncertainties into the definition and management of work-related disease. Indeed, Gilson and Hugh-Jones acknowledged that "such fine grades of assessment give a spurious appearance of accuracy." Moreover, the dyspnoeic index involved difficult tests, not suitable for the Pneumoconiosis Panels. For even the best test, there was a large amount of variability among individuals. Although precise grading of disability remained elusive, they suggested "using 20 per cent as the lowest limit of recognizable disability and thereafter recognizing only four grades of disability in increasing steps of 20 per cent."[67]

The physiologists' work—so breathtaking in its technical sophistication and apparently authoritative in its conclusions—remained politically and scientifically fraught. The 1951 deliberations of the Industrial Injuries Advisory Council (IIAC) over modifications to the National Injuries Act highlighted the uncertainties about disability, lung function, and diagnosis of CWP. For example, Charles L. Sutherland, senior medical officer in the Ministry of National Insurance, criticized the PRU's reliance on "complicated physiological tests." To Sutherland, Fletcher's dismissal of a pathological definition of pneumoconiosis in favor of lung function made no sense. "If a man is suffering from impaired lung function as a result of the action of dust we would expect that impaired lung function to be evident post mortem by demonstrable pathological changes. If the lung is normal from the aspect of morbid anatomy or histology it is difficult to see how the lung function in this case has been impaired by the action of dust." While Fletcher countered that "I should pay more attention to the observation of disturbed pulmonary function in life than I would to pathological changes after death unless they were extremely gross," he later admitted that "an abnormality of lung function is a very difficult thing to define."[68] By 1957, however, all exams at the Pneumoconiosis Medical Panel at Cardiff included lung function measurements.[69]

Cochrane, too, at least in retrospect, considered the physiology studies flawed, albeit for different reasons. Technically and conceptually, the validation of X-ray with disability frustrated him. Cochrane articulated the tension between laboratory-based and population-based research in his memoir:

> I was never entirely happy with this aspect of the research, which lay primarily in the hands of the Pneumoconoisis Research Unit's "eagle physiologists." . . . The "eagle survey" of pneumoconiosis related disability, which began just before I arrived at the unit, had immense prestige and distinguished personnel, but it looked at research through different spectacles from mine, focusing too deeply on the quality of its physiological techniques and, in my view, far too little on the selection of the subjects to be examined. The groups of miners investigated by the eagle physiologists were not representative of the situation generally. Too many of them were preselected because they had disability, and the kind of investigations that followed were never in a position to determine whether those with disability were disabled by pneumoconiosis or merely more subject to its effects.

According to Cochrane, the physiologists lacked sufficient commitment to developing portable instruments adapted to fieldwork: "I did not get the portable physiological equipment I sought for field tests of lung function, and the eagle physiologists remained in what seemed to me too rarified a laboratory stance."[70] Fletcher responded that the unit did prioritize adapting physiological tests to fieldwork: "the Eagle survey showed . . . that the breathing capacity was the best single test" of disability, simplified further to forced expiratory volume.[71] Despite the epistemological differences between basic science and epidemiology in the study of CWP, a consensus emerged among physicians—apparently confirmed by lung function tests— that category one simple pneumoconiosis was not disabling and should not be compensated.[72]

Through his writings—especially *Lung Function in Coalworkers' Pneumoconiosis*—and physiological experimentation, Gilson became an international authority on lung function. As PRU director, he fostered technological innovation in respiratory physiology and promoted spirometry as an objective measure of disability. By 1960, the debates about how best to test lung function temporarily settled on timed forced expiratory volume (FEV; forcible exhalation after full inspiration). After years of painstaking experimentation, PRU researchers developed their own instrument that relied less on the effort and motivation of subjects. Locally manufactured, this simple spirometer with an electronic timing device measured FEV in defined periods of time (e.g., seconds).[73] Although debate over pneumoconiosis, disability, and lung function testing would rage for decades, what emerged after nearly fifteen years of research at the unit framed scientific thinking for the rest of the twentieth century.[74] Via circuitous pathways, this simple instrument would enable and further authorize new lines of research on racial difference in lung function.

"Ethnic" Difference

Despite the elegant physiology research at the PRU, disability assessment remained contentious, and Gilson played an important role in international debates. Sponsored in part by the United Mine Workers of America, Gilson traveled to the coal-mining regions of the United States in 1955.[75] He was invited to numerous meetings on respiratory function to help develop tests and criteria for interpretation.[76] Meanwhile, the unit was changing. The epidemiology group split off in 1960, forming the Epidemiology Research Unit directed by Cochrane. The research direction of the PRU shifted to animal studies, asbestos-related disease, and "ethnic" difference in lung function.

As elsewhere, interest in racial and ethnic difference grew out of the problem of determining what "normal" references values to use when assessing disability. Earlier, Gilson and Hugh-Jones com-

mented that "it must be presumed that there is a considerable difference dependent on the constitution of the groups."[77] In Minneapolis, Myers's handbook *Vital Capacity of the Lungs* had already
established race as a "factor" to explain variability in lung function.[78]
The MRC questionnaire had also included race as a variable. But it
was not until the 1960s that PRU researchers began systematically
investigating group difference as part of their research program.
During the 1960s and 1970s, the international use of spirometric
measurement in biomedicine grew. Simultaneously, there was a
global resurgence in studies comparing lung function in racial and
ethnic groups that contributed to revitalizing mid-nineteenth-century American notions of racial difference in lung capacity (Figure
26). The goals of this research were varied but for the most part
oriented to bringing this technology into the clinic and deploying it
more broadly in epidemiological research.

During the twentieth and twenty-first centuries, the vast majority (83.6 percent) of studies worldwide comparing "whites" to "other
racial and ethnic groups" concluded that "white/European/Caucasian" spirometric values were higher than the majority of other
groups.[79] Moreover, claims of difference were made and accepted as

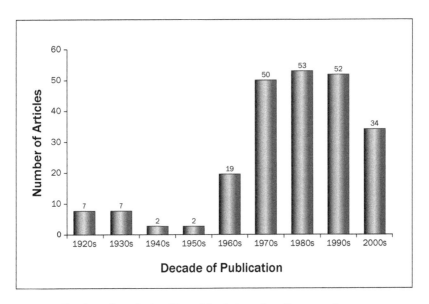

FIGURE 26. **Total number of scientific articles internationally comparing
"whites" to "other racial and ethnic groups" by decade of publication.**

fact despite the failure of the majority of researchers to define what they meant by the terms "race" and "ethnicity." In other words, they used "commonsense" understandings of race and ethnicity. Whether framed as "racial," genetic, or anthropometric, the most influential studies explained differences as innate.

Initially, comparative studies were incidental to the main focus of research at the PRU. But for John Cotes, they became critical to understanding lung physiology. To investigate ethnic and racial difference in lung function, the PRU turned to populations in the former British colonies of India, the West Indies, and Africa, as well as China and New Guinea.[80] In the early 1960s, for example, Gilson and his collaborators used indirect maximum breathing capacity and peak expiratory flow to measure lung function in male workers in ginneries and mills in Uganda, Kenya, and England.[81] Not surprising, given the labor conditions in Uganda and Kenya, they found lower lung function in African than in English workers. Setting European lung function as the standard of normal, researchers offered a tentative explanation for the lower MBC of African workers: "The difference can be explained partly by their small size (about 2 in. shorter sitting height), but this would only account for about 12 l./min.; the remainder is at present unexplained."[82]

During the 1920s, anthropologists studied the relation among racial type, physical measurements, environment, and the high rates of tuberculosis in Wales.[83] Yet, there is no evidence that PRU researchers viewed the Welsh as ethnically different. In fact, the Welsh served as a "white" standard in their studies. In an abstract for the 1964 *Proceedings of the Physiological Society,* Cotes and M. S. Malhotra, a visitor from the Defence Institute of Physiology and Allied Sciences in Madras, compared several parameters of lung function between Indians and "Europeans." (The category European was comprised of a convenience sample of Welsh factory workers.) Indians, they concluded, had low FEV, "due to a smaller vital capacity rather than to a higher airway resistance." According to Cotes and Malhotra, "muscle strength of the two groups of subjects" may differ.[84] Although this abstract was never published in full, it was cited extensively in the twentieth century as evidence of racial difference.

Aided by the unit's access to "normal populations," Cotes, Gilson, and others at the PRU published a standard that further reinforced the normativity of whiteness. "Average Normal Values for the Forced Expiratory Volume in White Caucasian Males" drew on the technologies developed at the PRU: apparatuses for testing lung function; Fletcher's grading scale of breathlessness; population-based sampling; and sophisticated statistical techniques. They combined regressions from their sample with those of the large American Veterans Administration Cooperative Study; Swedes; Dutch foundry workers; a sample of males in Berlin, New Hampshire; and the European Coal and Steel Community. This allowed them to create a homogeneous category termed "white Caucasian," constituted by subjects from "N.W. Europe and N. America," for whom "F.E.V.1 is related to age and height in an essentially uniform manner." Any ambiguities regarding the homogeneity of this category were left unstated, although PRU staff did call for more research on "the role of constitutional factors in determining the F.E.V."[85] With the establishment of a "normal" standard, lung function technology could be more fully exploited. Cotes pursued research on ethnicity and lung function during the 1960s and 1970s, with special attention to distinguishing the contribution of genetic and environmental factors in Indians, Bhutanese, Caribbeans, Chinese, and New Guineans.

The PRU's research on ethnicity and lung function reached a broad audience in Cotes's highly acclaimed textbook *Lung Function: Assessment and Application in Medicine,* first published in 1965 and now in its sixth edition. Drawing on a few studies from China and India, including his own, Cotes included a short section on "differences between racial groups" in the first edition. While Europeans throughout the world showed little difference, according to Cotes, there were "systematic variations" by race.[86] In the second edition, Cotes drew on American studies to rank populations. While Europeans were at the top, "inhabitants of the Indian subcontinent and the people of Polynesian stock appear to have the smallest volumes with the Negroid and Mongoloid peoples intermediate." There were many possible explanations for difference, such as the "relative sizes of the chest cage."[87]

In the third edition, Cotes references eighteen articles from the world literature on lung function and ethnicity and provides norms for people of Indian and African descent, noting that "the anatomical basis for this difference is not yet established."[88] In the fourth edition, he cites twenty-five references to racial difference and provides a more expansive explanation: "Some of the variation is environmental and relates to differences in altitude or in the level of habitual physical activity. However, after allowing for these factors material differences remain." Reflecting the focus on people of African descent so common in this literature, Cotes elaborates: "Australian Aborigines and Negro people, who have small lungs relative to stature, have longer legs and shorter bodies than people of Mongoloid, Indian, or European origin."[89]

In practice, physicians had difficulty incorporating race and ethnicity into their analysis of lung function. The situation changed drastically when, in 1974, Cotes's collaborator at the PRU, statistician Charles Rossiter, developed a seemingly simple solution. Working with Hans Weil, an American researcher at Tulane University on a sample of black and white male asbestos cement workers, Rossiter proposed applying a "scaling factor" (later called a "correction factor") of 13.2 percent to "normal" white values to adjust for observed "proportional" differences between blacks and whites. For these researchers, "genetic" or "constitutional" factors explained the differences. "It is possible that social or economic factors may have contributed to the differences observed," the authors conclude, "but the consistency with which the finding of a large ethnic difference in lung function occurs suggests that these factors may be unimportant." Generalizing their findings, they continued: "as the anthropometric evidence from other groups also agrees so closely with the lung function evidence from these asbestos cement workers, we believe that the results can be taken as representative of the ethnic differences throughout the U.S.A. and perhaps elsewhere until such time as further studies are published."[90] White lung function was the norm; black lung function needed "correction." Normal lung function in blacks would be set at roughly 13 percent below that of whites into the twenty-first century. They did not mention that this scaling factor was derived exclusively from male subjects. The consequences of this technological innovation would be felt most profoundly in the compensation system.

Conclusion

The PRU was a critical site for research on diseases that afflicted industrial workers in postwar Britain. It was also a site of technical innovation with the spirometer. In a context of industrial conflict, the instrument that Hutchinson had promoted to monitor the health and fitness of workers became a tool for negotiating who was normal, who was disabled, and who was worthy of compensation. For historically contingent reasons, spirometric measurement took on new racialized meanings at the PRU, adding to its scientific and cultural authority.

Basic physiological research conducted at the unit was not initially connected to race. Not until the 1960s did PRU researchers turn their attention to ethnic differences. There was nothing particularly cutting-edge in this initial research. Yet, through the technical development of a correction factor as a way to manage variability in lung function, the PRU became important in erasing the complexity of lung function. In collaborating with an American researcher and using an American sample of black and white industrial workers, research from the PRU contributed to and reinforced a now familiar refrain—that blacks and whites differ in the capacity of their lungs. The idea that white/European/Caucasian lung function should serve as a standard of "normal" deepened.

Not long after the establishment of the PRU in South Wales, South Africa launched its own PRU in Johannesburg. Located at the center of rich but low-yield deposits of gold embedded in silica-containing rock, a similarly talented group of scientists assembled to study the mechanics of lung function and to develop new methods to assess the disabling effects of silica dust. Again, race would loom large in physiology research in South Africa, although, as the next chapter will show, it would manifest in different ways than in the United States or Britain.

Diagnosing Silicosis
Physiological Testing in South African Gold Mines

The history of South Africa is steeped in racism.
This has affected all aspects of the body politic,
and underlies the development of the occupational
health system.

> JONATHAN E. MYERS AND IAN MACUN
> "The Sociologic Context of Occupational
> Health in South Africa"

Spirometric measurement became racialized in South Africa through different pathways than in Britain or the United States. Global knowledge exchanges, local histories, statutory segregation, and the biology of miners' phthisis (or silicosis) would shape the uses and meanings of spirometry in South Africa. With the embedding of racial preferences in the compensation system, long before apartheid spirometry became a tool for measuring lung capacity and gaining compensation exclusively for white miners. In South Africa, the spirometer was, for a time, racially coded "white."

As discussed in chapter 5, Eustace Cluver and colleagues deployed spirometric measurement in the early twentieth century to investigate the physical fitness of South Africa's "poor whites." Spirometry was also sometimes used in the gold mines during this same period. Lung capacity was not studied systematically, however, until the 1950s, when contentious debates over disability in gold miners led administrators, miners, and researchers at the newly established Pneumoconiosis Research Unit (PRU) in Johannesburg to use the apparatus to study lung physiology in relation to silicosis. With the burgeoning international interest in lung function as a marker of health, South African scientists, like their British and American counterparts, turned to comparative studies of lung capacity among racial groups. Thus, South African science became critical to building an "evidence base" for the belief in innate differences in lung capacity and the need for race correction.

The debates in South African occupational medicine during the first four decades of the twentieth century were similar to those taking place in other industrialized economies. Explicit racialized practices, however, structured the legal and medical edifice of occupational medicine—and the adoption of technological tools like the spirometer—to a greater extent in South Africa than in Britain. South African researchers published their findings on lung capacity and presented at international conferences. As this knowledge circulated globally, it erased the locally segregated context in which the "evidence" became racialized. Yet, new ways of thinking about race and lung capacity emerged in South Africa, despite the country's deeply entrenched apartheid structures of racial thought. For the first time since W. E. B. DuBois's and Kelly Miller's nineteenth-century critiques, mid-1980s South African occupational health physicians working closely with black trade unions contested the "fact" of racial difference and "race correction" of lung capacity measurements.

Building a Segregated Compensation System

The main reef of gold that prompted a worldwide gold rush was found in 1886 on the Witwatersrand plateau, located in the former Transvaal region of southern Africa (Figure 27).[1] Initially restricted to outcrop and open-cast mining, early-twentieth-century gold mining was an industrialized operation with a migrant workforce of white contract laborers from Europe, most of them retrenched from the depressed tin and copper mining industries in Cornwall; black African migrant workers from throughout southern Africa; and, between 1904 and 1910, Chinese indentured laborers.[2] By 1910, 10,000 "white underground employees," and "120,000 coloured underground employees" used approximately 5,550 dry rock drills in 87 mines, with an average depth of 1,100 feet, to produce 27 million tons of gold.[3] Over the coming century, South African–born whites would replace European migrant labor (Figure 28).

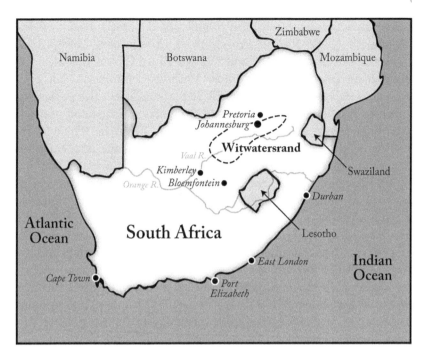

FIGURE 27. **Map of South Africa, dotted line indicates Witwatersrand plateau where gold fields were located.**

For the newly formed and politically unstable Union of South Africa, the gold industry's profitability was vital to nation building. In 1887, mine owners formed the formidable Chamber of Mines of Johannesburg.[4] Ruthlessly promoting the interests of the industry, the Chamber achieved strict cost containment through technological interventions, low wages, alliances with the emerging state—and complicated, changing, and contradictory racialized labor policies that would shape spirometry in South Africa decades later.

At the turn of the century, the health hazards of gold mining triggered a transnational crisis.[5] During the South African War of 1899–1902, previously healthy migrant miners, returning to Cornwall after short periods on the Transvaal mines, died at alarming rates. In response, the British government appointed a Royal Commission, headed by famed respiratory physiologist John S. Haldane, to determine the cause of sickness among the miners. The commission's *Report on the Health of Cornish Miners* identified a previously unrecognized accelerated form of silicosis, a fibrotic disease of the lungs with a long latency.[6] Pressured by white miners, Lord Milner, governor of the Transvaal and Orange River Crown Colonies, appointed the first Transvaal Miners' Phthisis Commission. The commission's medical examination of 1,201 miners, most from overseas, revealed 15.4 percent definite and 7.3 percent suspected cases of what was generically referred to as "miners' phthisis." The average age of those affected was thirty-five and a half years; after only five years of work, the majority of rock drillers were symptomatic.[7]

As historian Elaine Katz notes, the gold-mining industry addressed prevention in a piecemeal fashion. Unlike coal workers' pneumoconiosis, whose existence was denied for decades in Britain, the ravages of accelerated silicosis were not easily ignored. But its impact could be contained, in part through legislation that laid the foundation of a racially segregated system of occupational health.[8] In response to the militancy of skilled white and unskilled black workers, government initiatives between 1911 and 1919 addressed benefits, stages of disease, and technologies for diagnosing disease and disability.[9]

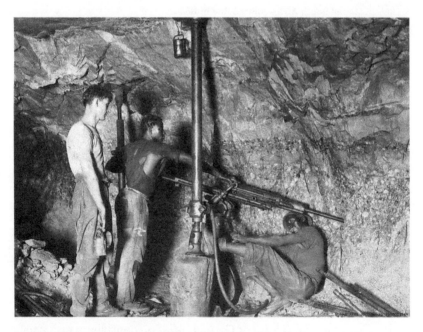

FIGURE 28. **Miners underground with a drill and stope support.**
Reproduced with permission of Museum Africa.

The 1911 Miners' Phthisis Allowances Act (No. 34) established a compensation fund and a board to oversee it. The 1912 Miners' Phthisis Act (No. 19) pioneered the use of X-ray, a new technology with the potential to diagnose respiratory disease. The 1916 Miners' Phthisis Act (No. 44) was particularly consequential in entrenching a racially discriminatory compensation system. Opening the problem of assessment that would bedevil the system, the 1916 act expanded awards to miners for two stages of silicosis—primary, which caused partial incapacity, and secondary, which caused total incapacity. With the establishment of the central Miners' Phthisis Medical Bureau to oversee medical examinations—but on a racially differentiated basis—this legislation built, almost invisibly, a color bar into the compensation system.[10]

The Bureau performed initial, periodical, and benefit exams and compensation certification for white miners. For black miners, part-time and overwhelmed medical practitioners working for mining companies conducted initial and periodical exams.[11] Theoretically, the Bureau supervised all the exams on the mines. In reality, doctors on the mines whose interests were deeply intertwined with those of the gold-mining industry monitored the health of black workers almost autonomously.[12]

In subtle ways, legislation allotted rights, benefits, and entitlement to medical examinations according to two (theoretically) mutually exclusive and racially determined categories of labor—"miners" and "native laborers."[13] "Miners," defined in the 1916 act as "any person of European descent, who, before or after the commencement of this Act has performed or performs as his regular occupation any class of work underground at a scheduled mine," were white. "Native laborers," defined in the 1911 Native Labour Regulation Act as natives working on or recruited to work on the mines, were black. The provisions of the 1916 act and subsequent updates focused almost exclusively on the rights and benefits of "miners." For example, "miners" were entitled to a monthly allowance for primary or secondary silicosis and tuberculosis.[14] On the other hand, disease in "Native labourers" was treated as an injury for which workers would receive a lump sum, not a monthly allowance, payable to the Director of Native Labour. Certificates of fitness to work were given directly to miners; for "Native labourers," they went to the director (Figure 29).

The act also established a spatially segregated system of medical examination. Physicians at the central bureau examined "miners";

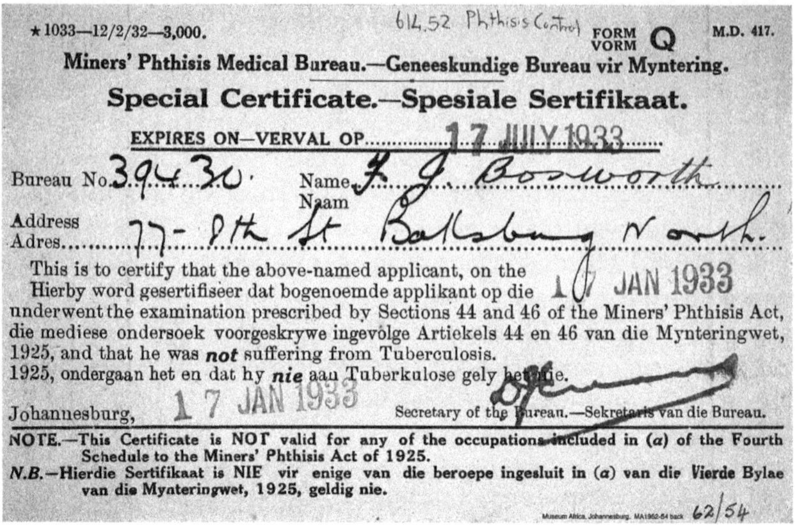

★1033—12/2/32—3,000. 614.52 Phthisis Control FORM VORM Q M.D. 417.

Miners' Phthisis Medical Bureau.—Geneeskundige Bureau vir Myntering.

Special Certificate.—Spesiale Sertifikaat.

EXPIRES ON—VERVAL OP 17 JULY 1933

Bureau No. 39430. Name / Naam F. J. Bosworth

Address / Adres 77 - 9th St Boksburg North.

This is to certify that the above-named applicant, on the
Hierby word gesertifiseer dat bogenoemde applikant op die 17 JAN 1933
underwent the examination prescribed by Sections 44 and 46 of the Miners' Phthisis Act, die mediese ondersoek voorgeskrywe ingevolge Artiekels 44 en 46 van die Mynteringwet, 1925, and that he was ***not*** suffering from Tuberculosis.
1925, ondergaan het en dat hy ***nie*** aan Tuberkulose gely het nie.

Johannesburg, 17 JAN 1933 Secretary of the Bureau.—Sekretaris van die Bureau.

NOTE.—This Certificate is NOT valid for any of the occupations included in (*a*) of the Fourth Schedule to the Miners' Phthisis Act of 1925.

***N.B.*—Hierdie Sertifikaat is NIE vir enige van die beroepe ingesluit in (*a*) van die Vierde Bylae van die Mynteringwet, 1925, geldig nie.**

Museum Africa, Johannesburg. MA1962-54 back 62/54

FIGURE 29. **Certificate to work issued by Miners' Phthisis Medical Bureau, 1933.** Reproduced with permission of Museum Africa.

mine doctors examined "Native labourers." Most black miners were not informed of their legal rights to compensation. Repatriation to South African reserves, homelands, or reserves in distant countries, rather than compensation, was the preferred method of handling sick black workers.[15] Compensation, medical surveillance, and research conducted by the central bureau reflected this categorization—irremediably distorting the knowledge that was internationally disseminated about the prevalence and pathogenesis of silicosis.

As historian Shula Marks has written, some officials objected to the neglect of black workers in the occupational system. The Inspector of Native Labour in Germiston West, for example, considered the six-month medical examination of black workers "really a farce." Other inspectors, such as W. Walker of Johannesburg, noticed that early silicosis in black men repatriated for tuberculosis went undiagnosed.[16] Despite such objections, this segregated system prevailed until the dismantling of apartheid in 1994. This was also the system in which spirometry developed as a medical technology in South Africa. In the late 1920s, physicians at the central bureau in Johannesburg used the spirometer to study vital capacity in silicotic and nonsilicotic miners. Vital capacity was "progressively reduced in silicotic cases," but individual variability and the "subjective factor" made its significance in diagnosis uncertain. For the next two decades, X-ray imaging would be the primary diagnostic technology on the mines.[17]

Race mattered in the sphere of X-ray technology. South African mines were the first to use X-ray technology on a widespread basis. The central bureau in Johannesburg had better machines with higher resolution, allowing for the diagnosis of more subtle, compensatable lesions, such as early-stage or ante-silicosis. On the other hand, medical doctors on the mines employed small X-rays, useful in detecting tuberculosis in "Native labourers"—but not silicosis. Interestingly, physicians and regulators considered X-ray imaging at regular intervals critical to solving phthisis and related tuberculosis in "Native labourers," for whom "ordinary clinical examination is often very difficult and may be misleading."[18] Although black workers on the mines received only cursory preemployment and periodical exams, there was a strong incentive for mine doctors to diagnose tuberculosis but to underdiagnose silicosis. Tuberculosis in blacks was managed primarily through repatriation. Moreover, to submit a claim for compensation, workers had to provide proof of work. Before the 1946 Silicosis Act, the Chamber of Mines did not even maintain records on black workers. As late as 1953, it was still developing systems for tracking the work history of blacks.[19]

The story of the spirometer is tightly connected to the importance placed on mining-related scientific research by the South African government. In 1912, the government and the Chamber of Mines jointly established the South African Institute of Medical Research (SAIMR). Scientists at the institute conducted highly acclaimed research on numerous health problems, including industrial hazards, pneumonia, and vaccines. Frequent exchanges of personnel among Europe, North America, and South Africa disseminated new methodologies and research findings. However, the definition, staging, and methods for assessing disability in gold miners remained fraught.[20] Hovering over technological innovation in South Africa were deeply entrenched notions of racial difference in disease. As historian Randall Packard noted, "Native labourers" were considered innately susceptible to respiratory disease, especially pneumonia and tuberculosis, but resistant to silicosis.[21]

Since the establishment of the central bureau, the statistics carefully compiled in government reports were collected systematically only on white miners seen in Johannesburg. Reports, addresses, and publications by Bureau members centered almost exclusively on white miners, and ignored black miners.[22] The major "Native" health problem in the mines was tuberculosis, to which the group was believed to be "so prone."[23] At international gatherings, such as the first International Silicosis Conference held in Johannesburg in 1930, scientists admired the world's most extensive database of industrial disease.[24] By 1922–23, its seventh year of operation, the Bureau had collected 47,518 medical and radiographic records on men "of European extraction."[25] It was not obvious to the international audience that the database was a white one, which neglected the majority of the workforce. The unacknowledged "whiteness" of this database nonetheless had profound ramifications for disease recognition, physiological research, disability assessments, and the application of the spirometer.

Despite purported progress in dust control, disease continued to ravage miners, both black and white. Concerned about contracting tuberculosis from "tubercular natives working underground," the Witwatersrand Phthisis Victims' Association publicized the miners' suffering and advocated for changes to the schedule of industrial disease.[26] Successive acts extended new benefits to white miners, modified intervals between examinations, and identified new stages of silicosis. But "miners" remained dissatisfied. Monthly allowances were inadequate; the Medical Bureau's examinations were meager; the statutory definition of compensable disease was unfairly restricted; and the rate of rejections was high. A system that invested so much power in bureau doctors—most of whom strongly sympathized with industry—to determine the ambiguous "capacity to work" was fiercely contested.

Diagnosing silicosis and assessing incapacity were not straightforward matters—either at the Bureau or on the mines. Both processes became increasingly contentious, culminating in 1950s debates over what constituted "pulmonary disability," or, in Afrikaans, borkswaal.[27] Was it a disease entity distinct from tuberculosis or silicosis—the only two occupational diseases currently recognized in South Africa—or was it functional impairment caused by one or both of them? As in Britain, both officials and unionists would look to science—and specifically to the spirometer—to arbitrate the conflict. Yet, until the ascendancy of black trade unions in the 1970s, black workers were largely excluded from the controversies over disease definitions, staging, and disability, to which the spirometer contributed.

Adjudicating *Borskwaal:*
Physiology Research and the Appeal of Technology

"As the great flywheel to regulate the Union's economy," gold mining dramatically expanded after the Second World War, triggering another labor crisis.[28] To maintain full capacity, more than a hundred thousand black workers were needed. Yet, with competition from the copper mines in Northern Rhodesia, recruitment was not easy. Despite the brutal defeat of the African Mine Workers Union after seventy thousand black miners struck in 1946, blacks did not flock to the mines for low-wage jobs. In refusing to work, they exerted control over their labor in ways that unsettled the industry. According to participants at a Gold Producers Committee of the Chamber of Mines meeting, "natives were prepared to remain unemployed in high-wage areas until jobs became available."[29] To the bitter opposition of white miners, the Chamber of Mines looked to Europe for workers.

Charged with conducting preemployment, periodical, and benefit exams, as well as ostensibly supervising examinations on the mines, the understaffed central bureau was overwhelmed. The Gold Producers Committee was increasingly dissatisfied with the functioning of the Bureau, as costs mounted owing to the large backlog of "native claimants" waiting at the Witwatersrand Native Labour Hospital before repatriation.[30] The high rates of rejection of workers' compensation claims outraged the Mine Workers Union; the union focused special attention—and fury—on the failure to recognize and compensate diseases ambiguously termed "other than silicosis or tuberculosis" among miners. Facing a new and ambiguously defined "disease" that could not be diagnosed with current tools, the situation at the Bureau exploded.

The discrepancy between radiography, clinical examination, and workers' experiences of disability bedeviled the compensation system in South Africa, as it did in Britain. Many irrefutably disabled men presented with radiographically negative respiratory disease—and no amount of statistical maneuvering could change that.[31] What was this entity termed "pulmonary disability"? Was it a distinct condition? Or was it the functional manifestation of other diseases, such as emphysema, bronchitis, or silicosis? If radiography, the best technological tool at the time, was not helpful in its assessment, how could this condition be reliably defined? New tools were required to navigate the terrain of disability. The need for an instrument that could detect altered lung function with numerical precision inspired innovation with the spirometer at the central bureau.

Beginning in 1946, a flurry of legislation attempted to resolve the ongoing crisis of silicosis on the South African mines. Two provisions of the 1946 Silicosis Act (No. 47) generated discussion of X-ray negative disability and "capacity to work." First, the act allowed for compensation of early-stage disease, even in the absence of functional incapacity. Second, it permitted compensated miners diagnosed with stage one or two silicosis to continue working. But the lack of visually detectable changes on X-ray made the diagnosis of early-stage disease difficult—and, as in Britain, it burdened physicians with the impossible task of predicting disease progression and assessing when it was no longer safe for a miner to work. Early-stage silicosis could, but did not always, progress to disabling disease, even after the afflicted left the industry. There were no reliable tools, including X-ray or periodical examination, to guide prognosis. As before, the various commissions of inquiry, the new acts addressing pulmonary disability, and later the use of the spirometer in the compensation system neglected "non-Europeans" or "Native labourers."

The Allan Commission, appointed in 1949, was the first commission of inquiry to take on the daunting issue of X-ray negative respiratory disease among miners. Composed of three physicians and two lawyers, the commission's charge was to assess the medical and legal issues regarding "any incapacitating diseases of a permanent or protracted nature (*other than* silicosis or tuberculosis) caused by mine work; the specific nature and relationship of these diseases to silicosis; and their legal redress in terms of compensation and further legislation."[32] In a memorandum, the Mine Workers Union argued that, because miners now spent more time underground, drilling more holes than in the past, they suffered from work-related diseases beyond just tuberculosis and silicosis. Together with testimony by miners whose claims were rejected, the memorandum informed the deliberations. Black workers, or even their paternalistic representatives, were notably absent from the discussion. (Not until the 1994 Leon Commission did black workers testify to a commission of inquiry on occupational disease.)[33] Because the Mine Workers Union could not provide statistical proof of their claims, the commission turned to the experts for evidence.[34]

In its report, the commission reviewed various international concepts of occupational disease, specifically noting Britain's recent experience in scheduling disease under the 1946 National Insurance (Industrial Injuries) Act. Based on postmortem statistics from the SAIMR, but also on nonstatistical medical judgment of experts, the commission found the incidence of most conditions other than tuberculosis and silicosis to be equivalent in miners and nonminers. Commission members were, however, "impressed by the fact that some miners suffer from a severe degree of respiratory disability in which X-ray findings give no clue to the underlying cause."[35]

The problem was not only that "respiratory disability" was undetectable on X-ray; it also did not exhibit distinctive clinical symptoms. Thus, neither clinical examination nor X-ray assisted in the diagnosis of this new condition. Despite the myriad definitional problems that emerged during the hearings, this elite body concluded unanimously, "there is strong presumptive evidence that there is a disabling respiratory condition occurring among miners, which is not recognizable by the usually accepted means"—that is, clinical or stethoscopic examination, work history, or hospital observation.[36] In response, the commission recommended compensation for miners with what it labeled "serious pulmonary disability." It outlined the necessary amendments to the Silicosis Act and called for more biological research. According to the provisions of the Silicosis Amendment Act of 1952, "'pulmonary disability' means an impairment of the cardio-respiratory functions" that "does not include silicosis or tuberculosis." It should be compensated. According to the 1952 act, there were two stages of disability to be assessed by the ability to perform light or moderate "manual work."[37] Despite their susceptibility to respiratory disease, according to the commission, short service on the mines protected "Native labourers" from disabling diseases that affect "civilized communities much more than primitive people."[38] Laying the groundwork for the discriminatory application of spirometry, "miners" with "pulmonary disability" and silicosis or tuberculosis would receive increased benefits; "Native labourers" with "pulmonary disability" would be treated as though they had silicosis.[39]

Parliament established the Pulmonary Disability Committee (PDC) within the central bureau, now called the Silicosis Medical Bureau (SMB), effective January 1, 1953, to facilitate the act. The

PDC would be responsible for all medical examinations related to pulmonary disability.[40] The establishment of a separate and parallel unit within the SMB, with jurisdiction over a controversial and ill-defined condition, however, produced even more conflict.[41] Despite assurances of the minister of mines, the PDC would survive for only three years.[42] The lack of a reliable method for assessing "pulmonary disability" threw the compensation system into another crisis.

The SMB and the Board of Appeal continued to frustrate the union. In narrowing the scope of its report to pulmonary disability, the Allan Commission had skirted the political problems in the central bureau, even though it complicated the commission's operations. Consequently, even before passage of the 1952 Silicosis Amendment Act, the governor-general appointed yet another commission of inquiry, the Beyers Commission. This time the charge was to examine the functioning of the SMB and the Board of Appeal. Appointed on October 23, 1951, the distinguished commission, composed of five physicians, was chaired by David O. K. Beyers. Taking evidence from a range of constituencies—the Mining Unions' Joint Committee, medical staff of the central bureau and the Board of Appeal, the medical superintendant of the Springkell Sanatorium (established by the Chamber of Mines for white miners), staff from the SAIMR, and uncertified disabled miners—the commission probed the methods, standards, duties, functions, and powers of the board.[43] Sympathetic to the white miners, the commission's report was a scathing attack on the SMB for its excessive reliance on X-rays and inadequate initial, periodical, and benefit exams.[44]

These findings set the stage for the spirometer by affirming the need for additional tests. According to the commission, examiners had failed to use "physiological or other valid tests to ascertain whether there is any incapacity for work, and if so, the degree of incapacity."[45] In a move important to the history of spirometry, the Beyers Commission called for the appointment of a full-time physiologist and for the establishment of a Pneumoconiosis Medical Research Committee to conduct research on pneumoconiosis, radiography, and physiology, with particular emphasis on "the techniques which might be clinically applied in the assessment of respiratory and cardiovascular efficiency."[46] The demand of the Mining Unions' Joint Committee to divide both silicosis and pulmonary disability into four stages necessitated special tests. The Gold Producers Committee supported the appointment of a physiologist and acquiesced to compensation for "pulmonary disability," but only in the specific circumstances "where the condition was due to the inhalation of mineral dust and was permanent."[47] In a small gesture to the black majority, the Beyers Commission wrote that "what has been said in regard to those examinations [of European miners] applies equally to Native labourers."[48] In practice, this would be an empty concession.

This expanded—yet confusing—definition of disability produced more legal and medical uncertainties. As claims mounted, another compensation crisis loomed. By the opening of the PDC on January 1, 1953, miners lodged four thousand claims for pulmonary disability. During 1952–53, the implications of this expanded definition were a major topic of discussion at the Gold Producers Committee meetings. As was the case with industry elsewhere, the committee's concern centered on extending compensation to diseases common in the general population—such as bronchitis and emphysema—that were not specific to miners. In this period, the inclusion of bronchitis and emphysema was still contentious in Britain; even a precision instrument like the spirometer might not bring resolution.

As McCulloch has described in depth, problems at the Bureau were personal, political, and structural. Composed of part-time physicians, all trained in South Africa, the PDC was at odds with most of the Bureau and the Gold Producers Committee in championing *borkswaal.*[49] The outspoken chair of the PDC, Gerritt Schepers, who was sympathetic to the Mine Workers Union, battled the chair of the SMB and the Board of Appeal over disability assessments. According to Schepers, blood and urine tests were essential, yet there was only one blood pressure apparatus at the Bureau. Schepers publicly castigated the central bureau for its assessment procedures, its definition of tuberculosis, the infrequency of periodical examinations, and underestimating disability.[50] Because "Natives" had short contracts on the mines, Schepers joined other experts in considering pulmonary disability, like silicosis, to affect primarily European miners. The main problem for "Native labourers," he believed, was tuberculosis.[51]

Mining magnates could not allow a report so sympathetic to (white) miners to stand. There were so many problems with the 1952 act's two definitions of pulmonary disability that efforts to amend it began almost immediately. In 1954, the minister of mines appointed yet another commission to reassess the findings of the Allan and

Beyers commissions, including issues related to staging. To do so, the commission, headed by Sarel François Oosthuizen, president of the South African Medical and Dental Council, would turn to scientific data, research, and technology to counter "vague impressions and opinions."

Composed of UK-trained physicians, many of them professors, the Oosthuizen Commission heard evidence from thirty-eight medical experts, including Cluver and members of the SMB, the PDC, the SAIMR, and the Chamber of Mines. The commission reviewed the international literature on industrial disease, notably the work on radiography, spirometry, and epidemiology at the Pneumoconiosis Research Unit in South Wales. (Recall Cluver's prior experience with the spirometer.) Three committee members traveled overseas for further technical discussions; the chair went to South Wales.[52] To study the methods and routines of the relevant institutions in South Africa, the commission visited the SMB, the PDC, the Witwatersrand Native Labour Association Hospital, the SAIMR, a few mines, and the Pulmonary Function Unit at Johannesburg General Hospital.

Among the experts testifying before the commission was Margaret Becklake, a young physiologist at the newly established Pulmonary Function Unit at the central bureau and an expert in lung function technologies. With the Mine Workers Union and the Mining Unions' Joint Committee declining to submit evidence, this was the first commission not to hear testimony from the unions. As was the case with previous commissions, discussion of "Native labourers" focused solely on tuberculosis. This commission relied on expertise and heard all evidence "in confidence," putatively allowing for frank discussion of the "various problems confronting the Committee."[53] Consequently, the final report was less sympathetic to white miners than those of past commissions.

For the Oosthuizen Commission it was politically untenable and biologically flawed to permit two different statutory definitions of pulmonary disability—one a distinct disease and the other a functional impairment. It had to be one or the other. Unable to conceptualize the problem of industrial disease outside of the lens of silicosis, the commission dismissed Schepers's view that pulmonary disability could be caused by multiple harmful agents in the mines, rather than a single agent. Reestablishing a narrow principle of specificity, it asserted that "inhalation of mineral dust is an essential requirement for pulmonary disability certification." Radiography, it conceded, could not assess disability. Bronchitis in miners was reduced to a complication of silicosis. In no uncertain terms, it settled on a single definition of pulmonary disability, one integral to the silicotic process. The new definition of silicosis would encompass four numerical stages and degrees of disability. A "standard for the measurement of incapacity" became more pressing.[54]

Because neither clinical evaluation nor work histories could be reliably quantified, the commission looked to pulmonary function tests for an "objective" assessment of stages of disability. Yet, the available pulmonary function tests were cumbersome, relied on patient cooperation, and required well-equipped laboratories. Importantly, the values considered "normal" were wide-ranging.[55] More research was needed to translate the values produced by the spirometer to staging by precise percentages. As time would show, even the spirometer would not solve this thorny measurement problem.

Lung Function Research in Johannesburg

Better research resources to support the operations of the central bureau were high on the agenda of the Oosthuizen Commission. One of the recommendations of its August 1954 report was to reorganize the SMB and immediately dismantle the PDC. A well-equipped Pulmonary Function Unit within the SMB, to conduct basic and applied physiological research on disability assessments, would replace the PDC. The unit's immediate tasks included assessing available lung function tests as screening tools for "pulmonary disability" and correlating pulmonary function tests with radiological findings and clinical examinations. "The investigation of lung function by physiological testing," commissioners wrote, "has not yet been fully exploited to ascertain what contribution such studies can make to the understanding of pulmonary disability in miners."[56] Given the unparalleled research "material" available at the central bureau, the Oosthuizen Commission supported the Beyers Commission's prior recommendation to form a Pneumoconiosis Research Unit, cosponsored by the SAIMR, the Department of Mines, and the Council for Scientific and Industrial Research, to study further the pathology, radiology, and pulmonary disability associated with pneumoconiosis. "The rest of the world expects this country to do more research," they asserted.[57]

Yet more legislation, in which spirometry would play a role, was on the horizon. The 1956 Pneumoconiosis Act (No. 57) incorporated a restricted definition of pulmonary disability. In repealing all medical provisions of the Silicosis Act of 1946 and eliminating pulmonary disability as a compensable disease distinct from tuberculosis and silicosis, respiratory disease caused by dust exposure on the mines was administratively redefined as "pneumoconiosis," now with four stages, all requiring evidence of permanent impairment. Another compensation crisis had been reined in, at least temporarily.[58] In Britain, "pulmonary disability" was understood as a physiological indicator of bronchitis and emphysema and was not compensated until the 1990s. In South Africa, the early recognition of pulmonary disability as distinct from silicosis and tuberculosis was progressive. Yet, it created complex medical and legal conflicts, tragically centered only on the health of white miners.

Amid these debates over pulmonary disease, a limited consensus emerged that disability could not be adequately evaluated by X-ray. This led, according to Margaret Becklake, to "an explosion of physiological techniques for the measurement of pulmonary function."[59] Becklake helped to establish the pulmonary function unit at the Bureau in 1954, one of whose goals was to develop a test "which could be completed in a reasonably short period of time and which would also give a fair discrimination between respiratory disability likely to have been caused by pneumoconiosis and/or disablement caused by other cardio-respiratory diseases." Efforts to adapt the technology for routine use were, however, temporarily abandoned, and the Bureau's research was turned over to the PRU.[60]

In 1956, a full-fledged pneumoconiosis research unit opened within the South African Council for Scientific and Industrial Research, with Alexander J. Orenstein, formerly chief medical officer on the Rand Mines and member of the Gold Producers Committee, as director.[61] Like the SAIMR, the unit was intimately connected to the gold-mining industry. (The South Wales PRU was, on the other hand, a government-sponsored research operation, not directly controlled by industry.) Funding came primarily from the Chamber of Mines and the government, with a contribution from the miners' union.

Patterned broadly after the South Wales PRU, the unit's goals were to investigate prevention, etiology, standardization, mechanisms, and disease treatment. Five interrelated projects formed the core of its research: etiology-pathology, statistics, dust, radiology, and clinico-physiology, directed by Margaret Becklake. As envisioned by the commissions of inquiry, the major goals of the clinico-physiology project of the PRU were: "(a) correlating respiratory function disturbances with radiological signs, (b) ascertaining whether any function test is reasonably accurate in discriminating between normal and disturbed lung function, (c) the relation of somatotype to susceptibility to lung distrubances [sic]." For Orenstein, it was important to find "one or two tests which could be carried out in the routine examinations of miners, both in preemployment and during employment examinations, which would be both valid and not too time-consuming."[62]

The clinico-physiological subcommittee was particularly excited about a longitudinal study to correlate physical attributes of miners with pulmonary lung function tests. (Physical measurements had been used as screening tools on European miners since 1916.)[63] For such technically demanding and innovative work, the young Becklake was an ideal project leader. A physiologist at the Pulmonary Function Unit of the Pneumoconiosis Bureau, she also worked in the Cardiopulmonary Unit of the Department of Medicine at the University of Witwatersrand.[64]

Spirometry was nearly absent from the biomedical literature in South Africa until Becklake began publishing on the basic science of lung function in the early 1950s. After completing her medical training at the newly established University of Witwatersrand in 1944, Becklake went to Hammersmith Hospital in London to work with Professor McMichael, the leading authority on functional residual capacity and the same McMichael who conducted lung volume tests on South Wales coal miners in the 1940s. Building on technologies developed for military use, postwar London was an exciting site for respiratory research. One of Becklake's major research questions was a basic physiological one: could the distribution of air in the lungs be used as a diagnostic test of emphysema and fibrosis? [65]

Taking Britain's interdisciplinary approach back to South Africa, Becklake—along with her technologically talented husband, cardiologist Maurice McGregor, and unit technicians—innovated with lung function apparatuses.[66] Influenced by Gilson and other PRU staff in South Wales, Becklake published widely on various aspects of lung function, including the effects of altitude, basic respiratory physiology, and statistical analysis of spirometry data. Importantly, she used the wealth of human material at the PRU, examining the use of lung function to identify silicosis in (white) miners.[67] Given resource constraints, Becklake sent the most complex data to Britain, where computers belonging to a restaurant chain performed the analysis.[68]

Understaffed and inadequately resourced, Becklake worked hard to create a laboratory for basic and applied lung function research on white miners at the central bureau. Some spirometers were made in the unit and others purchased overseas.[69] Drawing on tests developed at the South Wales PRU—Fletcher's dyspnoea scale, Hugh-Jones's exercise test, lung volumes, and maximum ventilatory ventilation (maximum breathing capacity), and the unit's epidemiologic approach to coal workers' pneumoconiosis—Becklake explored correlations between lung function and X-ray staging of disease. The findings of her first cautiously worded article, published after Becklake left South Africa for Canada in 1957, did not find a significant difference in lung function between radiologically normal miners and nonminers. According to the authors, nonminers were comparable in age, physique, and socioeconomic status, although their assessment of socioeconomic status was based on "our impression," not on data. Nor did researchers find a significant difference in bronchitis, emphysema, and bronchial spasm between miners and nonminers.[70] Thus, the study supported the narrowed definition of pulmonary disability in the 1956 Pneumoconiosis Act. Typical of the current racialized conventions, the study was restricted to "miners" who were seen at the Pneumoconiosis Bureau, thus excluding most black African workers. There is no mention of this exclusion in the scientific paper.

By the late 1950s, enthusiasm for lung function tests was mounting. The pulmonary division was now integral to a vibrant PRU, and it continued to conduct lung function tests on miners referred by the Bureau. The PRU submitted its project on lung function in radiologically normal miners and nonminers for publication; it initiated a project on somatotyping (relating lung function to various aspects of body build) to reduce the "'scatter' found in normal lung function"; and it began investigating new lung function tests appropriate for large-scale surveys.[71] A Miners' Chest Clinic, directed by Gerhard K. Sluis-Cremer, opened in August 1957, enabling further experimental investigation of lung function. Ominously for the industry,

Becklake's new studies suggested that older miners had lower lung function, perhaps owing to chronic bronchitis.

In the late 1950s, industry tightened control of research, and the functioning of the PRU was fraught. After the ascension of the National Party in 1948, many top scientists began to leave South Africa. This trend accelerated after the 1960 massacre at Sharpesville and the repression that gripped South Africa in its wake. By 1961, the country was becoming more isolated internationally. The reputation of South African research suffered, and recruiting qualified staff at the PRU was difficult.[72] While suppression of black labor demands continued, the white unions increased pressure for better medical examinations at the Bureau.

The PRU's physiology project continued for several years after Becklake's departure, under the uninspired leadership of B. van Lingren, whose main interest was somatotyping. By 1959, the PRU was poised to use the simple maximum breathing capacity as a screening test for miners. But there would be yet more change in the function of the PRU before routine use of lung capacity measurements could be implemented. After certifications for pulmonary disability declined, the miners' union voted no confidence in the Bureau in 1961.[73]

In the 1960s, the PRU shifted its research from the more politically sensitive pathological investigations of asbestos diseases to physiology and the "living workman." As the director explained, "the importance of detailed studies in lung physiology cannot be overestimated." An objective measurement of the extent of disability was key to the smooth functioning of the compensation system.[74] Attention to the living workman was not a humanitarian gesture. For the director, it meant the study of ergonomics, in order "to keep him an efficient unit in the industrial development of the country to the economy."[75] For nearly a decade, the physiology division focused on somatotyping and the technical aspects of spirometry as keys to solving the problem of the wide range of "normal" lung function. The unit was also overwhelmed performing routine lung function tests on cases referred by the certifying committee of the Bureau and the Miners' Chest Clinic.

A further boost to physiology research came with the 1962 Pneumoconiosis Compensation Act (No. 64), which mandated that impairment be expressed quantitatively. In calling for "further examinations, tests and observations to be carried out as the director deems necessary or as the committee may require," integrating lung function into the benefit examination became a more pressing issue.[76] The Bureau was not yet equipped for routine study, but it was testing a few volunteers in conjunction with the PRU. The majority of miners were invested in the technology. Only ninety-three of 3,160 miners refused lung function tests. With an "apparatus ordered from overseas" (a spirometer), the Bureau began examining twenty-five to thirty-five white miners a day.[77] Soon they would meet their statutory obligation. For five months in 1962 and 1963, the technical staff of the physiology division worked for the central bureau, effectively shutting down research in the division.[78] An automated system for statistically analyzing the more than thirty thousand Maximum Breathing Capacity tests already performed was desperately needed.[79] The lung function of black miners was not tested.

Epidemiological studies analyzing lung function assumed greater importance at the Bureau and the unit under the leadership of Sluis-Cremer. Until the late 1950s, Becklake authored most of the unit's publications on spirometry.[80] Since joining the PRU and the Bureau in 1956, Sluis-Cremer became experienced with epidemiological approaches to lung function testing. A contemporary of Becklake, Sluis-Cremer enjoyed a long career at the Pneumoconiosis Bureau (later the Miners' Medical Bureau). In 1962, he was appointed director of the Bureau and charged with its reorganization. In 1979, he became director of the Epidemiological Research Unit of the Bureau. In these positions, the prolific Sluis-Cremer contributed seminal papers on industrial disease and respiratory function, in white, and later "colored"—but not "Native"—workers. In the process, he would capitalize on the "wealth of human material" at the Bureau and gain worldwide recognition.[81]

"Everybody Will Go for Race Because It Summarizes Everything"

South African researchers contributed to the global resurgence in racial studies of lung function taking place during the 1960s and 1970s. With their growing expertise in spirometry in both black and white study populations, South African scientists drew on the "natural laboratory" in the mines to further entrench the idea of innate racial difference in lung capacity. In this endeavor, they turned to the South Wales PRU for innovative methods and to American research, including that from the 1920s, to explain racial difference.

The scientific, technical, and conceptual foundation of the resurgence of racial studies in South Africa was embedded in the racially exclusive battles of white miners and the racist legislation of the apartheid state. Still excluded from full access to compensation and preventive medicine, black miners now became objects of research on lung function designed to underscore difference. Yet, countering the seemingly inexorable march toward permanent racial separation in South Africa and hardened theories of biocultural difference in the 1980s, a small industrial medicine unit at the University of Cape Town worked with black trade unions to contest innate racial difference in lung capacity. In fact, this contestation represents one of South Africa's most important, yet largely unknown, contributions to the history of race and spirometry.

Hospitals throughout South Africa established pulmonary function units in the second half of the twentieth century. In the Western Cape, Eleanor Nash, a South African physician who trained in respiratory medicine in New York during the 1960s, established the Respiratory Clinic at the prestigious Groote Shuur Hospital, "full of enthusiasm for a new maneuver for measuring airway obstruction with the timed spirometer."[82] The University of Pretoria had already established its own pulmonary function laboratory, which collaborated closely with the Pneumoconiosis Bureau and the PRU in Johannesburg. Other medical institutions would follow suit. In 1974, the Diffuse Obstructive Pulmonary Syndrome unit opened at the University of Stellenbosch's medical school, under the direction of M. A. de Kock. After training with leading California pulmonologist Julius Comroe, de Kock established a lung function unit at Stellenbosch.[83]

The global web of difference constructed during this period cast people of African descent—whether in the United States, South Africa, the West Indies, or the Upper Volta (now Burkina Faso)—as icons of difference. Yet explanatory frameworks were complex. As Deborah Posel has written, apartheid was based on biocultural notions of difference, not strictly biological ones.[84] South African researchers' scientific explanations for difference in lung capacity also drew on biocultural explanations to convey a sense of immutable difference, reflecting—and informing—apartheid theorizing on race.

As spirometric measurement became widespread, the problem of "normal" values for black and white South Africans plagued the technology, as it did elsewhere in the world. Using innovative computer technology, researchers Zofia Johanssen and Leslie Erasmus at H.F. Verwoerd Hospital's Pulmonary Function Unit in Pretoria conducted the first comparative study of racial difference in South Africa, which they published in an American journal in 1968. Designed to assist with "predicting normal values for lung-function tests in the Bantu," Johanssen and Erasmus drew on studies of Polynesian rope workers, Indian males, and U.S. blacks.[85] Warning that "grossly erroneous conclusions may be reached unless prediction equations for lung-function tests for a given ethnic group are derived from studies from the same ethnic group," they invoked the now familiar refrain of racial difference in body trunk and limb length. They gave no indication that vital capacity might change over time, in response to improved nutrition or socioeconomic conditions. Black bodies were simply irremediably different from white bodies. Future research on prediction equations built on this study, and researchers across the globe would cite this paper fifty-one times into the twenty-first century.[86]

Several years later, researchers from the same unit collected anthropometric data on "Bantu" and "White South Africans." Confirming differences in limb length, they left unexplained the interesting *intra-ethnic* finding that South African whites had lower lung capacity than Welsh miners of "European descent."[87] Although observing difference *within* a racial group could have opened a different lens on the value of race-specific prediction equations and the homogeneity of racial groups, for historically contingent reasons, this observation was ignored. The primary focus on differences *between,* rather than *within,* racial groups continued in South African research—as it did globally.

Even as he continued epidemiological studies of pulmonary function in white miners, in the 1970s Sluis-Cremer marshaled the resources at the central bureau to generate "normal" values for blacks.[88] In a paper directed to mine medical officers, Sluis-Cremer wrote that ethnicity, along with other factors, such as age, smoking, altitude, and physical fitness, were "of particular importance," notably in "the Africans." Using a flawed and nearly incomprehensible study design, he presented "normal" values for blacks but provided no explanation for difference. In a study of children, however, Solomon R. Benatar of the Respiratory Clinic at the University of Cape Town was less circumspect. Advocating lung function measurement as a "routine part of the physician's and general practitioner's evaluation of patients with chronic respiratory symptoms," Benatar derived normal values from "Caucasian" and "Coloured (mixed race)" children in South Africa. Because "access to Black schools was not possible," black children were left out of his study. According to Benatar, explanations for differences in lung function between "Coloureds" and "Caucasians" included elastic recoil or smaller "sitting-to-standing height"—but not nutrition. Illustrating the global reach of American racial science, he wrote that "ethnic differences have been shown between White and Black American children of the same height and weight for age."[89]

Thus, despite gestures to environmental or socioeconomic explanations, the idea of fixed difference in lung function continued to solidify and to circulate transnationally. In 1978, for example, epidemiologist Janet Schoenberg and colleagues from Yale University, published separate reference values for blacks and whites. Differences were too variable for a scaling factor, they wrote. Invoking Benjamin Apthorp Gould's 1869 findings, they justified separate standards because "the lower FVC and FEV1 values among blacks are related to genetic rather than to environmental variables."[90] Rooted in the assumption of genetic equivalence between South African blacks and African Americans, Schoenberg's reference values were used widely in South Africa, from Cape Town to Stellenbosch to Johannesburg.[91]

Other powerful figures in the South African scientific establishment drew on the American context to promote innate racial difference in lung function. The same year that Benatar and Schoenberg published their papers, Professor de Kock organized an international conference on human respiratory disease at the newly built Tygerberg Hospital of Stellenbosch Medical School. Among the participants were Sluis-Cremer, Becklake, Benatar, and other researchers from South Africa, the United States, and Europe. Racial difference in lung function was not a topic of discussion, except in the introductory remarks by the esteemed Andries Brink, dean of the Stellenbosch Medical Faculty and president of the South African Medical Research Council, who highlighted the unique possibilities in South Africa to study ethnic difference:

Blacks in South Africa have been shown to have smaller values for vital capacity and other lung function measurements than Whites of comparable sex, age and standing height. Data from studies in Black men, women and children in the US also show close correspondence with these data and also with those found among Black people living under primitive conditions in a village in Upper Volta. Hence the difference between Blacks and Whites seems likely to have a genetic rather than an environmental basis. I am quoting Bouhuys [of Yale] when I say that anthropometric studies show that the difference may, in part, be related to the relatively longer length of the legs, and the shorter length of the trunk, in Blacks compared to Whites. However, there is no agreement whether this is the sole explanation, and a detailed study, using careful lung function measurements together with detailed anthropometric data might resolve this point.[92]

In the 1980s, the struggle to end apartheid intensified. The government declared two states of emergency, and political repression was severe. Black trade unions challenged the entrenched racial structures of occupational health in mining and secondary industries. New commissions of inquiry acknowledged the dearth of studies in occupational health. In this period, a few epidemiologists from the University of Cape Town began to conduct their own studies. One was Jonny Myers, physician, antiapartheid activist, and occupational health epidemiologist at the University of Cape Town.[93] Drawing on his work with black trade unions, Myers published a long paper in the May 1984 *South African Medical Journal* questioning the validity of using race- and ethnic-specific norms.[94] Ethnic-specific standards used in South African government, academic, and industrial settings, he noted, reflected the widespread belief "we adopted from America and other countries" that black lungs are smaller than those of whites.[95] Myers argued that his study of black South African stevedores demonstrated *higher* predicted values—despite a respiratory disease rate of 58 percent and radiological evidence of asbestosis of 30 percent.[96] In other words, a black population with high prevalence of respiratory disease had *higher* lung capacity than was predicted from normal values for their "race." Myers contested scaling factors, the definition of a normal subject, and simplistic interpretations of the effects of age on lung function. He questioned the low norms reported for blacks worldwide, and argued that living and working conditions could account for observable differences. Addressing the discriminatory consequences of "race correction" for black workers in compensation cases, he called for a universal standard.

The spirometer itself was not the subject of critique, and Myers held to the expectation that lung function measurements could find a firm scientific basis. He called for an examination of the assumptions that informed study design and interpretation. The comments of a researcher involved in the debate capture the importance of examining the social assumptions that inform research:

> If you don't take into account sociological or socio-economic factors, how can you make an adequate comparison? Because you are just assuming biological—you are assuming social equivalents in making this biological comparison. . . . Everybody will just go for race because it summarizes everything, all these other variables very neatly from a practical, pragmatic point of view. . . . It is a form of laziness . . . that race explains everything.[97]

Working with the nonracial National Union of Textile Workers in a study of byssinosis, occupational health physician Neil White found predicted values among African populations to be similar to those of European populations. Like Myers, he concluded that "the same reference values for pulmonary function" be used "regardless of subjects' ethnic descent."[98]

Myers's intervention was remarkable. Except for W. E. B. DuBois and Kelly Miller nearly a century earlier, the assumptions about racial difference embedded in routine methodology had been ignored. In December 1984, the *South African Medical Journal* published two responses. Noting Myers's "valuable service," the first response by J. C. A. Davies and Margaret Becklake proposed forming a working group to promote collaborative research on the relationship of stature and disease to "normal" lung function. With automation, they cautioned, "the source [of normal values] is often not known to the user, the choice having been left to the manufacturer."[99] On the other hand, S. C. Morrison and S. R. Benatar's response dismissed Myers's call for a universal standard and his argument for the relevance of social class to lung function. Myers's argument, they wrote, was "compassionate" but lacking in evidence and therefore invalid.[100] Myers countered that "in a situation of scientific uncertainty one either opts for standards based on apparent racial differences in FVC or, as I propose, for an interim standard based on a healthy population selected for optimal social and environmental characteristics. It would seem to be a question not just of compassion, but rather of a more appropriate starting-point to assume a universal standard."[101]

The debate continued in the *South African Medical Journal* from 1988 to 1989. Two years earlier, before the debate went public, researchers at the Pulmonary Unit at Tygerberg developed a machine into which all the specifications—including race-specific values *and* the interpretation of normality—would be built. The reference standards used in this innovation were those of Schoenberg and colleagues, derived from U.S. populations. With this development, the hardware, software, and interpretative dimensions of the technology were seamlessly integrated. As a representative from a South African spirometer manufacturer commented, "this country [South Africa] led the world in spirometry—and still does."[102]

In 1988, drawing on the natural laboratory of the mines in South Africa and its protectorate, Namibia, M.A. de Kock and colleagues at the University of Stellenbosch Medical School and Tygerberg Hospital used a computerized spirometer, the regression formulas of Schoenberg, and apartheid racial classification to develop "ethnic-specific" standards for lung function from a large study of Namibian uranium miners.[103] They noted both Gould's observations on vital capacity from 1869 and the worldwide studies that consistently demonstrated that blacks had lower lung capacity than other groups. They concluded: "arguments for uniform prediction formulae for all, proposed by Myers, are therefore not supported by the findings of the majority of investigators." Unconvinced that socioeconomic factors could explain difference, the researchers invoked a familiar call for more research on "elastic recoil in the different ethnic groups." Myers countered with a sharp critique of their methods and interpretations.[104]

Eventually, researchers and clinicians at the University of Cape Town adopted the standards of the European Coal and Steel Community, although the reference values of Schoenberg and colleagues continued, until recently, to be used at Tygerberg Hospital. North–South power dynamics are evident in this debate over reference values. According to one University of Cape Town physician, South Africans relied on American standards because "reference equations are put together by people who have time and money. . . . We should do our own reference equations but who would pay for it?"[105] Important studies in the 1990s by Jonathan Goldin, S.J. Louw, and G. Joubert did demonstrate that race was inextricably linked to socioeconomic circumstances in South Africa.[106] Still, the British Thoracic Society and the Association of Respiratory Technicians recommended discounting the European Coal and Steel Community Standards by 10 percent for people of African descent. Neil White's response to the recommendation emphasized the wide range of variation in lung function among Africans and the marked secular trends in median values. "I believe," he wrote, "that ethnic discounting contributes nothing useful to the accuracy of predictions." Correction "appeared to be an American practice," which was now globalizing. Was the 10 percent correction "a 'rule of thumb,' [or] a repetition of long-established but poorly substantiated dogma?" he queried.[107]

Concerned about possible discrimination in preemployment physical examinations, the 2000 Report of the Safety in Mines Research Advisory Committee came out in favor of race-specific standards: South African population-specific standards should be used for blacks and the European Coal and Steel Community reference values for whites. The recommendations, however, were "subject to the qualification that their [the prediction equations'] programming into spirometers does not preclude use of a single (sex-specific) equation for all mineworkers if a practitioner so chooses."[108] Some operators chose to use a single standard.

Conclusion

Beginning in the second decade of the twentieth century, legislation for silicosis produced a fraught, incoherent, and rigidly segregated compensation system that led to underdiagnosis of silicosis and overdiagnosis of tuberculosis in blacks, excluding blacks from the world's largest database of industrial disease. In segregated South Africa, the scientific literature erased the work experience of black miners in ways that were hard to "see." Later, as apartheid intensified, liberation movements swept the continent, and anxiety grew about overseas capital, the state and white unions looked to physiological research to defuse the growing sociopolitical and scientific crisis of compensation. Indeed, one outcome of this crisis was the establishment of a vibrant site of physiological research on lung function. For a period, spirometry embodied whiteness.

Beginning in 1954, researchers began to investigate spirometry in a systematic way. South Africa's massive database soon became a global contributor to racialized knowledge about lung function and occupational disease. Assuming difference, in the late 1960s, South

African researchers drew on U.S. racial science to produce "normal" predicted values in blacks and whites. By the early 1970s, despite the availability of alternative narratives, transnational exchanges among Britain, South Africa, and the United States—together with studies from India, China, and elsewhere—produced the "fact" of innate racial difference in lung function. Yet, while South Africa was important in racializing lung function measurements, for complex historical reasons it was also the first site of serious contestation of innate difference since W. E. B. DuBois's and Kelly Miller's writings in the late-nineteenth-century United States.

How Race Takes Root

Explaining these epidemiological mysteries
required speculation beyond the numbers and
statistics themselves; it required theories of
difference and of social change, and an active
racial imagination.

KEITH WAILOO
How Cancer Crossed the Color Line

The concept of race is virtually inseparable
from the idea of a hierarchy.

MIA BAY
The White Image in the Black Mind

When I asked physicians about the importance of the spirometer to their practice, I received a variety of responses. Some used spirometry as one element in the medical examinations. Others used the instrument's readings as a rigid cutoff to diagnose disease. One medical resident told me, "We don't ever really think about it [reference standards]. All we do is look at the FEV_1 and $FEV_1/FVC\%$, and if it's below the cutoff, we have a diagnosis." Few physicians knew which reference values had been built into the spirometer or how the machine handled race correction. One senior researcher insisted that she did not correct for race, even though a correction factor was built into the instrument. When discussing how physicians identified race, most of them acknowledged uncomfortably that they "eyeballed it" or told me, "You just knew it when you saw it."[1]

This book charts the socioscientific discourses and material practices by which race became embedded in spirometric measurement and the consequences of this racialization for our understanding of respiratory health and disease. As earlier chapters show, the racialization of the spirometer took place in continuous dialogue with other categories of difference—notably occupation, gender, and disability. Differences became hierarchically ordered through multiple and historically contingent paths. From the crude physiological studies in the mid-nineteenth-century American South to the more sophisticated epidemiological studies of the 1960s, the spirometer moved through myriad national contexts and social worlds, including biomedicine, life insurance, physical culture, the military, philanthropy, eugenics, anthropometry, and workers' compensation systems. In each domain, racialization enhanced the epistemic authority of the spirometer and of lung capacity, the entity it purported to measure. Over time, "race" became deeply but invisibly entrenched in the hardware and software of the machine itself. The remarkable adaptability of the spirometer allowed the powerful idea of race-as-difference to take root in a variety of social worlds and national contexts.

Despite its precision and popularity, spirometric knowledge has always been plagued with uncertainty about what constitutes "normality." In the 1980s and 1990s, consensus conferences in Europe, the United States, and South Africa attempted to standardize spirometry, including its use of race. With the exception of the South African conference, however, scientists tended to treat standardization as a technical problem, ignoring the social contexts that shaped the history and application of this technology and thereby enabling the early interpretative framework of spirometry to persist to the present day with little critical examination.

Seminal comparative studies published in the 1920s—many still cited today—gave the imprimatur of modern science to innate explanations for difference. In this work, prevailing understandings about racial difference in spirometric measurement cohered around a vaguely conceptualized but immutable "racial factor." Although researchers' explanations were speculative, rather than empirical, lung function in blacks became iconic of difference in this period—and has remained so.

Between 1930 and 1960, interest in comparative racial studies persisted in China and India but, for reasons that are unclear, not in the United States.[2] Researchers in China and India speculated about a broad range of explanations for difference, such as physical activity, climate, physiological adaptation, selection bias, and physique. Beginning in the 1960s, more methodologically sophisticated epidemiological studies brought more nuanced—though still speculative—explanations for difference: infections, tobacco smoke, pollution, climate, and nutrition were now included with anthropometric and inherent traits. Some studies suggested both genetics and environment factors; others favored one or the other. Most of the influential studies coming from the United States, however, emphasized innate difference between blacks and whites. With more robust studies, complex analytics, and new spirometric measures, American researchers derived separate standards for lung function in blacks and whites.[3] With support from South Africa studies on "the Bantu" (chapter 7), the black–white dichotomy came to dominate research worldwide.[4]

Harvard anthropologist and anthropometry expert Albert Damon's 1966 study of black and white army drivers lifted American racial thought and explanatory frameworks for lung function into prominence. Drawing on Benjamin A. Gould's nineteenth-century work, Damon raised environmentalist interpretations, only to rule them out:

> The difference in lung functions can therefore be regarded as truly functional or physiological. . . . As for aspects of the environment other than previous illness, it is difficult to imagine any that would specifically affect lung function but not body size, body build, or muscularity. The preceding arguments, by weakening the environmental hypothesis, strengthen the genetic hypothesis indirectly. . . . In the absence of definitive proof, as by family or twin studies, a genetic basis for an observed racial difference can be suspected when the difference is demonstrated at various ages . . . at diverse times and places; and in persons of varying physiological states. All these conditions have been met in the present case, Negro–white differences in vital capacity. . . . To sum up, the evidence favoring a genetic basis for the observed Negro–white difference . . . seems at least as strong as the evidence for an environmental basis, although both kinds of evidence leave much to be desired.[5]

As the first investigator to explicitly use the language of genetics, Damon's dismissal of environmentalist claims burrowed its way deep into the scientific literature. Cited sixty-three times into the 2000s, Damon's study helped to solidify a "modern," genetic framework for understanding racial differences in lung function.

American and British scientists set the standard in the global process of racializing lung capacity measurements: Americans compared blacks and whites, while the British scrutinized other populations.[6] The reasons for the dominance of these two nation-states are fairly obvious. Scientists in the United States and Britain have enjoyed disproportionate access to a research infrastructure—including complicated machinery, computers, and statistical technologies—as well as diverse comparison groups for investigation. Consequently, American and British researchers have been able to conduct more carefully "controlled" and scientifically credible studies than scientists in most other countries.

With access to a wide range of indigenous and immigrant groups, including the descendants of slaves, American researchers were in an especially privileged position to conduct direct comparisons of groups under so-called controlled conditions. British scientists used the residents of former colonies, such as those in India and the Caribbean, for their research. British studies, however, were less scientifically robust, because "white/European" comparison groups often resided in different countries. India, an important site for spirometric research, did not have resident "white/European" populations for comparison. Indian scientists resorted to standards published in the literature ("literature controls") for comparative claims—a much weaker study design. The fact that Indian researchers felt compelled to include international racial comparisons with their study of Indian regional groups demonstrates the power of race in establishing credibility in the field of lung capacity research. Studies with both strong and weak designs contributed to the growing consensus that whites had higher lung function than other racial and ethnic groups.

Explanatory frameworks in the 1960s and 1970s had similarities with—and divergences from—those that had come before.[7] Liberation movements were sweeping Africa, Asia, and Latin America; and the civil rights movement was transforming American society. As historians have demonstrated repeatedly, social conditions influence scientists and how they interpret their findings. In the aftermath of the Holocaust, scientists had generally repudiated eugenics. The 1950 and the 1951 revised versions of the UNESCO statements on "the Race Question" struggled with the scientific implications of racial thought—but, importantly, did not refute the notion of race as a scientifically demarcated, naturally occurring grouping.[8] In *How Cancer Crossed the Color Line,* historian Keith Wailoo explains how causal explanations for cancer changed in the 1940s, shifting from ideas of innate racial immunity to the environment. Similarly, in *Infectious Fear,* Samuel Roberts chronicles the rise of environmentalist explanations for tuberculosis post-1910, to which black physicians contributed in an important way, with ideas of innate difference in tuberculosis susceptibility disappearing by the 1940s.[9] Scientific and popular questioning about innate explanations may account for the disappearance of comparative lung function studies in the United States between 1930 and 1960. Individual diseases and physiologies, however, have their own micropolitics. In the case of lung function, which was less subject to popular scrutiny than cancer or tuberculosis, multifactorial explanations emerged in the 1960s but with the basic framework of innate difference intact. While researchers speculated about a long list of environmental and technical factors, the "fact" of innate racial difference in lung function persisted—even hardened—in this period.

By the 1970s, decades of technological innovation had produced a spirometer that was easier to use, less expensive, and better adapted to large-scale studies. In the same period, the expansion of U.S. government–funded pulmonary research, the global marketing of devices, and computerization brought more populations under scrutiny.[10] As spirometry expanded, however, new problems surfaced with reference values, apparatuses, the limits of normal, calibration, technique, study design, equipment, manufacture, interlaboratory consistency, sampling, and interpretation of findings. In 1969, a group of pulmonologists wrote that the "state of pulmonary function testing [has become] . . . more and more confusing."[11] Beginning in the mid-1970s, professional societies in Europe and the United States organized task forces, wrote manuals, and held workshops to rationalize the array of technical and biological factors that influence pulmonary function testing. Without clear standards, some scientists worried that manufacturers' recommendations would prevail.[12]

The role of race in lung function was just one of many factors that required ordering. The U.S. government–funded Epidemiological Standardization Project's 1978 report centered on standardization of questionnaires, pulmonary function tests, and radiography.[13] The 1979 Snowbird Statement from the American Thoracic Society

(ATS) issued minimum standards for the devices.[14] Other than the Standardization Project's recommendation to include race on questionnaires, neither report mentioned race. This situation changed in 1983, when the Statement of the American College of Chest Physicians claimed that it was "a reasonable approximation" to apply a correction factor of 12 percent for blacks—but only if there was "a precise definition of race."[15]

Still, confusion persisted. By the end of the 1970s, there were two options for taking the purportedly lower lung function of blacks into account: population-specific standards (based on the work of Schoenberg and her colleagues) or a scaling/correction factor (based on the work of Rossiter and Weill). The choice between the two options, however, was arbitrary. Importantly, both options established white lung capacity as the unmarked norm. The 1984 *Manual of Uniform Laboratory Procedures,* the "bible" of pulmonary function testing, selected reference values derived from Mormons in Utah as "representative of a group of healthy Caucasian North Americans of European ancestry," opting "not to attempt to adapt the reference values." Instead, it recommended that laboratories use "other available studies" for black patients. Some of the studies derived population-specific standards, and others used a scaling factor. Thus, this important pulmonary function manual provided no clear guidance on race correction.[16]

Despite this uncertainty, the U.S. government's long overdue surveillance of work-related disease among cotton dust workers and coal miners made a scaling factor a statutory requirement. The 15 percent correction factor for the Cotton Dust Standards of the Occupational Safety and Health Administration (OSHA) for African Americans was justifiable, according to engineer and occupational medicine researcher Henry Glindmeyer, because previous investigators had demonstrated that "blacks of the same standing height as Caucasians generally have slightly longer legs and a slightly shorter thorax."[17] Demonstrating what science and technology studies theorists Geoffrey Bowker and Susan Leigh Star call "the inertia of standards," a scaling factor remains in effect for African American cotton-exposed workers.[18]

Because "abnormality" can vary up to 20 percent, cutoffs for normal and correction factors profoundly influenced the awarding of compensation. Many scientists questioned the accuracy of a single scaling factor or population-specific standards. Still, by 1990, nearly half of American pulmonary training programs adjusted in some way for race and ethnicity, while half used no adjustment.[19] The 1993 report of a working party of the European Coal and Steel Community (ECSC) revised its 1983 standards, recommending that ethnicity be taken into account: "Either reference values for the appropriate ethnic group can be consulted or a correction factor can be applied to the corresponding reference values for white people."[20]

In 2005, the ATS/European Respiratory Society working group settled on the U.S. population-based reference values derived by John Hankinson from the National Health and Nutrition Examination Survey (NHANES III). Between 1988 and 1994, NHANES III randomly sampled U.S. Census–defined populations—Caucasians, Mexican Americans, and African Americans—using self-report to determine race and ethnicity. In using separate reference values for these three groups, NHANES III obviated the need for a correction factor, considered "less suitable and arbitrary."[21] For other groups, correction factors would remain in effect. Older machines in physicians' offices also continued to use a variety of older reference standards. Following ECSC and ATS guidelines, the medical device company Vitalograph programmed correction factors into spirometers marketed in Europe and Hankinson's standards into spirometers marketed in the United States.[22]

Although using self-report for racial and ethnic identification might seem less problematic than relying on observer identification, NHANES III standards continued the racialization of spirometry, now with seemingly stabilized groups and an apparently scientifically rigorous foundation. NHANES III should, however, be viewed with caution. Although useful in studying the effects of discrimination, self-report is a sociopolitical act that does not represent a stable racial or ethnic "essence." However we try to fix them, racial and ethnic identities are fluid, changing continuously over time and place. Hankinson's reference values are based on U.S census categories that have changed every decade in American history.[23] Conducted decades ago, the survey's racial and ethnic identifications are dated.

As sociologist Ann Morning writes, global census terms are heterogeneous: some countries rely on notions of ancestry; others rely on concepts of ethnicity or nationality; a few, such as he United States, employ both race and ethnicity. The United States is among only 15 percent of countries whose census employs the language of race. And the United States alone treats race as conceptually distinct from—

rather than interchangeable with—ethnicity. In the U.S. Census, only Hispanics are considered an ethnic group. In the 2000 census, 11 percent of Mexican immigrants (the largest Latino immigrant group in the United States) declined to select a race, and 45 percent checked the category "some other race."[24] A similar pattern of racial/ethnic self-identification likely prevailed for Mexican Americans participating in NHANES III, suggesting that the standards were based on a limited subset of Latinos. Morning cautions against the use of census categories for health studies:

> The United States' unique conceptual distinction between race and ethnicity may unwittingly support the longstanding belief that race reflects biological difference and ethnicity stems from cultural difference. In this scheme, ethnicity is socially produced but race is an immutable facet of nature. Consequently, walling off *race* from *ethnicity* on the census may reinforce essentialist interpretations of race and preclude understanding of the ways in which racial categories are also socially constructed.[25]

As socially constructed, not genetically homogeneous, designations, census categories are important for monitoring the biological and health effects of racial and ethnic discrimination. On the other hand, the use of unstable categories in studies of fixed genetic differences in disease or physiology conveys a deceptive sense of biological permanence.[26]

With the exception of the work of some South Africans who called for a universal standard, the 1920s studies on racial difference in lung function were never refuted. Neither was Damon's 1966 study, nor Gould's 1869 study. Despite the many modifications of the spirometer, the interpretative framework for racial difference has shown remarkable continuity over time. With complex new genomic technologies and renewed cultural enthusiasm for race-based medicine, another era in the use of race in spirometry—still centered on African Americans—looms. In a 2010 issue of the *New England Journal of Medicine*, Rajesh Kumar and colleagues reported an inverse association between African ancestry and lung function, using Ancestry Informative Markers (AIMs), one of the latest genomic methodologies.[27] Asserting a "genetic component" to lung function, the authors entered the long-standing debate over the accuracy of prediction equations and race correction. "Easily" and "inexpensively" obtained estimates of ancestry, they argued, should be incorporated into "standard race-based models" of lung function.[28] In noting that their findings could be the result of "factors other than genetic variation, such as premature birth, prenatal nutrition, socio-economic status, and other environmental factors," they—like many of their predecessors—gestured to more complex explanations, but failed to investigate them.

The *New England Journal of Medicine* also published an accompanying editorial. Coauthors pulmonologist Paul Scanlon and geneticist Mark Shriver, owner of a company that develops AIMs, drew on the long history of pulmonary function testing and used the idea of genetic difference to endorse race correction: "For the present, the practice of 'race correction' or 'ethnic adjustment' of predicted lung-function values derived from reference equations still provides the best estimate of normal lung-function."[29] This article has reinvigorated interest in lung capacity and blackness. A recent update of the Web site Spirexpert run by pulmonologist Philip Quanjer, author of both ECSC task force reports, added Kumar's article to the evidence that differences in lung capacity are genetic.[30] Citing "recent findings suggest[ing] that African ancestry influences lung function in African American adults," a report in the *Journal of Allergy and Clinical Immunology* draws on a familiar explanatory framework: "Our findings suggest that African ancestry is associated with lower FEV1 and FVC in Puerto Rican children independently of SES [social and economic status] and health care access, ETS [environment tobacco smoke] and allergen exposure, and Vitamin D level. Genetic variants predominantly found in West African subjects, early-life environmental/lifestyle factors that might be correlated with African ancestry but were unmeasured in this study (e.g., maternal nutrition), or both might influence lung development and growth during childhood."[31] The authors lay out a program of research: admixture mapping and genome-wide association studies to identify specific genetic variants. The Eve Consortium, a collaborative effort to study the genetics of racial difference in asthma, plans to extend its work to the genetics of racial difference in lung function. Like nineteenth-century research, the focus of investigation remains people of African descent.

As legal scholar Dorothy Roberts has written, "genomic scientists have not discovered race in our genomes. They are taking already accepted racial categories and telling us a new way, based on computer-generated genetic differences, to verify them scientifically."[32]

This new way extends to the shaping of genomic tools, such as AIMs and Structure by traditional concepts of race, all under "the banner of health, medicine, and science."[33] The issue of intent is complicated. Some scientists are working hard to rethink racial categories, while others defend them in the name of social justice.[34] Regardless of intent, the use of race-based tools in studies of lung function research reinforces the concept of inherent difference among racial and ethnic groups. Importantly, crude understandings of race produce impoverished understandings of racial disparities.

Is this the best we can do? Whereas health is simultaneously a biological, genetic, and social state of being, racial disparities are a social problem. How we think about, use, and understand race and ethnicity in scientific research or clinical practice on lung function (and other health conditions) is a social dilemma. Seeking quick fixes or technical solutions—such as race correction—to complex social problems of health and disease is misguided and harmful, even if well-intentioned, especially when it comes to race.[35] As Wailoo has written, "those who have claimed that racial categories are proxies for biological or genetic differences are proved to have erred many times in history."[36]

I suggest that the available evidence does not allow us to answer the question of whether certain groups have lower lung function than "whites/Caucasians/Europeans." The vast majority of studies establishing this "fact" have never even defined what they mean by race. Moreover, homogenizing traits relevant to lung function in people of African descent ignores the fact that continental Africa contains vast genetic heterogeneity. It also ignores the long-established evidence that there is more genetic heterogeneity within conventional categories of race than between them. In other words, the vast majority of variability in lung function represents individual, not group, variation.

We cannot get answers to questions we do not ask. A more productive question is: how can we better understand the social context of respiratory physiology in states of health and disease? To begin this discussion, we need to reimagine the relationship between race and health in ways that view the body as a complex developmental system in continuous interaction with the environment. How, then, is the external environment embodied to produce poor health? In this regard, a recent study showed that lung cancer mortality is higher in highly segregated regions.[37]

The history of the racialization of spirometry has almost com-pletely erased the social determinants of respiratory function. Scat-tered through the scientific literature is evidence for the influence of social class.[38] Yet few studies seriously investigate the social and environmental aspects of lung function. For example, there has been surprisingly little work on the connections between occupation, race, and lung function. As historian Karl Figlio observes, occupation is an "index of social class [that] also indexes all those features of class-based life which have health consequences."[39] More than twenty-five years ago, Malcolm Steinberg and Margaret Becklake wrote that so-cial and economic status should be considered when analyzing lung function in groups.[40] If some differences in lung function do exist, a more fruitful line of investigation would consider lung function as the embodied legacy of slavery, imperialism, and racism, rather than a reflection of a genetic essence.[41]

Additional evidence for the social dimensions of lung function is accumulating, including temporal changes in lung function among Africans and African Americans—and the data points in different directions. Over the twentieth century, lung function has increased among black Africans and decreased among African Americans.[42] Yet, despite clear evidence for social and environmental contribu-tions to lung function, vast resources are being invested in studying the genetics of respiratory difference.[43]

Considering race, class, and gender as deeply intertwined and the lungs as sensitive indicators of lived experience, we can ask how global inequality affects respiratory health.[44] What are the health consequences of the racialization of labor, when blacks have histori-cally performed the most hazardous jobs in low-wage occupations? We know that groups are differentially exposed to respiratory haz-ards according to race, class, and gender, both in occupational and in nonoccupational settings. There is compelling evidence that air pollution affects lung function growth, and racial and ethnic minori-ties in the United States are exposed to disproportionate levels of environmental—including respiratory—pollutants.[45] There is also convincing data that Vitamin A promotes lung development, and maternal supplementation enhances the lung function of offspring.[46] In societies where race is often the answer to medical uncertainty, it is not surprising that the lung function literature has largely overlooked environmental and socioeconomic differences as possible explanations for difference.[47] Given that race is entrenched in lung function technology, the past will likely continue to shape explanations of difference—albeit in new, more technologically complex forms—unless we think more critically.

Racialized science produces racialized results. To ascribe racial disparities in lung function (and in disease more broadly) to genetic difference is to ascribe pathology to entire groups of people. The near absence of careful analyses of the social, political, and economic context of race and respiratory health in the literature leaves Cartwright's, Gould's, and Hoffman's views unrefuted. It is time to forge a new path—one that takes our common humanity as its starting point. As a South African trade unionist emphatically declared, "We do not want separate standards."[48] Separate standards are not only scientifically flawed, they also produce racialized and unequal understandings of human variation.

Notes

Introduction

1. Erin Texeira, "Racial Basis for Lawsuits: Owens Corning Seeks More Stringent Standards for Blacks," *Baltimore Sun,* March 25, 1999, 1A. As a manufacturer of asbestos products, Owens Corning Corporation has been the target of hundreds of thousands of lawsuits by exposed workers in the United States.
2. Caitlin Francke, "Lawyers Debate Trying Asbestos Lawsuits in City," *Baltimore Sun,* April 10, 1999, B4.
3. Lung function is the term most commonly used in contemporary medicine. Historically, lung function, lung capacity, and vital capacity have been used almost interchangeably. To the extent possible, I will refer to each in its historical context. There are many spirometric measures of lung function, the most common being forced vital capacity (FVC), which refers to the volume of air expired after maximal inspiration, and forced expiratory volume in one second (FEV1), which measures timed air flow.
4. Jim Fite, "Will the Asbestos Companies Ever Learn?" *Baltimore Sun,* March 27, 1999, http://www.whitelung.org/news/sunlte.html, accessed July 27, 2011.
5. Texeira, "Racial Basis for Lawsuits," 1A.
6. The company filed a preliminary motion that opposed moving African American plaintiffs to the active docket. Framed in legal language, the motion noted that pulmonary function tests of plaintiffs "do not conform to the standards set forth in ATS Guidelines . . . [and] therefore cannot provide a valid basis for a finding of clinical non-malignant changes" (*Anthony S. Bradford et al. v. A. C. & S., Inc. et al.,* Case No. 98228505CX1618, November 16, 1998, Measley Publications, Inc. Doc #990402-014).
7. Anonymous, "Judge Denies Attempt to Bar Some Blacks from Asbestos Suit," *Providence Journal,* March 26, 1999, A5.
8. Lundy Braun, Melanie Wolfgang, and Kay Dickersin, "Defining Race/Ethnicity and Explaining Difference in Research Studies on Lung Function," *European Respiratory Journal* 41 (2013): 1362–70.
9. Texeira, "Racial Basis for Lawsuits," 1A.
10. Michael Omi and Howard Winant, *Racial Formation in the United States: From the 1960s to the 1990s* (London: Routledge, 1994).
11. American Thoracic Society, "Lung Function Testing: Selection of Reference Values and Interpretive Strategies," *American Review of Respiratory Disease* 144 (1991): 1202–18; British Thoracic Society and the Association of

Respiratory Technicians and Physiologists, "Guidelines for the Measurement of Respiratory Function," *Respiratory Medicine* 88 (1994): 165–94; R. Pellegrino, G. Viegi, V. Brusasco, R. O. Crapo, R. Burgos, R. Casaburi, et al., "Interpretative Strategies for Lung Function Tests," *European Respiratory Journal* 26 (2005): 948–68.

12. American Thoracic Society, "Lung Function Testing," 1202–18.

13. Lyle Palmer, "UK Biobank: Bank on It," *Lancet* 369 (2007): 1980–82.

14. American Thoracic Society, "Standardization of Spirometry, 1994 Update," *American Journal of Respiratory and Critical Care Medicine* 152 (1995): 1107–36; Thomas L. Petty, "John Hutchinson's Mysterious Machine Revisited," *Chest* 121 (2002): 2195–235.

15. "Lack of Exercises Leaves Half of Chinese Secondary School Students Overweight: Survey," *People's Daily Online,* June 12, 2006; Peter Hessler, "The Wonder Years," *New Yorker* (March 31, 2008): 68–76.

16. http://www.thoracic.org/chapters/world-spirometry-day.php, accessed January 2, 2013.

17. Spirometry can help diagnose diseases like asthma, emphysema, asbestosis, silicosis, and chronic obstructive pulmonary disease.

18. A. J. Ghio, R. O. Crapo, and C. G. Elliott, "Reference Equations Used to Predict Pulmonary Functions," *Chest* 97 (1990): 400–403.

19. P. H. Quanjer, ed., "Report of the Working Party on Standardisation of Lung Function Tests: European Community for Coal and Steel," supplement, *Bulletin Européen de Physiopathologie Respiratoire* 19, no. S5 (1983): 7–95. See also Quanjer's Web site.

20. Braun, Wolfgang, and Dickersin, "Defining Race/Ethnicity," 1362–70.

21. H. J. Schunemann, J. Dorn, B. J. Grant, W. Winkelstein, and M. Trevisan, "Pulmonary Function Is a Long-term Predictor of Mortality in the General Population: 29-Year Follow-up of the Buffalo Health Study," *Chest* 118 (2000): 656–64; P. G. Burney and R. L. Hooper, "The Use of Ethnically Specific Norms for Ventilatory Function in African-American and White Populations," *International Journal of Epidemiology* 4 (2012): 782–90.

22. See Christopher Crenner, "Racial and Laboratory Norms," *Isis,* forthcoming 2014 for a discussion of normal values in the first half of the twentieth century.

23. Anonymous interview, July 26, 2001, Providence, Rhode Island.

24. R. Pellegrino et al., "Interpretative Strategies for Lung Function Tests," 948–68. For a survey of North American respiratory medicine programs, see Ghio, Crapo, and Elliott, "Reference Equations Used to Predict Pulmonary Functions." The preferred population-specific standards in the United States for "Caucasians," "African Americans," and "Mexican Americans" are those derived from National Health and Nutrition Examination Survey III (NHANES III 1983–1992) by Hankinson; see J. L. Hankinson, J. R. Odencrantz, and K. B. Fedan, "Spirometric Reference Values from a Sample of the General U.S. Population," *American Journal of Respiratory Critical Care Medicine* 159 (1999): 179–87. Population-specific equations require separate studies of each group. In Europe, a "conversion factor" is applied to the standards of the European Coal and Steel Community reference values; see Ph. H. Quanjer, G. J. Tammeling, J. E. Cotes, O. F. Pedersen, R. Peslin, and J. C. Yernault, "Lung Volumes and Forced Ventilatory Flows. Report Working

Party Standardization of Lung Function Tests, European Community for Steel and Coal. Official Statement of the European Respiratory Society," *European Respiratory Journal* 16 (1993): 5–40.

25. Charles Rossiter and Hans Weill, "Ethnic Difference in Lung Function: Evidence for Proportional Differences," *International Journal of Epidemiology* 3 (1974): 55–61.

26. Historically, reference standards in the United States were derived from three population-based studies—healthy nonsmokers in Oregon, healthy adults in Tucson, Arizona, and Mormons in Salt Lake City. These standards are built into the equipment (Ghio, Crapo, and Elliott, "Reference Equations Used to Predict Pulmonary Functions"). In Europe, the European Community for Coal and Steel (ECCS) reference values are commonly used (Quanjer et al., "Lung Volumes and Forced Ventilatory Flows"). Other countries developed their own population-based standards. Yet, the problems with applying individual values to reference standards continue. For example, Baur et al. argue that "the normal range of lung function parameters derived from the standard deviation within populations is too wide for the assessment of individual values" (X. Baur, P. Degens, R. Heitmann, C. Hillenbach, W. Marek, V. Rausch, and W. T. Ulmer, "Lung Function Testing: The Dilemma of Predicted Values in Relation to the Individual Variability," *Respiration* 63 [1996]: 123).

27. I thank Amy Slaton for pushing me on this point.

28. A variety of spirometers and standards are used in South Africa. There is a rigid cutoff of 10 percent for qualification for compensation, according to the *Deed of Trust Creating Asbestos Relief Trust* (2003), 32, http://www.asbestos trust.co.za, accessed January 17, 2013. According to the medical director of the Trust, they do not correct for race.

29. Mary C. Townsend, *ACOEM Position Statement: Spirometry in the Occupational Health Setting—2010 Update* (Elkgrove Village, Ill.: American College of Occupational and Environmental Medicine, 2010), 14.

30. Yossef Aelony, "Ethnic Norms for Pulmonary Function Tests," *Chest* 99 (1991): 1051.

31. Roscoe C. Young and Jean G. Ford, "Standards for Assessment of Lung Function and Respiratory Health in Minority Populations: Some Challenges Linger into the New Millennium," *Journal of Health Care for the Poor and Underserved* 12 (2001): 152–61.

32. See, for example, John V. Pickstone, *Medical Innovations in Historical Perspective* (London: Palgrave Macmillan, 1992); Carsten Timmermann and Julie Anderson, eds., *Devices and Designs: Medical Technologies in Historical Perspective* (Houndmills, UK: Palgrave Macmillan, 2006).

33. David Skinner and Paul Rosen, "Opening the White Box: The Politics of Racialised Science and Technology," *Science as Culture* 10 (2001): 296.

34. For recent books in STS addressing race, see Jenny Reardon, *Race to the Finish: Identity and Governance in an Age of Genomics* (Princeton, N.J.: Princeton University Press, 2004); Amade M'Charek, *The Human Genome Diversity Project: An Ethnography of Scientific Practice* (Cambridge: Cambridge University Press, 2005); Steven Epstein, *Inclusion: The Politics of Difference* (Chicago: University of Chicago Press, 2007); Ian Whitmarsh, *Biomedical Ambiguity: Race, Asthma, and the Contested Meaning of Genetic Research in*

the Caribbean (Ithaca, N.Y.: Cornell University Press, 2008); Evelynn Hammonds and Rebecca Herzig, *The Nature of Difference: Sciences of Race in the United States from Jefferson to Genomics* (Cambridge: MIT Press, 2009); Ann Morning, *The Nature of Race: How Scientists Think and Teach about Human Difference* (Berkeley: University of California Press, 2011); Alondra Nelson, *Body and Soul: The Black Panther Party and the Fight against Medical Discrimination* (Minneapolis: University of Minnesota Press, 2011); Michael Montoya, *Making the Mexican Diabetic: Race, Science, and the Genetics of Inequality* (Berkeley: University of California Press, 2011); Catherine Bliss, *Race Decoded: The Genomic Fight for Social Justice* (Palo Alto, Calif.: Stanford University Press, 2012); Anne Pollock, *Medicating Race: Heart Disease and Durable Preoccupations with Difference* (Durham, N.C.: Duke University Press, 2012); Jonathan Kahn, *Race in a Bottle* (New York: Columbia University Press, 2012).

35. Troy Duster, "Buried Alive: The Concept of Race in Science," in *Genetic Nature / Culture: Anthropology and Science Beyond the Two-Culture Divide,* ed. Alan H. Goodman, Deborah Heath, and M. Susan Lindee (Berkeley and London: University of California Press, 2003), 258–77.

36. Keith Wailoo, *Drawing Blood: Technology and Disease Identity in Twentieth-Century America* (Baltimore: Johns Hopkins University Press, 1997), 189; Keith Wailoo, *Dying in the City of the Blues: Sickle Cell Anemia and the Politics of Race and Health* (Chapel Hill: University of North Carolina Press, 2000).

37. I thank Anne Fausto-Sterling for helping me sharpen the idea of race as embedded in the machine.

38. See Hamilton Cravens, Alan I. Marcus, and David M. Katzman, eds., *Technical Knowledge in American Culture: Science, Technology, and Medicine since the Early 1800s* (Tuscaloosa and London: University of Alabama Press, 1996).

39. Hamilton Cravens, "The Case of Manufactured Morons: Science and Social Policy in Two Eras, 1934–1966," in ibid., 154.

40. Stephen Jay Gould, *The Mismeasure of Man* (New York: W. W. Norton, 1981). See also Nancy Stepan, *The Idea of Race in Science: Great Britain, 1800–1960* (London: Macmillan, 1982).

41. Stanley Joel Reiser, *Medicine and the Reign of Technology* (Cambridge: Cambridge University Press, 1978); Karl E. Rothschuh, *History of Physiology* (Huntingdon, N.Y.: Robert E. Krieger Publishing Company, 1973).

42. M. Norton Wise, "Introduction," in M. Norton Wise, ed., *The Values of Precision* (Princeton, N.J.: Princeton University Press, 1995).

43. Cravens, Marcus, and Katzman, "Introduction to Chapter 5," in Cravens, Marcus, and Katzman, *Technical Knowledge in American Culture,* 92; Edward T. Layton, "The Inventor of the Mustache Cup: James Emerson and Populist Technology, 1870–1900," in *Technical Knowledge in American Culture,* 93–109.

44. Wise, "Introduction."

45. Reiser, *Medicine and the Reign of Technology;* Merriley Borell, "Instrumentation and the Rise of Modern Physiology," *Science & Technology Studies* 5 (1987): 53–62; Frederic L. Holmes and Kathryn M. Olesko, "The Images of Precision: Helmholtz and the Graphical Method in Physiology," in Wise, *The Values of Precision,* 198–221; H. Otto Sibum, "Exploring the Margins of

Precision," in *Instruments, Travel and Science: Itineraries of Precision from the Seventeenth to the Twentieth Century* (London: Routledge, 2002), 216–42; Michael Adas, *Machines as the Measure of Men* (Ithaca, N.Y.: Cornell University Press, 1990).

46. As Lorraine Daston and Peter Gallison have written ("The Image of Objectivity," *Representations* 40 [1992]: 81–128), objectivity has a history. See also Lorraine Daston, "Objectivity and the Escape from Perspective," *Social Studies of Science* 22 (1992): 597–618.

47. Amy Slaton, "Go/No Go: Measurement as Gatekeeping in U.S. Manufacturing," unpublished manuscript.

48. For more on this argument, see Crystal Biruk, "Seeing like a Research Project: Producing 'High-Quality Data' in AIDS Research in Malawi," *Medical Anthropology* 31 (2010): 347–66.

49. Vron Ware and Les Back, *Out of Whiteness: Color, Politics, and Culture* (Chicago: University of Chicago Press, 2002), 149.

1. "Inventing" the Spirometer

1. Bruce Haley, *The Healthy Body and Victorian Culture* (Cambridge: Harvard University Press, 1994), 11.

2. In Charles Dicken's *Bleak House*, the polluted fog, which hovered over London in the mid-nineteenth century, was the overarching metaphor for all that ailed society, both physically and socially. One French traveler compared Manchester to an active volcano, as noted in Anthony Wohl, *Endangered Lives: Public Health in Victorian Britain* (Cambridge: Harvard University Press, 1983), 208.

3. Friedrich Engels, *The Condition of the Working Class in England* (Oxford: Oxford University Press, 1993); E. J. Hobsbawm, *The Age of Revolution, 1789–1848* (New York: New American Library, 1962); E. P. Thompson, *The Making of the English Working Class* (New York: Vintage Books, 1963); Gareth Stedman Jones, *Outcast London: A Study in the Relationship between Classes in Victorian Society* (New York: Pantheon Books, 1971, 1984); Wohl, *Endangered Lives;* Mary Poovey, *Making a Social Body: British Cultural Formation, 1830–1864* (Chicago: University of Chicago Press, 1995).

4. Anthony Wohl, introduction to Andrew Mearns, *The Bitter Cry of Outcast London* (New York: Humanities Press, 1970).

5. Engels, *The Condition of the Working Class in England*, 107, 165. Engels remarks specifically on the problem of finding adults "fit" for military service (168, 208).

6. Wohl, *Endangered Lives*, 264–65. Phthisis refers generally to diseases of the respiratory system, most often tuberculosis or, in mining and other manufacturing districts, silicosis.

7. Lorraine Daston, ed., *Biographies of Scientific Objects* (Chicago: University of Chicago Press, 2000). In the introduction, Daston points to salience, embeddedness, productivity, and emergence as approaches to "the historicicity of scientific objects."

8. The stethometer was a small instrument that recorded the upward and outward movements of the chest.

9. E. A. Spriggs, "John Hutchinson, the Inventor of the Spirometer—His North Country Background, Life in London, and Scientific Achievements," *Medical*

History 21 (1977): 357–64; John H. Arnett, "The Vital Capacity of the Lungs: Early Observations and Instruments, *Medical Life* 43 (1936): 1–8; Clifford Hoyle, "The Brompton Hospital. A Centenary Review," *Chest* 14 (1948): 269–86; George Williamson, "Report on Mr. Hutchinson's Spirometer, as Applied to Recruits and Young Soldiers," *Medical Times* 16 (1847): 255–56. Hutchinson worked at Britannia when insurance companies began systematically to use medical examiners. See Theodore Porter, "Precision and Trust: Early Victorian Insurance and the Politics of Calculation," in W. Norton Wise, ed., *The Values of Precision* (Princeton, N.J.: Princeton University Press, 1995), 173–97.

10. In his first publication in the *Journal of the Statistical Society of London* 7 (1844): 193–212, Hutchinson refers to his research "with the instruments I constructed." His failure to credit others who had built similar devices undoubtedly contributed to his legacy as inventor.

11. Biographers have puzzled over the reasons for Hutchinson's departure from England to Australia. Some suggest alcoholism, marital problems, the allure of the discovery of gold, or health problems, but ultimately, his motives remain unknown. We know little about Hutchinson's life or why he became interested in spirometry in the first place. See Bryan Gandevia, "John Hutchinson in Australia and Fuji," *Medical History* 21 (1977): 365–83.

12. See H. Beigel, "On Spirometry," *Lancet* 1 (January 30, 1864): 119–20, for early questioning of Hutchinson's status as inventor.

13. Spriggs, "John Hutchinson, the Inventor of the Spirometer"; Stanley Joel Reiser, *Medicine and the Reign of Technology* (Cambridge: Cambridge University Press, 1978), 91–95.

14. A hogshead is a crate or barrel that holds fifty-four British imperial gallons (sixty-three U.S. gallons) of liquid.

15. Edmund Goodwyn, *The Connexion of Life with Respiration; or an Experimental Inquiry into the Effects of Submersion, Strangulation, and Several Kinds of Noxious Airs, on Living Animals: With an Account of the Nature of the Disease They Produce; Its Distinction from Death Itself; and the Most Effectual Means of Cure* (London: J. Johnson, 1788), 21–47.

16. William Clayfield of Bristol was a gentleman chemist and philosopher, wine merchant, and co-owner with his brother of Clayfield's Colliery. See W. D. A. Smith, "Clayfield's Mercurial Airholder," *History of Anaesthesiology Society* 4 (1988): 32–36; William Clayfield, "Description of a Mercurial Air-Holder, Suggested by an Inspection of Mr. Watt's Machine for Containing Factitious Airs," in Humphry Davy, *Researches, Chemical and Philosophical; Chiefly concerning Nitrous Oxide, or Diphlogisticated Nitrous Air, and Its Respiration* (London: printed for J. Johnson by Biggs and Cottle, Bristol, 1800): 573–76. See also Christopher Lawrence, *Medicine in the Making of Modern Britain, 1700–1920* (London: Routledge, 1994), 29; Leon S. Gottlieb, "Thomas Beddoes, M.D., and the Pneumatic Institution at Clifton, 1798–1801," *Annals of Internal Medicine* 63 (1965): 530–33.

17. The gasometer is a device for measuring and storing gas.

18. Davy, *Researches, Chemical and Philosophical*, 409–11.

19. Ibid, 7.

20. Karl E. Rothschuh, *History of Physiology, trans. Guenter B. Risse* (Huntingdon, N.Y.: Robert E. Krieger, 1973), 172.

21. Arnett, "The Vital Capacity of the Lungs."
22. Thackrah provides no description or illustration of the instrument in his book. The *Oxford English Dictionary* equates the pulmometer with the spirometer.
23. C. Turner Thackrah, *The Effects of Arts, Trades, and Professions, and of Civic States and Habits of Living, on Health and Longevity: With Suggestions for the Removal of Many of the Agents Which Produce Disease, and Shorten the Duration of Life*, 2d ed. (London: Longman, Rees, Orme, Brown, Green, & Longman; Simpkin & Marshall, 1832; reprint, Edinburgh and London: E. & S. Livingstone Ltd., 1957); A. Meiklejohn, *The Life, Work and Times of Charles Turner Thackrah, Surgeon and Apothecary of Leeds (1795–1833)* (Edinburgh and London: E. & S. Livingston Ltd., 1957). For a discussion of Thackrah's importance to the field of occupational health, see George Rosen, *The History of Miners' Diseases: A Medical and Social Interpretation* (New York: Schuman's, 1943), 200–206.
24. John Hutchinson, "Contributions to Vital Statistics, Obtained by Means of a Pneumatic Apparatus for Valuing the Respiratory Powers with Relation to Health," *Journal of the Statistical Society of London* 7 (1844): 193–212, 193.
25. W. H. Bodkin, "Pneumatic Apparatus for Valuing the Respiratory Powers," *Lancet* 1 (1844): 390–91; John Hutchinson (delivered by Lieutenant-Colonel Sykes), "Lecture on Vital Statistics, Embracing an Account of a New Instrument for Detecting the Presence of Disease in the System," *Lancet* 1 (1844): 567–70, 594–97; P. J. Bishop, "A Bibliography of John Hutchinson," *Medical History* 21 (1977): 384–96.
26. Hutchinson, "Lecture on Vital Statistics," 567.
27. Ibid., 568. The men he studied were sailors, soldiers, fire-brigade, metropolitan and Thames police, paupers, mixed-class, pugilists, giants, dwarfs, printers, draymen, and gentlemen.
28. Editor, "Obituary: The Late Dr. John Hutchinson," *Medical Times and Gazette* 1 (1862): 200–201.
29. The technical features of Hutchinson's device were very similar to Clayfield's. Hutchinson never cites Clayfield, but he must have been aware of his instrument, since it was the frontispiece of Davy's book, which Hutchinson does reference.
30. W. H. Bodkin, "On a Pneumatic Apparatus for Valuing the Respiratory Powers with Relation to Health by John Hutchinson," *Transactions of the Society for the Encouragement of Arts, Manufactures, and Commerce* 55 (1845): 199–203.
31. Ibid, 199. For debates over the stethoscope and its use in clinical diagnosis, see Reiser, *Medicine and the Reign of Technology*.
32. John Hutchinson, "On the Capacity of the Lungs, and on the Respiratory Functions, with a View of Establishing a Precise and Easy Method of Detecting Disease by the Spirometer," *Medico-Chirurgical Transactions* 29 (1846): 137–252.
33. W. P. Bain, "On a Portable Spirometer," *British Medical Journal* 1 (February 5, 1870): 129.
34. Dividing lung function into parts that were or were not controlled by the will converged with philosophical debates over free will. See Mary Poovey,

"Figures of Arithmetic, Figures of Speech: The Discourse of Statistics in the 1830s," *Critical Inquiry* 19 (1993): 256–76, 268.

35. Julius Jeffreys, *View upon the Statics of the Human Chest, Animal Health, and Determination of Blood to the Head* (London: Longman, Brown, Green & Longmans, 1843). Jeffreys is best (and most controversially) known as inventor and advocate for an apparatus called the respirator, designed to warm and humidify the air entering the lungs of those with pulmonary ailments.

36. Ibid., 3.

37. William B. Carpenter, *Principles of Human Physiology, with Their Chief Applications to Pathology, Hygiene, and Forensic Medicine,* 5th ed. (London: John Churchill, 1855), 280; William Senhouse Kirkes, *Handbook of Physiology* (London: Taylor, Walton & Maberly, 1848), 152.

38. Jeffreys, *View upon the Statics of the Human Chest,* x.

39. Ibid., 6.

40. Andrew Marshall, *Striving for the Comfort Zone: A Perspective on Julius Jeffreys* (Dallas: Windy Knoll Publications, 2004), 65–67; David Zuck, "Julius Jeffreys and the Physiology of Lung Volumes," *Proceedings of the History of Anaesthesia Society* 10 (1990): 55–61.

41. Reiser, *Medicine and the Reign of Technology,* 93–95.

42. Hutchinson, "Contributions to Vital Statistics," 194.

43. John Hutchinson (presented by Dr. Cursham), "On the Capacity of the Lungs, and on the Respiratory Movements with the View of Establishing a Precise and Easy Method of Detecting Disease by the Spirometer," *Lancet* 1 (1846): 631.

44. John Hutchinson, *The Spirometer, the Stethoscope, and the Scale-Balance; Their Use in Discriminating Diseases of the Chest, and Their Value in Life Offices; with Remarks on the Selection of Lives for Life Assurance Companies* (London: John Churchill, 1862), 2.

45. Owsei Temkin, "Basic Science, Medicine, and the Romantic Era," *Bulletin of the History of Medicine* 37 (1963): 97–129; Rothschuh, *History of Physiology,* 180–87.

46. The term "capacity," for example, carried meanings as diverse as "holding power," a volume or "containing space," ability, or possibility *(Oxford English Dictionary).*

47. For a discussion of the relationship between mechanistic and vitalist explanation in British physiology, see June Goodfield-Toulmin, "Some Aspects of English Physiology," *Journal of the History of Biology* 2 (1969): 283–320; Theodore M. Brown, "Physiology and the Mechanical Philosophy in Mid-Seventeenth-Century England," *Bulletin of the History of Medicine* 51 (1977): 25–54; Theodore M. Brown, "From Mechanism to Vitalism in Eighteenth-Century English Physiology," *Journal of the History of Biology* 7 (1974): 179–216. For a discussion of the various meanings of vitalism, see E. Benton, "Vitalism in Nineteenth-Century Scientific Thought: A Typology and Reassessment," *Studies in the History of the Philosophical Sciences* 5 (1974): 17–48, and Jacalyn Duffin, "Vitalism and Organicism in the Philosophy of R.-T.-H. Laennec," *Bulletin of the History of Medicine* 62 (1988): 525–45.

48. Tore Frangsmyr, J. L. Heilbron, and Robin E. Rider, eds., *The Quantifying Spirit in the Eighteenth Century* (Berkeley: University of California Press, 1990).

49. Stedman Jones, *Outcast London*, 20.
50. Reiser, *Medicine and the Reign of Technology*.
51. Ibid., 93–95.
52. Hutchinson, "Lecture on Vital Statistics," 596.
53. Bain, "On a Portable Spirometer," 129.
54. Beigel, "On Spirometry," 119. For enthusiastic responses to the spirometer, see Alexander Rattray, "A Combined Spirometer, Aspirator, and Aeroscope," *Lancet* 100 (December 28, 1872): 915.
55. "Machine-made Diagnoses," *British Medical Journal* 1 (1895): 36; quoted in Reiser, *Medicine and the Reign of Technology*, 223.
56. Hutchinson, *The Spirometer, the Stethoscope, and the Scale-Balance*, 74.
57. To collect data for this analysis, I hand-searched the Index of Patents in the British Public Library. The increase in patents during the 1880s is partly the result of a change in patent law, which lowered the price of an application. The 1880s surge in patents is somewhat specific, however, because overall patent applications continued to increase in the 1890s, while spirometry-related ones declined.
58. Somerville Scott Alison, *The Physical Examination of the Chest in Pulmonary Consumption* (London: John Churchill, 1861), 351–52.
59. Robert Mann Lowne. Spirometers. British Patent No. 3343, filed December 21, 1870.
60. His family-operated company, Lowne Instruments, opened in 1855 and did not close until 2002 (Sue Hayton, "Lowne Instruments," http://gihs.gold.ac.uk/gihs25.html#lowne).
61. Charles Roberts, *A Manual of Anthropometry or a Guide to the Physical Examination and Measurement of the Human Body* (London: J. & A. Churchill, 1878).
62. "Medical Spirometer," *Lancet* 135 (February 1, 1890): 251; W. F. Stanley, "Note on a New Spirometer," *Journal of the Anthropological Institute of Great Britain and Ireland* 20 (1891): 28–30.
63. Ian Hacking, "How Should We Do the History of Statistics?" in *The Foucault Effect: Studies in Governmentality*, ed. Graham Burchell, Colin Gordon, and Peter Miller (Chicago: University of Chicago Press, 1991), 187.
64. Poovey, "Figures of Arithmetic, Figures of Speech," 256–76; Wohl, *Endangered Lives*, 257. For a history of statistical debates in the first half of the nineteenth century, see Victor L. Hilts, "Aliis Exterendum, or, the Origins of the Statistical Society of London," *ISIS* 69 (1978): 21–43; Lawrence Goldman, "The Origins of British 'Social Science': Political Economy, Natural Science and Statistics," *Historical Journal* 26 (1983): 587–616; Ian Hacking, "Biopower and the Avalanche of Printed Numbers," *Humanities in Society* 5 (1982): 279–95; Theodore M. Porter, *The Rise of Statistical Thinking 1820–1900* (Princeton, N.J.: Princeton University Press, 1985); and Mary Poovey, *A History of the Modern Fact: Problems of Knowledge in the Sciences of Wealth and Society* (Chicago: University of Chicago Press, 1998), 307–28.
65. Poovey, *Making a Social Body;* Stedman Jones, *Outcast London*.
66. William Augustus Guy, "Medical Statistics," *Cyclopaedia of Anatomy and Physiology* 5 (1849), 801–2.
67. Hutchinson, "On the Capacity of the Lungs," 150.
68. Ibid., 158.

69. For more on Quetelet, see Porter, *The Rise of Statistical Thinking*, 100–107. The table was such a convincing experimental device that Hutchinson even used one to organize stethoscopic sounds in *The Spirometer, the Stethoscope, and the Scale-Balance.*

70. Hutchinson, *The Spirometer, the Stethoscope, and the Scale-Balance*, 18.

71. Charles Dickens, *Bleak House,* ed. George Ford and Sylvère Monod (New York: W.W. Norton, 1977), 15n4. See Edward J. Wood's *Giants and Dwarfs* for a bibliography of famous giants and dwarfs (London: Richard Bentley, 1868).

72. W.H. Bodkin, "Society of Arts. 29 May 1844," *Lancet* 1 (1844): 390–91.

73. Hutchinson, "Lecture on Vital Statistics," 570; see also Thomas Lewis, "On the Vital Capacity of the French Giant," *British Medical Journal* 2 (September 16, 1865): 297.

74. Poovey, "Figures of Arithmetic, Figures of Speech."

75. Editor, "Obituary: The Late Dr. John Hutchinson," 200–210.

76. Hutchinson, "Lecture on Vital Statistics," 569.

77. Merriley Borrell, "Instrumentation and the Rise of Modern Physiology," *Science and Technology Studies* 5 (1987): 53–62; Frederic Holmes and Kathryn Olesko, "Images of Precision: Helmholtz and the Graphical Method in Physiology," in Wise, *The Values of Precision*, 198–221.

78. Hacking, "Biopower and the Avalanche of Printed Numbers," 280.

79. J. Cleeland and S. Burt, "Charles Turner Thackrah: A Pioneer in the Field of Occupational Health," *Occupational Medicine* 45 (1995): 285–97.

80. Georges Dreyer and George Fulford Hanson, *The Assessment of Physical Fitness by Correlation of Vital Capacity and Certain Measurements of the Body* (New York: Paul B. Hoeber, 1921).

81. Michael Anton Budd, *The Sculpture Machine: Physical Culture and Body Politics in the Age of Empire* (New York: New York University Press, 1997), 15.

82. Hutchinson, "Contributions to Vital Statistics," 204, 202. In a humorous note, he remarks that the low vital capacity of Stephen Hales was owing to his gentlemanly status. The nature of labor distinguished the bodies of the Thames and Metropolitan police—upper-body strength in the case of the Thames police who rowed throughout the day and leg speed for the Metropolitan police who spent their days chasing thieves.

83. Peter Linebaugh, *The London Hanged: Crime and Civil Society in the Eighteenth Century* (Cambridge: Cambridge University Press, 1992); Thompson, *The Making of the English Working Class*, 265.

84. Engels, *The Condition of the Working Class in England*, 168, 208.

85. Hutchinson, "On the Capacity of the Lungs," 160.

86. Porter, "Precision and Trust," 189–91.

87. Hutchinson, "On the Capacity of the Lungs," 178.

88. John Syer Bristowe, *A Treatise on the Theory and Practice of Medicine,* 2d American ed. (Philadelphia: Henry C. Lea, 1879), 339.

89. Hutchinson, "On the Capacity of the Lungs," 195.

90. Hutchinson, "Contributions to Vital Statistics," 193, 206.

91. See Georges Dreyer, "Investigations on the Normal Vital Capacity in Man and Its Relation to the Size of the Body: The Importance of This Measurement as a Guide to Physical Fitness under Different Conditions and in Different Classes of Individuals," *Lancet* 2 (1919): 233.

92. Bishop, "A Bibliography of John Hutchinson"; Herbert Davies, "A Course of Lectures on the Physical Diagnosis of Diseases of the Chest," *Lancet* 1 (1850): 39–41.

93. Bishop, "A Bibliography of John Hutchinson"; Arnett, "The Vital Capacity of the Lungs."

94. The funding structure of German universities allowed for rapid institutionalization of physiology, technical innovation, a proliferation of instrument makers, and the export of these research skills and instrumentation. See Gerald L. Geison, "Social and Institutional Factors in the Stagnancy of English Physiology, 1840–1870," *Bulletin of the History of Medicine* 46 (1972): 30–58.

95. G. O., "The Spirometer as a Means of Diagnosis," *Boston Medical and Surgical Journal* 36 (June 30, 1847): 437.

96. "Dr. Mattson on the Curability of Consumption," *Boston Medical and Surgical Journal* 43 (January 8, 1851): 449–57.

97. William Pepper, "The Spirometer; Its Use in Detecting Disease of the Lungs," *American Journal of the Medical Sciences* 25 (April 1853): 312.

98. E. Andrews, "Vital Capacity," *Peninsular Journal of Medicine and the Collateral Sciences* 1 (June 1854): 532.

99. S. W. Mitchell, "Improved Spirometer," *American Journal of the Medical Sciences* (1859): 378–79; S. W. Mitchell, "On the Inhalation of Cinchonia, and Its Salts," *Proceedings of the Academy of Natural Sciences of Philadelphia* 10 (1858): 21–28.

100. W. E. Bowman, "A Cheap Spirometer," *British American Journal* 3 (1862): 200–201.

101. The first edition was published in 1842 in Britain and in 1843 in the United States.

102. Carpenter, *Principles of Human Physiology,* 280–82. The Americans favored muscular power.

103. Ibid., 3d ed., (London: John Churchill, 1846), viii.

104. I reviewed the extensive collection of physiology and medical textbooks from the mid-nineteenth century to the turn of the century in the Wellcome Library for the History and Understanding of Medicine. Most textbooks, handbooks, and physiology manuals throughout the nineteenth century, including those written by American authors, such as Winfield Hall who published in Britain, discussed Hutchinson's work.

105. E. Fletcher Ingals, *Diseases of the Chest, Throat and Nasal Cavities,* 2d ed. (New York: William Wood & Company, 1892), 19.

106. Lawrence, *Medicine in the Making of Modern Britain,* 45.

107. Jonathan Reinarz, "Mechanizing Medicine: Medical Innovation and the Birmingham Voluntary Hospitals in the Nineteenth Century," in Carsten Timmermann and Julie Anderson, eds., *Devices and Designs: Medical Technologies in Historical Perspective* (Houndmills, Basgingstoke: Palgrave Macmillan, 2006), 37–60. See also Christopher Lawrence, "Incommunicable Knowledge: Science, Technology and the Clinical Art in Britain 1850–1914," *Journal of Contemporary History* 20 (1985): 503–20, on the relationship between technology and clinical practice.

108. Hutchinson, *The Spirometer, the Stethoscope, and the Scale-Balance,* 64. In the United States, his call was taken up by physicians involved in

insurance medicine, as we will see in the next chapter. See William Gleitsmann, "Life Insurance Companies and Pulmonary Phthisis," *Medical and Surgical Reporter* 34 (1876): 1–5.

2. Black Lungs and White Lungs

1. Thomas Jefferson, "Notes on the State of Virginia," in *Race and the Enlightenment: A Reader,* ed. Emmanuel Eze (Malden, Mass., and London: Blackwell Publishing, 1997), 98. Enlightenment thinking about race played out differently in India. See Mark Harrison, *Climates and Constitutions: Health, Race, Environment and British Imperialism in India, 1600–1850* (Oxford: Oxford University Press, 1999).
2. Stephen Jay Gould, *The Mismeasure of Man* (New York: W.W. Norton, 1996).
3. Samuel Cartwright, "Report on the Diseases and Physical Peculiarities of the Negro Race," *New Orleans Medical and Surgical Journal* 7 (1851): 691–715.
4. Samuel A. Cartwright, "Slavery in the Light of Ethnology," in *Cotton Is King and Proslavery Arguments,* ed. E. N. Elliott (Geo. M. Loomis, 1860), 695–96. I am grateful to Walter Johnson for his unpublished manuscript, "River of Dark Dreams," where I first noted the use of the spirometer by Cartwright. See also James Denny Guillory, "The Pro-Slavery Arguments of Dr. Samuel A. Cartwright," *Louisiana History* 9 (1968): 209–27, and Dorothy Roberts, *Fatal Invention: How Science, Politics, and Big Business Re-create Race in the Twenty-First Century* (New York: New Press, 2012).
5. Cartwright, "Slavery in the Light of Ethnology," 701.
6. Ibid., 696.
7. Mia Bay, *The White Image in the Black Mind: African-American Ideas about White People, 1830–1925* (Oxford: Oxford University Press, 2000), 165.
8. Ibid., 33.
9. Ibid., 36; emphasis added.
10. Ibid., 61.
11. Ibid., 62. See also Editor, "James McCune Smith," *Journal of the National Medical Association* 44 (1952): 160; James McCune Smith, "Civilization: Its Dependence on Physical Circumstances," *Anglo-African Magazine* (1859): 5–17.
12. John S. Haller Jr., *Outcasts from Evolution: Scientific Attitudes of Racial Inferiority, 1859–1900* (Urbana: University of Illinois Press, 1971), 19–34.
13. Charles J. Stillé, *History of the United States Sanitary Commission Being the General Report of Its Work during the War of the Rebellion* (Philadelphia: J. B. Lippincott & Co., 1866); Ezra B. McCagg, "The United States Sanitary Commission," read November 5, 1884, *Journal of Civil War Medicine* 5 (2001), 2–14; George Fredrickson, *The Inner Civil War: Northern Intellectuals and the Crisis of the Union* (New York: Harper & Row, 1965), 98–112; Haller, *Outcasts from Evolution,* 20.
14. Jane Tuner Censer, ed., *The Papers of Frederick Law Olmsted,* vol. 4, *Defending the Union: The Civil War and the U.S. Sanitary Commission 1861–1863* (Baltimore: Johns Hopkins University Press, 1986), 1–61.
15. Ibid., 51.
16. Stillé, *History of the United States Sanitary Commission,* 460.
17. Benjamin Apthorp Gould, *Investigations in the Military and Anthropological Statistics of American Soldiers* (New York: Arno Press, 1979), 221. See

Records of the United States Sanitary Commission, New York Public Library, Manuscripts and Archives Division, Box 100, for original questionnaires (hereafter NYPL Manuscripts and Archives).

18. A. Hunter Dupree, "The National Academy of Sciences and the American Definition of Science," in *The Organization of Knowledge in Modern America, 1860–1920,* ed. Alexandra Oleson and John Voss (Baltimore: Johns Hopkins University Press, 1979), 343; Seth Chandler, "Benjamin Apthorp Gould," *Proceedings of the American Academy of Arts and Sciences* 32 (1897): 355–60, 358.

19. Gould, *Investigations in the Military and Anthropological Statistics of American Soldiers,* 221. In *Intensely Human: The Health of the Black Soldier in the American Civil War* (Baltimore: Johns Hopkins University Press, 2008), Margaret Humphreys notes that many other physicians recognized this opportunity for understanding racial difference.

20. Gould, *Investigations in the Military and Anthropological Statistics of American Soldiers,* v–vi.

21. Ibid., 221.

22. Agassiz was one of the founders of the National Academy of Sciences (Dupree, "The National Academy of Sciences and the American Definition of Science").

23. The mid-nineteenth-century United States was still largely rural, and many people held a variety of occupations simultaneously.

24. Gould, *Investigations in the Military and Anthropological Statistics of American Soldiers,* 469.

25. Ibid., 471. In *Shades of Citizenship: Race and Census in Modern Politics* (Palo Alto, Calif.: Stanford University Press, 2000), Melissa Nobles analyzes scientific views of racial mixture in 1850 census categories.

26. Lucius Brown to Benjamin Apthorp Gould, May 7, 1896, Box 133, Records of the United States Sanitary Commission, NYPL Manuscripts and Archives.

27. Brown to Gould, February 24, 1868, Box 133, Records of the United States Sanitary Commission, NYPL Manuscripts and Archives.

28. Gould, *Investigations in the Military and Anthropological Statistics of American Soldiers,* 223. Subsequent references are given in the text.

29. Matthew Frye Jacobson, *Whiteness of a Different Color: European Immigrants and the Alchemy of Race* (Cambridge: Harvard University Press, 1998); David R. Roediger, *Working toward Whiteness: How America's Immigrants Became White: The Strange Journey from Ellis Island to the Suburbs* (New York: Basic Books, 2005); Nell Painter, *The History of White People* (New York: W. W. Norton, 2010). Scholars differ in their periodization. Painter speaks in terms of "great enlargements of whiteness." All agree that during the late nineteenth and early twentieth centuries, immigration from Southern and Eastern Europe reconfigured notions of race and racial difference.

30. James Allen Young, "Height, Weight, and Health: Anthropometric Study of Human Growth in Nineteenth-Century American Medicine," *Bulletin of the History of Medicine* 53 (1979): 214–43.

31. Paul Steiner, *Medical History of a Civil War Regiment: Disease in the 65th US Colored Infantry* (Claxton, Mo.: Institute of Civil War Studies, 1977). In *Intensely Human,* Humphreys argues that modern medicine provides evidence for biological differences in lung volumes related to susceptibility to pneumonia among blacks.

32. Stillé, *History of the United States Sanitary Commission*, 467.
33. Sanford Hunt, "The Negro as a Soldier," *Anthropological Review* 17 (1869): 48, 54.
34. Jedediah H. Baxter, *Statistics, Medical and Anthropological of the Provost-Marshal-General's Bureau Derived from Records of the Examination for Military Service in the Armies of the United States during the Late War of the Rebellion of over a Million Recruits, Drafted Men, Substitutes, and Enrolled*, 2 vols. (Washington, D.C.: U.S. Government Printing Office, 1875).
35. Ibid., 1:vii.
36. John Hutchinson, *The Spirometer, the Stethoscope, and the Scale-Balance; Their Use in Discriminating Diseases of the Chest, and Their Value in Life Offices; with Remarks on the Selection of Lives for Life Assurance Companies* (London: John Churchill, 1852), 5.
37. Baxter, *Statistics, Medical and Anthropological*, 4. According to Humphreys, physicians who filled out the surveys may have held less derogatory views toward blacks (*Intensely Human*, 9).
38. Ibid., 30–48. Subsequent references are given in the text.
39. John Harley Warner, "The Fall and Rise of Professional Mystery: Epistemology, Authority and Emergence of Laboratory Medicine in Nineteenth-Century America," in *The Laboratory Revolution in Medicine*, ed. Andrew Cunningham and Perry Williams (Cambridge: Cambridge University Press, 1992). In *Intensely Human*, Humphreys notes that completion of the Provost-Marshall-General's questionnaire was highest in New England, although she does not comment on Gould's sample (146).
40. W. E. B. DuBois, *Black Reconstruction in America, 1860–1880* (repr. New York: Atheneum, 1975), discussed in Anthony Bogues, *Black Heretics, Black Prophets: Radical Political Intellectuals* (New York and London: Routledge, 2003), 84. Bogues argues that by viewing the mass exodus of slaves from plantations as a general strike, DuBois reconceptualizes slaves as a social category.
41. Charles Darwin, "On the Races of Man," reprinted from *The Descent of Man and Selection in Relation to Sex*, in *The Idea of Race*, ed. Robert Bernasconi and Tommy L. Lott (Indianapolis: Hackett Publishing Company), 55.
42. Ibid., 59.
43. John S. Haller Jr., "Race, Mortality, and Life Insurance: Negro Vital Statistics in the Late Nineteenth Century," *Journal of the History of Medicine and Allied Sciences* 25 (1970): 255.
44. John S. Haller Jr., *Outcasts from Evolution: Scientific Attitudes of Racial Inferiority, 1859–1900* (Urbana: University of Illinois Press, 1971).
45. Charles Gayaree, "The Southern Question," *North American Review* 125 (1877): 497.
46. John S. Haller Jr., "The Physician versus the Negro: Medical and Anthropological Concepts of Race in the Late Nineteenth Century," *Bulletin of the History of Medicine* 44 (1970): 154–67; Eugene R. Corson, "The Future of the Colored Race in the United States from an Ethnic and Medical Standpoint," *New York Medical Times* 15 (1887): 225–30; Edward A. Balloch, "The Relative Frequency of Fibroid Processes in the Dark-Skinned Races," *Medical News* 64 (1894): 29–35; R. M. Cunningham, "The Morbidity and Mortality of Negro Convicts," *Medical News* 64 (1894): 113–17.

47. W. J. Burt, "On the Anatomical and Physiological Differences between the White and Negro Races, and the Modification of Diseases Resulting Therefrom," *St. Louis Courier of Medicine* 8 (1882): 422.
48. Cunningham, "The Morbidity and Mortality of Negro Convicts," 115. The same strategy of using prisoners to justify lower lung capacity in blacks can be found in Smillie and Augustine's 1926 paper (see chapter 5).
49. M. V. Ball, "The Mortality of the Negro," *Medical News* 64 (1894): 389–90.
50. Quoted in George W. Stocking, "The Turn-of-the-Century Concept of Race," *Modernism / Modernity* 1, no. 1 (1994): 9.
51. Frederick L. Hoffman, *Race Traits and Tendencies of the American Negro* (New York: American Economic Association, 1896).
52. Francis J. Sypher, "The Rediscovered Prophet: Frederick L. Hoffman (1865–1946)," http://www.cosmos-club.org/journals/2000/sypher.html; accessed January 5, 2000. I thank Sam Roberts for bringing this article to my attention. See also Megan J. Wolff, "The Myth of the Actuary: Life Insurance and Frederick L. Hoffman's *Race Traits and Tendencies of the American Negro*," *Public Health Reports* 121 (2008): 84–91.
53. Frederick L. Hoffman, "Vital Statistics of the Negro," *Arena* 29 (1892): 529–42.
54. Agents working on commission sold industrial insurance. Agents visited the homes of policyholders each week to collect fees.
55. Haller, "Race, Mortality, and Life Insurance," 251.
56. Frederick L. Hoffman, *History of the Prudential Insurance Company of America (Industrial Insurance), 1875–1900* (Newark: Prudential Press, 1900); "The Colored Race in Life Assurance," *Lancet* 2 (1898), 902; Haller, "Race, Mortality, and Life Insurance."
57. Frederick L. Hoffman, "The Negro in the West Indies," *Publications of the American Statistical Association* 4 (1895): 181–200.
58. Hoffman, *Race Traits and Tendencies of the American Negro*, viii.
59. Haller, "Race, Mortality, and Life Insurance," 255.
60. Hoffman, *Race Traits and Tendencies of the American Negro*, 162.
61. Ibid., 164.
62. George W. Stocking, *Race, Culture, and Evolution: Essays in the History of Anthropology* (New York: Free Press, 1968); Stocking, "The Turn-of-the-Century Concept of Race"; Roediger, *Working toward Whiteness*.
63. DuBois, *Black Reconstruction in America*, 4. One theme that characterizes opposition to Radical Reconstruction was "the great difference between the two races in physical, mental and moral characteristics" (President Andrew Johnson, quoted in ibid., 342).
64. The reality was more complicated because, whether enslaved, "free," or incarcerated, blacks worked in Southern mines and industries in both the antebellum and postbellum period. Many artisans in the South were black. The divisions between black and white labor, though, led to separate labor union organization. See, for example, Jacqueline Jones, *The Dispossessed: America's Underclasses from the Civil War to the Present* (New York: Basic Books, 1993); Ronald Lewis, *Black Coal Miners in America: Race, Class, and Community Conflict 1780–1980* (Lexington: University Press of Kentucky, 1987); Sterling D. Spero and Abram L. Harris, *The Black Worker: The Negro and the Labor Movement* (New York: Atheneum, 1969); Philip S. Foner and Ronald L. Lewis, eds., *Black Workers: A Documentary History from Colonial*

Times to the Present (Philadelphia: Temple University Press, 1989); DuBois, *Black Reconstruction in America;* Eric Foner, "Reconstruction and the Crisis of Free Labor," in *Politics and Ideology in the Age of the Civil War* (Oxford: Oxford University Press, 1980), 97–127.

65. Frederick L. Hoffman, "The Mortality from Consumption in Dusty Trades," *Bulletin of the Bureau of Labor,* no. 79 (November 1908): 728–29.

66. See the Frederick L. Hoffman Collection, Rare Book and Manuscript Library of Columbia University, New York, hereafter referred to as FLH papers.

67. Frederick L. Hoffman,"Racial Aspects of the Tuberculosis Problem," *Association of Tuberculosis Clinics NYC* 4 (April 27, 1917), Box 14, Folder 423, FLH papers.

68. Frederick L. Hoffman, "The Problem of Negro–White Intermixture and Intermarriage," *Eugenics in Race and State* 2 (1923): 175–87.

69. Frederick L. Hoffman, "What America Has Done for Haiti," *Stone and Webster Journal* 55 (July 1929), Box 14, FLH papers.

70. Gary N. Calkins, "Book Review: Race Traits and Tendencies of the American Negro," *Political Science Quarterly* 11 (1896): 754–57; "How to Figure the Extinction of a Race," *Nation* 64 (1867): 246–48; W. J. McGee, "Book Review: Race Traits and Tendencies of the American Negro," *Science* 5 (1897): 65–69; Frederick Starr, "The Degeneracy of the American Negro," *Dial* 22 (1897): 17–18.

71. Miles Melander Dawson, "Hoffman's Statistical Study of the Negro," *Publications of the American Statistical Association* 5 (1896): 142–48; Starr, "The Degeneracy of the American Negro," 17–18; McGee, "Book Review," 65–68.

72. Calkins, "Review of Race Traits and Tendencies of the Negro," 756.

73. "How to Figure the Extinction of a Race," 246.

74. Rudolph Matas to Frederick L. Hoffman, April 21, 1897, Correspondence File, FLH papers.

75. Samuel Kelton Roberts, *Infectious Fear: Politics, Disease, and the Health Effects of Segregation* (Chapel Hill: University of North Carolina Press, 2009), 68.

76. Ibid., 52–53.

77. See http://www.math.buffalo.edu/mad/special/miller_kelley.html for biographical details; accessed December 10, 2012.

78. Kelly Miller, "A Review of Hoffman's Race Traits and Tendencies of the American Negro," in *Occasional Papers,* no. 1 (Washington, D.C.: American Negro Academy, 1897), 6.

79. Ibid., 16.

80. Ibid., 19.

81. Ibid., 21.

82. W. E. B. DuBois, "The Study of the Negro Problems," in *Writings by W. E. B. DuBois in Periodicals Edited by Others,* vol. 1, *1891–1909,* ed. Herbert Aptheker (Millwood, N.J.: Kraus-Thompson, 1982), 47.

83. Ibid., 48.

84. Frederick Hoffman, "The Life Story of a Statistician, 1865–1884," Box 9, No. 29, FLH papers.

85. George Fredrickson, *The Black Image in the White Mind: The Debate on Afro-American Character and Destiny, 1817–1914* (Middletown, Conn.: Wesleyan University Press, 1987), 249–52; Roberts, *Infectious Fear,* 52–53.

86. Frederick Hoffman to John F. Dryden, November 12, 1909, and November 24, 1909, Box 1, No. 1, FLH papers.

87. Burton J. Bledstein, *The Culture of Professionalism: The Middle Class and the Development of Higher Education in America* (New York: W. W. Norton, 1976).
88. Hoffman's professional memberships included the National Association for the Study and Prevention of Tuberculosis (founded in 1904); the American Association of the Academy of Science; Royal Anthropological Institute; American Public Health Association; Committee on Anthropology and chairman of the Subcommittee on Race in Relation to Disease (Civilian Records) of the National Research Council; and the American Statistical Society (president in 1911); Hoffman was one of only ten laypeople among the 156 original members (Julius Lane Wilson, "History of the American Thoracic Society. Part I. The American Sanatorium Association," *American Review of Respiratory Disease* [1979]: 119, 177–84). See also FLH papers.
89. Alice Hamilton, *Exploring the Dangerous Trades: The Autobiography of Alice Hamilton* (Boston: Little, Brown & Company, 1943).
90. Roberts, *Infectious Fear*, 55.
91. Ibid., 57–62.
92. Alexander Rattray, "The Spirometer in Diagnosis," *Pacific Medical and Surgical Journal* 22 (1879): 110–17.
93. Audrey B. Davis, "Life Insurance and the Physical Examination: A Chapter in the Rise of American Medical Technology," *Bulletin of the History of Medicine* 55 (1981): 392–406.
94. One such innovation was based on the model of a Chinese paper lantern (G. W. Fitz, "A Portable Dry Spirometer," *Boston Society of Medical Sciences* 5 [1900–1901]: 340).
95. Joseph Jones, "Vital Capacity of the Lungs and the Vacuum Pneumatic Spirometer," *Journal of the American Medical Association* 11 (1888): 13.
96. James Allen Young, "Height, Weight, and Health: Anthropometric Study of Human Growth in Nineteenth-Century American Medicine," *Bulletin of the History of Medicine* 53 (1979): 214–43; Nicholas Hudson, "From 'Nation' to 'Race': The Origin of Racial Classification in Eighteenth-Century Thought," *Eighteenth-Century Studies* 29, no. 3 (1996): 247–64. See Audrey Davis, *Medicine and Its Technology: An Introduction to the History of Medical Instrumentation* (Westport, Conn.: Greenwood Press, 1981), 185–201, for a discussion of the spirometer in the life insurance industry.
97. Morton Keller, *The Life Insurance Enterprise, 1885–1910: A Study in the Limits of Corporate Power* (Cambridge: Belknap Press of Harvard University Press, 1999), 9; Thomas L. Stedman, "The Medical Relations of Life Insurance, *Medical Record* (December 10, 1904): 938–39; Editor, "A Department of Insurance Medicine, *Medical Record* 80 (1911): 17–18.
98. Editorial, *Medical Examiner and Practitioner* 10 (1900): 196–97.
99. William Gleitsmann, "Life Insurance Companies and Pulmonary Phthisis," *Medical and Surgical Reporter* 34 (1876): 4.
100. Rattray, "The Spirometer in Diagnosis."

3. The Professionalization of Physical Culture

1. David R. Roediger, *Working toward Whiteness: How America's Immigrants Became White: The Strange Journey from Ellis Island to the Suburbs* (New York: Basic Books, 2005), 50.
2. W. S. Tyler, *History of Amherst College during Its First Half Century, 1821–1871* (Springfield, Mass.: Clark Bryan and Company, 1873).

3. Ibid., 458.
4. J. Edmund Welch, *Edward Hitchcock, M.D. Founder of Physical Education in the College Curriculum* (Greenville, N.C.: East Carolina College, 1966), 71.
5. Quoted in Nathan Allen, *Physical Culture in Amherst College* (Lowell, Mass.: Stone & Huse, Book Printers, 1869), 3–4.
6. The committee included prominent health reformer and physician Nathan Allen, lawyer Henry Edwards, and Colonel Alexander H. Bullock (Tyler, *History of Amherst College*, 410–11). Allen suggested the name.
7. There are three Edward Hitchcocks, two of whom are confusingly referred to as Edward Hitchcock Jr. The first Edward Hitchcock was president of Amherst. His son, Edward Hitchcock, M.D., became the first professor of hygiene and physical training. His son, Edward Hitchcock Jr., would head the physical education department at Cornell University.
8. Welch, *Edward Hitchcock, M.D.*, 1–9. Welch argues that gymnastics in particular was seen as "foreign."
9. Allen, *Physical Culture in Amherst College*, 10–11.
10. Matthew Frye Jacobson, *Whiteness of a Different Color* (Cambridge: Harvard University Press, 1999); Roediger, *Working toward Whiteness;* Nell Painter, *The History of White People* (New York: W. W. Norton, 2010), 145.
11. E. P. Frost, M. K. Pasco, and A. H. Howland, "Testimony in Favor of the Gymnasium," quoted in Welch, *Edward Hitchcock, M.D.*, 269.
12. Tyler, *History of Amherst College*, 413.
13. James C. Whorton, *Crusaders for Fitness: The History of American Health Reformers* (Princeton, N.J.: Princeton University Press, 1984); Harvey Green, *Fit for America: Health, Fitness, Sport, and American Society* (New York: Pantheon Books, 1986); Gerald Gems, Linda Borish, and Gertrud Pfister, *Sports in American History: From Colonization to Globalization* (Champaign, Ill.: Human Kinetics, 2008).
14. Thomas Higginson, "Saints and Their Bodies," *Atlantic Monthly*, March 1858, 586.
15. Ibid., 590.
16. According to Painter, Amherst was the first college to teach Anglo-Saxon.
17. Reports and letters to Nathan Allen; Welch, *Edward Hitchcock, M.D.*
18. Edward Hitchcock, Personal Diary, Series 5, Travel, Subseries A, Trip to France and England 1860, Box 15, Folder 4, Edward and Mary Judson Hitchcock Papers, Archives and Manuscript Collection, Amherst College (hereafter EMJH Papers).
19. Edward Hitchcock, Personal Diary, Series 5, Travel, Subseries A, Trip to France and England 1860, Box 15, Folder 4. Travel to England 1860; Letter from Richard Owen to Edward Hitchock, July 24, 1869, EMJH Papers.
20. Edward Hitchcock and Edward Hitchcock Jr., *Elementary Anatomy and Physiology, for Colleges, Academies, and Other Schools* (New York: Ivison, Phinney, Blakeman & Co.; Chicago: S. C. Griggs & Co., 1864).
21. Welch, *Edward Hitchcock, M.D.*, 155; "Death of Dr. Hitchcock. Veteran Amherst Professor," *Springfield Republican* (February 16, 1911), OSB2, Bound Obituaries, EMJH Papers.
22. Edward Hitchcock to Burges Johnson, December 6, 1906; Series 4, Professional Correspondence, Subseries B, Outgoing Correspondence, Box 14, Folder 28; Burges Johnson, "'Old Doc' Hitchcock: Creator of a System of

Physical Education," *Outlook* (April 27, 1907): 955–61, 958, EMJH Papers. The data for 1861–62 includes lung capacity.

23. Edward Hitchcock, "Second Report of the Professor of Physical Education and Hygiene to the Trustees of Amherst College, 1862–3," Papers connected with the Department of Physical Education, vol. 1, Collection of the Physical Education Department, Archives and Special Collections, Amherst College, hereafter referred to as CPED (uncataloged).

24. In 1863, E. H. Sawyer established the Sawyer Prize for excellence in physical training. Over the years, numerous donors supported other prizes.

25. Tyler, *History of Amherst College*, 412.

26. Welch, *Edward Hitchcock, M.D.*, 74–100.

27. Edward Mussey Hartwell, "A Preliminary Report on Anthropometry in the United States," in *Papers on Anthropometry* (Boston: American Statistical Society, 1894), 1–15.

28. Welch, *Edward Hitchcock, M.D.*, 42.

29. Dio Lewis, *Weak Lungs and How to Make Them Strong* (Boston: Ticknor and Fields, 1863), 259–60.

30. Edward Hitchcock, "Report [to the Trustees] of 1866–67 (handwritten)," Papers Connected to the Physical Education Department, vol. 1: 1861–79, CPED (uncataloged).

31. Edward Hitchcock, "Report to Trustees, 1879–80," Papers Connected to the Physical Education Department, vol. 2, CPED.

32. Edward Hitchcock, "To the Trustees of Amherst College, 1884–5," Papers Connected to the Department of Physical Education, vol. 2, CPED.

33. Hartwell, "A Preliminary Report on Anthropology in the United States." Nathan Allen's *Physical Culture at Amherst*, commissioned by the Board of Trustees, was the first U.S. publication on anthropometry in students.

34. "Physical Culture," *New York Sunday Tribune*, February 18, 1883.

35. Green, *Fit for America*, 103, 135.

36. Edward Hitchcock, "Hygiene at Amherst College. Experience of the Department of Physical Education and Hygiene in Amherst College for the Past Sixteen Years," paper read at meeting of the American Public Health Association in Chicago, September 26, 1877, CPED (uncataloged).

37. Edward Hitchcock, *A Report of Twenty Years Experience in the Department of Physical Education and Hygiene in Amherst College* (Amherst: Press of C. A. Bangs & Co., 1881).

38. Edward Hitchcock, "The Average Man as a Rational Basis for Physical Education," address to students of the summer session of the gymnasium department of the school for Christian workers (Springfield, Mass.: Press of Weaver, Shipman & Co., July 1988).

39. Edward Hitchcock, *The Need of Anthropometry* (Brooklyn: Rome Brothers, 1887), 6. In *The History of White People*, Painter writes that height was a "fetish" among nineteenth-century race theorists.

40. C. Roberts to Edward Hitchcock, March 22 (no year), box labeled "Anthropometric Study (Misc Belonging to Edward Hitchcock), 9/8/97."

41. Francis Galton, "Anthropometric Statistics from Amherst College, Mass. U.S.A.," *Journal of the Anthropological Institute* 18 (1889): 192.

42. Hitchcock and Hitchcock, *Elementary Anatomy and Physiology*, 268.

43. Edward Hitchcock, "A Report of Twenty Years Experience in the Department

of Physical Education and Hygiene in Amherst College, to the Board of Trustees, Physical Culture in Amherst College," June 27, 1881 (Amherst: Press of C.A. Bangs and Co., 1881), CPED.

44. With the rise of spectator sports, interest in gymnastics exhibitions declined after 1888. See Bruce Lanyon Bennett, "The Life of Dudley Allen Sargent, M.D. and His Contributions to Physical Education," Ph.D. diss., University of Michigan, 1947, 49.

45. Martha Verbrugge, *Able-Bodied Womanhood: Personal Health and Social Change in Nineteenth-Century Boston* (Oxford: Oxford University Press, 1988).

46. Kim Townsend, *Manhood at Harvard: William James and Others* (Cambridge: Harvard University Press, 1998). I thank Corey Walker for suggesting this book.

47. Dudley Allen Sargent, *An Autobiography*, ed. Ledyard W. Sargent (Philadelphia: Lea and Febinger, 1927), 103.

48. Ibid., 146; Bennett, "The Life of Dudley Allen Sargent," 26–28.

49. Sargent, *An Autobiography*, 149.

50. Bennett, "The Life of Dudley Allen Sargent," 34–40; Edward Hitchcock Jr., "Physical Examinations," *Physical Education* 1 (February 1893): 221–28.

51. Doug Bryant, "William Blaikie and Physical Fitness in Late Nineteenth Century America," *Iron Game History* 2, no. 3 (1992): 3–6; Carolyn de la Peña, *The Body Electric: How Strange Machines Built the Modern American* (New York: New York University Press, 2003), 64. The key elements of the Sargent system were: the taking of personal and family histories, examination of heart and lungs, muscular strength tests, physical measurements (compared to a standard), use of apparatuses to strengthen weak muscles, and developmental exercises (Bennett, "The Life of Dudley Allen Sargent," 32–33).

52. His contract stipulated that he "will patent no apparatus and seek no income from that source." This caused much bitterness in later years (Bennett, "The Life of Dudley Allen Sargent," 44).

53. Sargent, *An Autobiography*, 206; Roberta Park, "The Rise and Demise of Harvard's B.S. Program in Anatomy, Physiology, and Physical Training: A Case of Conflicts of Interest and Scarce Resources," *Research Quarterly for Exercise and Sport* 63 (1992): 246–60.

54. D.A. Sargent, "The Physical Proportions of the Typical Man," *Scribner's Magazine* 2 (1887): 6.

55. Ibid.; D.A. Sargent, "Strength Tests and the Strong Men of Harvard," *American Physical Education Review* 2 (1897): 108–19; D.A. Sargent, "The Physical Test of a Man," *American Physical Education Review* 26 (April 1921): 188–94.

56. Bennett, "The Life of Dudley Allen Sargent," 48.

57. D.A. Sargent, "The Harvard Summer School of Physical Training: Its Aims, Its Methods and Its Work," *Boston Medical and Surgical Journal* 134 (February 20, 1896): 181–88.

58. D.A. Sargent, "The System of Physical Training at the Hemenway Gymnasium," in *Physical Training: A Full Report of the Papers and Discussion of the Conference Held in Boston in November, 1889*, ed. Isabel C. Barrows (Boston: George H. Ellis, 1899), 67.

59. Roberta Park, "1989 C.H. McCloy Research Lecture: Health, Exercise, and the Biomedical Impulse, 1870–1914," *Research Quarterly for Exercise and Sport* 61 (1990): 128.

60. Roberta J. Park, "Science, Service, and the Professionalization of Physical Education: 1885–1905," *International Journal of the History of Sport* 24 (2007): 1674–700.

61. Mabel Lee, *A History of Physical Education and Sports in the U.S.A.* (Indianapolis: Wiley, 1983), 110–20.

62. D. A. Sargent, Edw. Hitchcock, and Wm. G. Anderson, *The Report of the Committee upon the Method of Physical Measurement* (Brooklyn: Rome Brothers, 1887).

63. Hitchcock, *The Need of Anthropometry*, 6.

64. Welch, *Edward Hitchcock, M.D.*, 178.

65. Park, "Science, Service, and the Professionalization of Physical Education," 1684.

66. Ibid.

67. Anthropometry flourished in physical anthropology, where it was used explicitly to describe racial difference.

68. Park, "The Rise and Demise of Harvard's B.S. Program."

69. Gail Bederman, *Manliness and Civilization: A Cultural History of Gender and Race in the United States, 1880–1917* (Chicago: University of Chicago Press, 1996).

70. Green, *Fit for America*, 181; Wm. W. Hastings, *A Manual for Physical Measurements. Boys and Girls* (Springfield, Mass.: International Young Men's Christian Association Training School, 1902), viii.

71. Hastings, *A Manual for Physical Measurements*, xi.

72. Edward Hitchcock, "To the Trustees of Amherst College: Annual Report for 1980–1981," Box (not numbered), vol. 2 (uncataloged), Papers Connected to the Department of Physical Education, CPED.

73. Welch, *Edward Hitchcock, M.D.*, 90–91; Japanese anthropometry by Dr. S. A. Leland; Box (unnumbered), "Anthropometry by Age (Studies), Japanese, Misc. Ed. Insts.," CPED. (Amherst College has the raw data.)

74. Edward Hitchcock, "A Comparative Study of the Average Measurements of Amherst, Mt. Holyoke and Wellesley Colleges," Box (unnumbered), "Anthropometric Study (misc belonging to Edward Hitchcock)," Folder 1, CPED.

75. Welch, *Edward Hitchcock, M.D.*, 173.

76. 1887 Amherst College Program of the Exercises and the Students Competing in the Annual Ladd Prize Exhibition, Anthropometry at Amherst College, bound volume, CPED.

77. E. Hitchcock and H. H. Seelye, *An Anthropometric Manual* (Amherst: J. E. Williams, Book and Job Printer, 1887), 3.

78. Paul Phillips, "An Anthropometric Study of the Students of Amherst College to Determine the Norms for Different Heights at Each Age from Seventeen to Twenty-Two Years," n.d. (circa 1904), Uncataloged box, "Anthropometric Study (misc belonging to Edward Hitchcock), Japanese Anthropometry by Dr. S. A. Leland," CPED; Box (unnumbered), "Anthropometry by Age (Studies), Japanese, Misc. Ed. Insts.," CPED.

79. E. Hitchcock and H. H. Seelye, *An Anthropometric Manual*, 3d ed. (Amherst: Press of Carpenter & Morehouse, 1893).

80. Hitchcock and Seelye, *An Anthropometric Manual* (1887), 32.

81. Edward Mussey Hartwell, "The Nature of Physical Training and the Best Means of Securing Its Ends," in Barrows, *Physical Training*, 16.

82. D. A. Sargent, "The System of Physical Training at the Hemenway Gymnasium," in Barrows, *Physical Training*, 72–73.

83. Sargent, "The Physical Test of a Man," 190.

84. Jay W. Seaver, *Anthropometry and Physical Examination: A Book for Practical Use in Connection with Gymnastic Work and Physical Education* (New Haven: Press of the O. A. Gorman Co., 1896), 10–11. Racial differences in the trunk to limb ratio, owing to the longer limbs and shorter trunks of people of African descent, remain a major explanation for racial differences in lung capacity.

85. Sargent, "The Harvard Summer School of Physical Training," 181.

86. Dudley Allen Sargent, *Health, Strength, and Power* (New York and Boston: H. M. Caldwell Co., 1904).

87. Dudley Sargent, "Relation of Height, Weight, and Strength to the Cephalic Index," *Scientific American Supplement* 49 (June 23, 1900): 20463–65.

88. Park, "Health, Exercise, and the Biomedical Impulse," 128.

89. "Physical Education of Girls," *Journal of Health*, no. 1 (1829): 14.

90. Sargent laid out an entirely different set of exercises for women than for men in *Health, Strength, and Power*. Girls and boys could engage in the same exercises until puberty. Reflecting the ambivalent attitude toward the education of women, and in a time of the "rest cure," participation in physical training activities could not be taken for granted. At the same time, there is no evidence that women physical educators questioned the racial nature of the project of anthropometry. See Martha Verbrugge, *Active Bodies: A History of Women's Physical Education in Twentieth-Century America* (Oxford: Oxford University Press, 2012).

91. Bennett, *The Life of Dudley Allen Sargent*, 83–117; Paula Rogers Lupcho, "The Harvard Summer School of Physical Education," *Journal of Physical Education, Recreation and Dance* 65 (March 1994): 43–48.

92. Sargent, "The Harvard Summer School of Physical Training," 181.

93. Leadership of the professional societies was dominated by men, until 1931, when Mabel Lee became president of the American Association of Physical Education.

94. Barrows, *Physical Training*, 79.

95. Hastings, *A Manual for Physical Measurements*, xv–xvii.

96. Verbrugge, *Active Bodies*, 9.

97. Hitchcock Jr., "Physical Examinations." Hitchcock estimates that, at the time of his writing, physical educators had collected anthropometric data on fifty thousand subjects between the ages of sixteen and twenty-three.

98. Gladys Palmer, "The Physical Measurements of Hollins Freshman, 1920–1927," *American Statistical Association* 24 (1929): 40–49.

99. Edith Pasmore and Frank Weymouth, "The Relation of Vital Capacity to Other Physical Measurements in Women," *American Physical Education Review* (1924): 166–75; Abby H. Turner, "The Vital Capacity of College Women," *American Physical Education Review* 32 (1927): 593–603; B. W. DeBusk, "Height, Weight, Vital Capacity and Retardation," *Pedagogical Seminary* 20 (1913): 89–91; W. P. Bowen, "The spirometer as a scientific instrument," *American Physical Education Review* 11 (1906): 141–48.

100. S. W. Mitchell, "On the Inhalation of Cinchonia, and Its Salts," *Proceedings of the Academy of Natural Sciences of Philadelphia* 10 (1858): 21–28.

101. See James M. Edmonson and F. Terry Hambrecht, *The Centennial Edition of George Tiemann & Co. American Armamentarium Chirurgicum* (San Francisco: Normal Publishing & the Printers' Devil, 1989).
102. Turner, "The Vital Capacity of College Women."

4. Progress and Race

1. Donald E. Hall, "On the Making and Unmaking of Monsters: Christian Socialism, Muscular Christianity, and the Metaphorization of Class Conflict," in *Muscular Christianity: Embodying the Victorian Age*, ed. Donald E. Hall (Cambridge: Cambridge University Press, 1994), 45–65.
2. E. P. Thompson, *The Making of the English Working Class* (New York: Vintage Books, 1963).
3. Michael Anton Budd, *The Sculpture Machine: Physical Culture and Body Politics in the Age of Empire* (New York: New York University Press, 1997); Daniel Pick, *Faces of Degeneration: A European Disorder, c. 1848–1918* (Cambridge: Cambridge University Press, 1989); Nancy Stepan, *The Idea of Race: Britain, 1800–1950* (Hamden, Conn.: Archon Press, 1982).
4. David Kirk, *Defining Physical Education: The Social Construction of a School Subject in Postwar Britain* (London: Falmer Press, 1992), 50.
5. J. A. Mangan, *Athleticism in the Victorian and Edwardian Public Schools: The Emergence and Consolidation of an Educational Ideology* (Cambridge: Cambridge University Press, 1981).
6. Ibid.; Trevor Hearl, "The Fitness of the Nation—Physical and Health Education in the Nineteenth and Twentieth Centuries," in *The Proceedings of the 1982 Annual Conference of the History of Education Society of Great Britain*, ed. Nicholas Parry and David McNair (Leister: History of Education Society, 1983), 8–9; Peter C. McIntosh, *Physical Education in England* (London: Bell, 1968); Kirk, *Defining Physical Education*. Hughes's *Tom Brown's Schooldays* was one of the most widely read books in 1858 in England, as discussed in Roberta Park, "Sport, Gender and Society in a Transatlantic Victorian Perspective," *International Journal of the History of Sport* 24 (2007): 1570–603.
7. Hearl, "The Fitness of the Nation," 46–69; Emmett A. Rice, *A Brief History of Physical Education* (New York: A. S. Barnes & Co., 1926), 128–33.
8. J. D. Campbell, "Training for Sport Is Training for War: Sport and the Transformation of the British Army, 1860–1914," *International Journal of the History of Sport* 17 (2000): 21–58.
9. Kirk, *Defining Physical Education*, 191.
10. McIntosh, *Physical Education in England*, 33–40.
11. Ibid.; Fred Eugene Leonard, *A Guide to the History of Physical Education* (Philadelphia: Lea & Febinger, 1923), 203–8; J. W. MacKail, *The Life of William Morris* (London and New York: Longmans, Green & Co., 1901); Rice, *A Brief History of Physical Education*.
12. MacKail, *The Life of William Morris*, 33.
13. Ibid., 28–66.
14. Archibald MacLaren, *A System of Physical Education: Theoretical and Practical* (Oxford: Clarendon Press, 1869), 11.
15. Ibid., 36; MacIntosh, *Physical Education in England*, 95.
16. Archibald MacLaren, *A Military System of Gymnastic Exercise for the Use of Instructors* (London: His Majesty's Stationery Office, 1862), 5–7. The

first cohort of twelve noncommissioned officers (NCOs), accompanied by their commander, Major Hammersley (later a colonel), attended a six-month course at Oxford. Returning to the military center Aldershot, where an Oxford model gymnasium had been built and a normal school established, this group, called "the apostles," formed the core of the Army Gymnastic Staff.

17. E. A. L. Oldfield, *History of the Army Physical Training Corps* (Aldershot: Gale and Polden, 1955), 1–4.

18. MacLaren *A System of Physical Education,* 11.

19. Ibid., 24.

20. Archibald MacLaren, *Training in Theory and Practice,* 2d ed. (London: MacMillan & Co., 1874); McIntosh, *Physical Education in England,* 92–98.

21. MacLaren, *A System of Physical Education,* 49.

22. Ibid., 24; emphasis added.

23. Ibid., 72–73.

24. Rice, *A Brief History of Physical Education,* 131.

25. MacLaren, *A System of Physical Education,* 496–97, 500–504; McIntosh, *Physical Education in England,* 97.

26. MacLaren, *A System of Physical Education,* 73.

27. Mangan, *Athleticism in the Victorian and Edwardian Public Schools,* 48–54.

28. McIntosh, *Physical Education in England,* 96; Rice, *A Brief History of Physical Education,* 131.

29. George Stocking, *Victorian Anthropology* (New York: Free Press, 1987); Francis Galton, *The Narrative of an Explorer in Tropical South Africa* (London: John Murray, 1853).

30. Biographical information comes from Francis Galton, *Memories of My Life* (London: Methuen & Co., 1908); Karl Pearson, *Life, Letters and Labours of Francis Galton,* vol. 2 (Cambridge: Cambridge University Press, 1924); Nicholas Wright Gilham, *A Life of Sir Francis Galton: From African Exploration to the Birth of Eugenics* (Oxford: Oxford University Press, 2001); Theodore Porter, *The Rise of Statistical Thinking, 1820–1900* (Princeton, N.J.: Princeton University Press, 1986); and "Obituary, Sir Francis Galton," *Journal of the Royal Statistical Society* 74 (1911): 314–20. Dates differ for some of his awards.

31. Porter, *The Rise of Statistical Thinking, 1820–1900,* 294–96.

32. Stocking, *Victorian Anthropology,* 238–73.

33. Pearson, *Life, Letters and Labours of Francis Galton,* 2:334.

34. Galton, *Memories of My Life,* 244.

35. Francis Galton, "Proposal to Apply for Anthropological Statistics from Schools," *Journal of the Anthropological Institute* 3 (1874): 308–11; Galton, *Memories of My Life,* 245; Pearson, *Life, Letters and Labours of Francis Galton,* 2:336–37.

36. John Venn, "Cambridge Anthropometry," *Journal of the Anthropological Institute of Great Britain and Ireland* 18 (1889): 140–54.

37. Francis Galton, "The Anthropometry Laboratory," *Fortnightly Review* 31 (1882): 332–38; Francis Galton, "Anthropometry at Schools," *Journal of Preventive Medicine* 14 (1906): 93–98.

38. Stocking, *Victorian Anthropology.*

39. "Report of the Anthropometric Committee," *Report of the British Associa-*

tion for the Advancement of Science 51 (1881): 225–72; John M. Eyler, *Victorian Social Medicine: Ideas and Methods of William Farr* (Baltimore: Johns Hopkins University Press, 1979), 29, notes that the reports of the Anthropometric Committee of the British Association for the Advancement of Science became more theoretical after Galton assumed the chairmanship from Farr in 1880. Prior to this, reports focused on relationships between occupational and social groups and anthropometric measurements.

40. "Report of the Anthropometric Committee," *Report of the British Association for the Advancement of Science* 47 (1877): 232; "Report of the Anthropometric Committee," *Report of the British Association for the Advancement of Science; Report* 53 (1883): 254. Coxeter was an instrument maker who supplied the University College and Middlesex Hospital, London, with spirometers, beginning in the 1850s. Coxeter's spirometer, comprised of two flexible airtight bags with a stopcock, was an adaptation of Hutchinson's water-filled spirometer. Designed to fold easily into a pocket, the instrument was ideal for fieldwork, although it was mostly used for medical applications.

41. Ernest Hart, "Abstract of a Lecture on the International Health Exhibition of 1884: Its Influence and Possible Sequels," *British Medical Journal* 2 (December 6, 1884): 1115–22. In exhibitions following Hyde Park's Great Exhibit of 1851, displays of machines and laboratories related to health and hygiene were a response to British fears of research decline relative to Germany, the United States, and France, and a testament to Anglo-Saxon superiority. See *The Health Exhibition Literature*, vol. 9, *Health in Relation to Civic Life* (Charing Cross, S.W.: William Clowes and Sons, 1884).

42. Francis Galton, "On the Anthropometric Laboratory at the Late International Health Exhibition," *Journal of the Anthropological Institute of Great Britain and Ireland* 14 (1885): 205.

43. Galton, "Anthropometric Laboratory," in *International Health Exhibition* (London: William Clowes and Sons, 1884), 4.

44. Francis Galton, "Retrospect of Work Done at My Anthropometric Laboratory at South Kensington," *Journal of the Anthropological Institute* 21 (1892): 282–83; Galton, *Memories of My Life*, 250–51.

45. Galton, *Memories of My Life*, 252.

46. Galton, "On the Anthropometric Laboratory at the Late International Health Exhibition"; Francis Galton, "Some Results of the Anthropometric Laboratory," *Journal of the Anthropological Institute of Great Britain and Ireland* 14 (1885): 275–87.

47. Galton, "On the Anthropometric Laboratory at the Late International Health Exhibition."

48. Francis Galton, "Outfit for an Anthropometric Laboratory," March 1883, www.galton.org.

49. Venn, "Cambridge Anthropometry."

50. "A Descriptive List of Anthropometic Apparatus, Designed under the Direction of Mr. Francis Galton, and Manufactured and Sold by the Cambridge Scientific Instrument Company," 1887; see www.galton.org.

51. Galton, "Some Results of the Anthropometric Laboratory," 278.

52. Richard A. Soloway, *Demography and Degeneration: Eugenics and the Declining Birthrate in Twentieth-Century Britain* (Chapel Hill: University of North Carolina Press, 1990), 23.

53. Venn, "Cambridge Anthropometry," 146. Venn recognized that these distinctions might eliminate some qualified men from the top category. Even poll-men (the lowest category) were highly distinguished in relation to "the masses" (144–45). Galton, after all, was just a poll-man, having suffered nervous breakdowns and poor health as a student.

54. Ibid., 147.

55. Ibid., 149.

56. "A Morning with the Anthropometric Detectives: An Interview with Mr. Francis Galton, F. R. S.," *Pall Mall Gazette,* November 16, 1888, 1–2.

57. Francis Galton, *Anthropometric Laboratory: Notes and Memoirs* (London: Richard Clay and Sons, 1890), 5.

58. Francis Galton, "Physical Tests in Competitive Examinations," *Journal of the Society of Arts* 39 (1890): 21.

59. Francis Galton, "On the Advisability of Assigning Marks for Bodily Efficiency of Candidates for the Public Services," *Report of the British Association for the Advancement of Science* 59 (1889): 472.

60. Francis Galton, "On the Principle and Methods of Assigning Marks for Bodily Efficiency," *Nature* 40 (1889): 649–52.

61. Ibid., 649.

62. Galton, *Anthropometric Laboratory,* 8, http://www.galton.org/books/anthro-lab-memoirs/index.html; accessed December 13, 2012. Although Galton acknowledges the relationship between height and lung capacity, I have not found any direct reference to Hutchinson in his writings.

63. Civil-service reform, codified first in the Northcote–Trevelyan Report of 1854, reflected the interests of the rising bourgeoisie. Competitive examination to counter the influence of hereditary privilege for civil-service candidates was a key provision. The literary examination—rooted in the "liberal"/classical education of public schools—ensured that the civil service remained in the hands of a gentleman elite. As G. R. Searle writes in *The Quest for National Efficiency: A Study in British Politics and Political Thought, 1899–1914,* "the intention of the civil service reforms was to root out the abuses of the old aristocratic methods of administration. . . . Yet the effect was to exclude not only the grossly incompetent, the extravagant and the corrupt, but also powerful administrators of the Chadwick camp" (Berkeley: University of California Press, 1971), 21.

64. Francis Galton, "Marks for Physical Efficiency," *Times,* March 28, 1890, 4F.

65. Ibid.

66. Galton, "Physical Tests in Competitive Examinations," 20.

67. Searle, *The Quest for National Efficiency.*

68. Francis Galton, "Our National Physique: Prospects of the British Race, Are We Degenerating?" *Daily Chronicle,* July 29, 1903. In "Hereditary Improvement" published in *Fraser's Magazine* 7 (1873): 116–30, Galton elaborated on his ideas in *Hereditary Genius,* equating race to heredity and advancing his notion of "race improvement"; Gilham, *A Life of Sir Francis Galton,* 195.

69. Galton, "On the Anthropometric Laboratory at the Late International Health Exhibition," 207; Galton, "Anthropometry at Schools," read at the Royal Institute of Public Health, London Congress, 1905, Francis Galton Papers, University College London, Special Collections, 137/15 (hereafter referred to as Galton Papers).

70. "Anthropometric Tables and Pamphlets Sent to Francis Galton by E. Hitchcock," Folder 137/16, Galton Papers.

71. "Lectures on Heredity and Nurture," South Kensington Museum, November 26, December 3, December 10, 1887, Folder, 137/6, Galton Papers.

72. Manuscript of part of Francis Galton's Rede Lecture, 36, Folder 137/5, Galton Papers.

73. Jay Seaver to Francis Galton, January 31, 1890, Folder 194/5, Galton Papers.

74. Francis Galton, "Useful Anthropometry," in *Proceedings of the American Association for the Advancement of Physical Education, at Its Sixth Annual Meeting Held in Boston, Mass., April 3 and 4, 1891* (Ithaca, N.Y.: Andrus & Church, 1891), 51–52.

75. "Race" had many meanings that changed over time and place. Regarding Galton's specific uses of race, see Stepan, *The Idea of Race*, 128.

76. Galton, "On the Principle and Methods of Assigning Marks for Bodily Efficiency."

77. Pick, *Faces of Degeneration*, 215.

78. Budd, *The Sculpture Machine;* no author, "The Man," *Times*, November 26, 1906, 11; *The Times Digital Archive*, accessed December 20, 2012.

79. Pick, *Faces of Degeneration*, 201. See also Gareth Stedman Jones, *Outcast London: A Study in the Relationship between the Classes in Victorian London* (Oxford: Clarendon Press, 1971).

80. No author, "The Physique of the Army," *Times*, April 23, 1892, 14, *The Times Digital Archive*, accessed December 2012.

81. Searle, *The Quest for National Efficiency*, 54, 82. According to Searle, Radical Liberals and many Conservatives opposed the ideals of national efficiency (101).

82. For debate, see Soloway, *Demography and Degeneration;* Searle, *The Quest for National Efficiency;* and David J. Kevles, *In the Name of Eugenics: Genetics and the Uses of Human Heredity* (Cambridge: Harvard University Press, 1998).

83. Pick, *Faces of Degeneration*, 200.

84. Soloway, *Demography and Degeneration*, 38–47.

85. Robert Farquharson, "Physical Deterioration," *Times*, December 26, 1903, 8, *The Times Digital Archive*, accessed December 20, 2012.

86. George Shee, "The Deterioration in the National Physique," *Nineteenth Century and After* 53 (1903): 805.

87. Soloway, *Demography and Degeneration*, 42; *Report of the Inter-departmental Committee on Physical Deterioration*, vol. 1, *Report and Appendix* (London: His Majesty's Stationery Office, 1904), 1–2, Appendix I.

88. *Report of the Inter-departmental Committee on Physical Deterioration*, 1:v.

89. The committee found urbanization, overcrowding, air pollution, and poor conditions of work, alcoholism, and depletion of the "best types" in rural areas, as well as low birthrates among "superior types," to be the main causes of decline in physique. Committee recommendations included government and philanthropic schemes focused on mothers and children, such as physical training programs in cities and schools.

90. *Report of the Inter-departmental Committee on Physical Deterioration*, 1:14.

91. Pick, *Faces of Degeneration;* Searle, *The Quest for National Efficiency;* Kevles, *In the Name of Eugenics*.

92. *Report of the Inter-departmental Committee on Physical Deterioration*, 1:7.
93. See Appendix II for details on Cunningham and Gray's proposal for an Anthropometric Survey (ibid., 102–3). The committee thought the survey would prove the "condition of the rural population as a reservoir of national strength" (35).
94. Ibid., 8.
95. Ibid., 9. Other measurements and tests included height; weight; head length, breadth, and height; breadth of shoulders and hips; and vision.
96. Based on experience with the Irish, who often refused to participate in surveys, the committee anticipated resistance to such measurements (ibid., 11–12).
97. Ibid., 99; Soloway, *Demography and Degeneration*, 45.
98. Part of Francis Galton's Rede Lecture, 40–41, Folder 137/5, Galton Papers.
99. Simon Szreter, "The GRO and the Public Health Movement in Britain, 1837–1914," *Social History of Medicine* 4 (1991): 435–63.

5. Globalizing Spirometry

1. Following devastating critiques summarized in the Flexner Report, the influential study of medical education, most colleges that educated blacks and females closed. See Earl H. Harley, "The Forgotten History of Defunct Black Medical Schools in the 19th and 20th Centuries and the Impact of the Flexner Report," *Journal of the National Medical Association* 98 (2006): 1425–29; Andrew Cunningham and Perry Williams, eds., *The Laboratory Revolution in Medicine* (Cambridge: Cambridge University Press, 1992).
2. Joel D. Howell, *Technology in the Hospital: Transforming Patient Care in the Early Twentieth Century* (Baltimore: Johns Hopkins University Press, 1995), 18; Stefan Timmermans and Marc Berg, *The Gold Standard: The Challenge of Evidence-Based Medicine and Standardization in Health Care* (Philadelphia: Temple University Press, 2003), 30–54; Christopher Crenner, "Race and Laboratory Norms," *Isis*, forthcoming, 2014.
3. Elizabeth Fee, *Disease and Discovery: A History of the Johns Hopkins School of Hygiene and Public Health, 1916–1939* (Baltimore: Johns Hopkins University Press, 1987).
4. Crenner, "Race and Laboratory Norms."
5. Howell, *Technology in the Hospital*, 2.
6. See Irving Fisher *National Vitality, Its Wastes and Conservation* (New York: Arno Press, 1976), for examples of narratives linking national vitality to efficiency in the United States.
7. John Harley Warner, "The Fall and Rise of Professional Mystery," in Cunningham and Williams, *The Laboratory Revolution in Medicine*, 110–40.
8. Many of Peabody's publications feature patients' biographies. A society at Harvard Medical School was named after Peabody. See http://hms.harvard.edu/content/dr-francis-weld-peabody (accessed December 18, 2012).
9. Oglesby Paul, *The Caring Physician: The Life of Dr. Francis W. Peabody* (Boston: Francis A. Countway Library of Medicine, 1991), 36; Clark T. Sawin, "Book Review, *The Caring Physician: The Life of Dr. Francis W. Peabody*," *New England Quarterly* 66 (1993): 150–52.
10. Francis W. Peabody and John A. Wentworth, "Clinical Studies of the Respiration. IV. The Vital Capacity of the Lungs and Its Relation to Dyspnea," *Archives of Internal Medicine* 20 (1917): 463.

11. Francis W. Peabody, "Cardiac Dyspnea," *American Journal of Medical Science* 155 (1918): 101.
12. I take the notion of taming uncertainty in public health from Deborah Lupton.
13. Crenner, "Race and Laboratory Norms."
14. Peabody and Wentworth, "Clinical Studies of the Respiration. IV," 448.
15. Ibid., 449.
16. Francis W. Peabody and Cyrus C. Sturgis, "Clinical Studies of the Respiration. VII. The Effect of General Weakness and Fatigue on the Vital Capacity of the Lungs," *Archives of Internal Medicine* 28 (1921): 509.
17. Christen Lundsgaard and Donald D. Van Slyke, "Relation between Thorax Size and Lung Volume in Normal Adults," *Journal of Experimental Medicine* 27 (1918): 65–87.
18. Howard F. West, "Clinical Studies on the Respiration. VI. A Comparison of Various Standards for the Normal Vital Capacity of the Lungs," *Archives of Internal Medicine* 25 (1920): 306.
19. Ibid., 316.
20. J. A. Myers, "Studies on the Respiratory Organs in Health and Disease. IV. A Comparison of Vital Capacity Readings and X-ray Findings in Pulmonary Tuberculosis," *American Review of Tuberculosis* 5 (1922): 894.
21. Ibid., 892. Some present-day researchers offer longitudinal studies on individuals as a better substitute for prediction equations.
22. J. A. Myers, *Vital Capacity of the Lungs: A Handbook for Clinicians and Others Interested in the Examination of the Heart and Lungs Both in Health and Disease* (Baltimore: Williams & Wilkins Company, 1925). As Crenner writes in "Race and Laboratory Norms," handbooks were an outcome of normal values research in this period.
23. Myers, *Vital Capacity of the Lungs*, 90. See also Howell, *Technology in the Hospital*, for discussions of record keeping and ideas about efficiency imported from the business world (30–68).
24. M. C. R., "Georges Dreyer, C.B.E., F.R.S.," *Lancet* 2 (1934): 514–15; "Obituary Notices of Deceased Members, Georges Dreyer, 1873–1934," *Journal of Pathology and Bacteriology* 39 (1934): 707–34; S. R. Douglas, "Georges Dreyer, 1873–1934," *Obituary Notices of Fellows of the Royal Society* 1 (1935): 568–76; Margrete Dreyer, *Georges Dreyer: A Memoir by His Wife* (Oxford: Basil Blackwell, 1937).
25. M. C. R., "Georges Dreyer, C.B.E., F.R.S.," 514.
26. FD1/3756, Public Record Office (PRO), Georges Dreyer, "For Normal Vital Capacity in Man and Its Relation to the Size of the Body," confidential memo to the Medical Research Council, June 1919, 1.
27. J. A. Gillies, *A Textbook of Aviation Physiology* (Oxford: Pergamon Press, 1965).
28. W. H. Wilmer, "The Early Development of Aviation Medicine in the United States," *Military Surgery* 77 (1935): 115–34.
29. Georges Dreyer, "Biological Standards and Their Application in Medicine," *Harvey Society Lectures*, no. 13, in Collected Papers from the Department of Pathology, University of Oxford, vol. 4, 25, 191901934, Wellcome Library; *Science* 50 (1919): 434.
30. Georges Dreyer and E. W. Ainley Walker, "Iatro-Mathematics: A Plea for a More General Appreciation of the Value of Applied Mathematics and Exact

Quantitative Methods in Biological Science," in *Contributions to Medical and Biological Research* (New York: Paul B. Hoeber, 1919) 40–51.

31. Dreyer, "For Normal Vital Capacity in Man and Its Relation to the Size of the Body," 1–6; Sally Horrocks and David Smith, "Implications of the History of Medicine for the History of Diet and Body Dimensions," in *The Biological Standard of Living in Comparative Perspective*, ed. John Komlos and Joerg Baten (Stuttgart: Steiner, 1998), 497–508.

32. Correspondence between Sir Walter Fletcher, Georges Dreyer, and Hobson between June and September 1919, FD1/3756, PRO.

33. FD1/3756, PRO, Medical Research Committee, "Standards of Physique and Physical Fitness," Department of Pathology, University of Oxford, December 1919, 1–2.

34. FD1/3756, PRO, F. C. Hobson to Sir Walter Fletcher, September 10, 1919; Hobson to Fletcher, October 2, 1919; Hobson to Fletcher, October 10, 1919; October 28, 1919. They give no indication in correspondence why they purchased spirometers from Paris.

35. Georges Dreyer, "The Normal Vital Capacity in Man and Its Relation to the Size of the Body," *Lancet* 2 (1919): 227–34; Dreyer and L. S. T. Burrell, "The Vital Capacity Constants Applied to the Study of Pulmonary Tuberculosis," *Lancet* 2 (1920): 1212–16; Georges Dreyer and L. S. T. Burrell, "The Vital Capacity Constants Applied to the Study of Pulmonary Tuberculosis," *Lancet* 2 (1922): 374–76.

36. Georges Dreyer, *The Assessment of Physical Fitness by Correlation of Vital Capacity and Certain Measurements of the Body* (New York: Paul B. Hoeber, 1921), 1.

37. Ibid.

38. Ibid., 2.

39. Ibid., ix–x.

40. For details of the debates, see Horrocks and Smith, "Implications of the History of Medicine for the History of Diet and Body Dimensions"; David Smith and Sally Horrocks, "Defining Perfect and Not-So Perfect Bodies: The Rise and Fall of the 'Dreyer Method' for the Assessment of Physique and Fitness, 1918–1926," in *Weighty Issues: Fatness and Thinness as Social Problems*, ed. Jeffery Sobal and Donna Maurer (Hawthorne, N.Y.: Aldine de Gruyter, 1999), 75–94.

41. FD1/3763, PRO, Anthropometric Standards Committee, Karl Pearson to Walter Fletcher, October 26, 1922; Walter Fletcher to Karl Pearson, November 14, 1922.

42. Lucy D. Cripps, Major Greenwood, and Ethel M. Newbold, "A Biometric Study of the Inter-Relations of 'Vital Capacity' Statures, Stem Length and Weight in a Sample of Healthy Male Adults," *Biometrika* 14 (March 1923): 325.

43. Alfred A. Mumford and Matthew Young, "The Interrelationships of the Physical Measurements and the Vital Capacity," *Biometrika* 15 (August 1923): 124.

44. Ibid., 123.

45. "'Vital Capacity' of School Children," *Times*, July 12, 1922, 7.

46. "'Vital Capacity,' Value of Physical Training at School," *Times*, January 6, 1926, 17.

47. Charles Cameron, "The Vital Capacity in Pulmonary Tuberculosis," *Tubercle* 3 (1922): 353–62, 385–99.
48. Ibid., 397.
49. "Vital Capacity in Pulmonary Tuberculosis," *Journal of the American Medical Association* 79 (1922): 246.
50. Louis I. Dublin, "The Work of Dreyer in Relation to Life Insurance Examinations," *Journal of the American Statistical Association* 18 (June 1922): 226.
51. Eugene Lyman Fisk, "Books and Reports Reviewed: The Assessment of Physical Fitness," *American Journal of Public Health* 12 (1922): 623.
52. Dreyer's handbook was especially well known in India.
53. "Eustace Henry Cluver," *SA Medical Journal* 62 (1982): 144; Ann Cluver Weinberg, *Looking for Goodness: Exploring Eustace Cluver and His Family, 1657–1982* (Johannesburg: Sapler Press, 2008).
54. The South African Air Force became a permanent arm of the military on February 1, 1920: http://www.saairforce.co.za/the-airforce/history/saaf/south-africa-aviation-corps; accessed December 21, 2012.
55. E. H. Cluver, "Tests for Determination of Physical Fitness," *Medical Journal of South Africa* (April 1923): 228–33; H. Graeme Anderson, *The Medical and Surgical Aspects of Aviation* (London: Oxford University Press, 1919).
56. William Beinart and Saul Dubow, eds., *Segregation and Apartheid in Twentieth-Century South Africa* (London and New York: Routledge, 1995); Morag Bell, "American Philanthropy, the Carnegie Corporation and Poverty in South Africa," *Journal of Southern African Studies* 26 (2000): 481–504.
57. E. G. Malherbe, "The Carnegie Poor White Investigation: Its Origins and Sequels," Carnegie Corporation Grant Files Series 1, Poor White Study 295.7, 1973, Columbia University Rare Books and Manuscripts Library (hereafter CURBML). Malherbe, who had helped convince Carnegie to fund the project, subsequently studied the poor white problem in the American South.
58. "The Poor White Problem," *Cape Times,* October 14, 1927, Poor White Study 295.5, 1927–29, Carnegie Corporation Grant Files Series 1, CURBML.
59. E. H. Cluver, "Physical Tests Applied to the White Population of the Union," *South African Medical Journal* 9 (1935): 825–26.
60. Ibid., 826.
61. E. H. Cluver and E. Jokl, "A Survey of Physical Efficiency in South Africa," *South African Journal of Science* 37 (1941): 384–408; Ernst Jokl and E. H. Cluver, "Physical Fitness," *Journal of the American Medical Association* 116 (1941): 2383–89; E. H. Cluver, E. Jokl, E. Jooste, and T. W. de Jongh, "The Growth of Physical Efficiency," *South African Journal of Science* 38 (1942): 198–202; E. H. Cluver, "The Attainment and Economic Value of Human Physical Efficiency, *South African Journal of Science* 38 (1942): 69–80.
62. Jokl and Cluver, "Physical Fitness," 2383.
63. Cluver and Jokl, "A Survey of Physical Efficiency in South Africa," 406.
64. Jokl and Cluver, "Physical Fitness," 2385.
65. Cluver and Jokl, "A Survey of Physical Efficiency in South Africa," 400.
66. Ibid., 403.

67. Ibid., 405.

68. E. H. Cluver, E. Jokl, C. Goedvolk, and T. W. de Jongh, *Training and Efficiency: An Experiment in Physical and Economic Rehabilitation* (Johannesburg: South African Institute for Medical Research, 1941).

69. "Vital Discovery on Poor White Problem," *Johannesburg Sunday Times,* May 31, 1941.

70. Timmermans and Berg, *The Gold Standard,* 8; Geoffrey Bowker and Susan Leigh Star, *Sorting Things Out: Classification and Its Consequences* (Cambridge: MIT Press, 2000).

71. John S. Haller, "The Physician versus the Negro: Medical and Anthropological Concepts of Race in the Late Nineteenth Century," *Bulletin of the History of Medicine* 44 (1970): 154–67.

72. Howell, *Technology in the Hospital.*

73. May G. Wilson and Dayton J. Edwards, "Diagnostic Value of Determining Vital Capacity of Lungs of Children," *Journal of the American Medical Association* 78 (1922): 1108.

74. Ibid., 1110.

75. Ibid. Researchers have cited Wilson and Edwards sixteen times in influential publications on this topic, once as recently as 1989. See, for example, J. B. Pool and A. Greenough, "Ethnic Variation in Respiratory Function in Young Children," *Respiratory Medicine* 83 (1989): 123–25. Wilson and Edwards did not cite Gould, although researchers writing on lung capacity later in the century would.

76. Other commission members were Harry Pratt Judson, president of the University of Chicago, and Roger S. Green, consul general at Hankow and later resident director of the China Medical Board.

77. Between 1908 and 1915, there were three commissions appointed first by John D. Rockefeller and then the Rockefeller Foundation to examine education in China. The third commission recommended establishing two medical schools, one in Peking and the other in Shanghai, but ultimately the foundation concentrated resources on Peking. See Francis Peabody, "The Department of Medicine at the Peking Union Medical College," *Science* 56 (1922): 317–20; John Z. Bowers, "The Founding of Peking Union Medical College: Policies and Personalities," *Bulletin of the History of Medicine* 45 (1971): 305–21, 409–28.

78. Mary Brown Bullock, *An American Transplant: The Rockefeller Foundation and the Peking Union Medical College* (Berkeley: University of California Press, 1980).

79. Francis W. Peabody, "The Clinical Importance of the Vital Capacity of the Lungs," in *Addresses and Papers Dedication Ceremonies and Medical Conference* (Concord, N.H.: Rumford Press, 1922), 208–27.

80. Ibid., 219–20.

81. Bullock, *An American Transplant,* 14.

82. Hunan-Yale medical school was established in 1917 by Yale-in-China, originally known as the Yale Foreign Missionary Society, with grants from the Rockefeller Foundation.

83. John H. Foster and P. L. Hsieh, "The Vital Capacity of the Chinese: An Occupational Study," *Archives of Internal Medicine* 32 (1923): 335–42; John H. Foster, "A Study of the Vital Capacity in Chinese," *Chinese Medical Journal* 38 (1924): 285–94. Foreigners included hospital physicians, teachers

at the College of Yale-in-China, local businessmen, and sailors for the
USS *Quiros.*

84. Foster and Hsieh, "The Vital Capacity of the Chinese," 336, 342.

85. Myers, *Vital Capacity of the Lungs,* 32.

86. This claim is based on searches for each paper in the Web of Science, as
of June 2013.

87. Henry Morton Robinson, "What John D. Rockefeller Has Done for Me,"
Popular Science Monthly (July 1929): 22.

88. John Ettling, *The Germ of Laziness: Rockefeller Philanthropy and Public Health in the New South* (Cambridge: Harvard University Press, 1981),
35–38; Charles Wardell Stiles, "Early History, in Part Esoteric, of the Hookworm (Uncinariasis) Campaign in Our Southern United States," *Journal of
Parasitology* 25 (1939): 283–308.

89. As Ettling shows, this was a politically delicate campaign. Popularly
known as dirt-eating, chalk-eating, ground-itch, sore feet of coolies, and so
on, human hookworm infection is caused by two main species, *Anclyostoma*
Dubini and *Necator* Stiles (Stiles, "Early History, in Part Esoteric, of the
Hookworm [Uncinariasis] Campaign").

90. Irving Fisher, *National Vitality, Its Wastes and Conservation* (New York:
Arno Press, 1976), 623, 744. Treatment for hookworm infection in the 1920s
involved injection with the toxic chemical carbon tetrachloride.

91. W. G. Smillie and D. L. Augustine, "Hookworm Infestation: The Effect of
Varying Intensities on the Physical Condition of School Children," *American
Journal of Diseases of Children* 31 (1926): 151.

92. Charles Wardell Stiles, "Soil Pollution and Hookworm Disease in the
South—Their Results and Their Prevention," in *Transactions of the Medical
Association of the State of Alabama, April 21–24, 1908* (Montgomery, Ala.:
Medical Association of the State of Alabama, 1908), 484; Charles Wardell
Stiles, "Hookworm Disease in Relation to the Negro," *Southern Medical
Journal* 2 (1909): 1124–28. For a discussion of changing explanations for the
origins of hookworm in relation to labor, see Alan Marcus, "Physicians Open
a Can of Worms: American Nationality and Hookworm in the United States,
1893–1909," *American Studies* 30 (fall 1989): 104–21.

93. George Rosen, "Some Recollections of Wilson G. Smillie, M.D. (1886–
1971)," *American Journal of Public Health* 62 (1972): 431–34; F. L. Roberts,
"Vital Capacity of Children Infected with Hookworm," *American Journal of
Public Health* 15 (1925): 774–80.

94. John Farley, *To Cast Out Disease: A History of the International Health
Division of the Rockefeller Foundation, 1913–1951* (Oxford: Oxford University
Press, 2004), 82–83; Stiles, "Soil Pollution and Hookworm Disease in the
South."

95. F. L. Roberts, "Vital Capacity of Children Infected with Hookworm,"
American Journal of Public Health 15 (1925): 774–80.

96. Smillie and Augustine, "Hookworm Infestation," 161–62.

97. W. G. Smillie and D. L. Augustine, "Vital Capacity of the Negro Race,"
Journal of the American Medical Association 87 (1926): 2055–58. Although
not from an elite New England family, Smillie's early career trajectory and
investment in scientific medicine were similar to Peabody's. Ultimately, he
ended up in public health rather than medicine (see Rosen, "Some Recollections of Wilson G. Smillie").

98. Smillie and Augustine, "Vital Capacity of the Negro Race," 2055. See also David McBride, *From TB to AIDS: Epidemics among Urban Blacks since 1900* (Albany: State University of New York Press, 1991).

99. Smillie and Augustine, "Vital Capacity of the Negro Race," 2055.

100. Ibid.

101. Ibid., 2058.

102. Frank L. Roberts and James A. Crabtree, "Vital Capacity of the Negro Child," *Journal of the American Medical Association* 88 (1927): 1950–53. For discussion of difference in stem length between white and black children, see Smillie and Augustine, "Hookworm Infestation," 160.

103. S. L. Bhatia, "The Vital Capacity of the Lungs," *Indian Medical Gazette* 64 (1929): 520.

104. C. H. McCloy, "Vital Capacity of Chinese Students," *Archives of Internal Medicine* 40 (1927): 694.

105. Ibid., 699.

106. Andrew Morris, *Marrow of the Nation: A History of Sport and Physical Culture in Republican China* (Berkeley: University of California Press, 2004), 52.

107. Ibid., 61.

108. According to the Web of Science (accessed April 5, 2010), McCloy was not cited after 1932.

109. Timmermans and Berg, *The Gold Standard*, 9.

6. Adjudicating Disability in the Industrial Worker

1. J. A. Myers, *Vital Capacity of the Lungs: A Handbook for Clinicians and Others Interested in the Examination of the Heart and Lungs Both in Health and Disease* (Baltimore: Williams & Wilkins Company, 1925), 37.

2. L. Teleky, "The Compensation of Occupational Disease," *Journal of Industrial Hygiene and Toxicology* 23 (1941): 353–73.

3. Scheduling refers to the official designation of a disease as compensatable.

4. Arthur McIvor and Ronnie Johnston's *Miner's Lung: A History of Dust Disease in British Coal Mining* chronicles the medicalization of coal workers' pneumoconiosis in Britain, emphasizing workers' perspectives (Aldershot: Ashgate Publishing Limited, 2007).

5. Roger Williams and David Jones, *The Cruel Inheritance: Life and Death in the Coalfields of Glamorgan* (Pontypool, Gwent: Village Publishing, 1990), 16.

6. McIvor and Johnston, *Miner's Lung,* 63–90.

7. Andrew Meiklejohn, "History of Lung Diseases of Coal Mines in Great Britain: Part I, 1800–1875," *British Journal of Industrial Medicine* 8 (1951): 127–36; "Part II, 1875–1920," *British Journal of Industrial Medicine* 9 (1952): 93–98; "Part III, 1920–1950," *British Journal of Industrial Medicine* 9 (1952): 208–20; A. G. Heppleston, "Coal Workers' Pneumoconiosis: A Historical Perspective on Its Pathogenesis," *American Journal of Industrial Medicine* 22 (1992): 905–23.

8. See Charles Rosenberg, "The Tyranny of Diagnosis: Specific Entities and Individual Experience," *Milbank Quarterly* 80 (2002): 237–60, for a history of disease as specific entities.

9. McIvor and Johnston, *Miner's Lung,* 66.

10. Meiklejohn, "History of Lung Diseases of Coal Mines in Great Britain: Part II"; Heppleston, "Coal Workers' Pneumoconiosis."

11. Mark Bufton and Joseph Melling, "'A Mere Matter of Rock': Organized Labour, Scientific Evidence and British Government Schemes for Compensation of Silicosis and Pneumoconiosis among Coalminers, 1926–1940," *Medical History* 49 (2005): 155–78.

12. Paul Weidling, ed., *The Social History of Occupational Health* (London: Croom Held, 1985); David Rosner and Gerald Markowitz, *Deadly Dust: Silicosis and the Politics of Occupational Disease in Twentieth-Century America* (Princeton, N.J.: Princeton University Press, 1991).

13. For examples of the South Wales Miners' Federation (known as the Fed) positions, see South Wales Miners' Federation (Anthracite District), *The Prevention of Silicosis and Anthracosis*, n.d. (circa the 1930s), South Wales Miners' Library; "Workmen's Compensation," *Colliery Workers' Magazine* 2 (August 1924): 197, South Wales Miners' Library. See also C. L. Sutherland, "Legislation and Pneumoconiosis," *Postgraduate Medical Journal* 25 (1949): 651; Norman Tattersall, "The Occurrence of Clinical Manifestations of Silicosis among Hard Ground Workers in Coal Mines," *Journal of Industrial Hygiene and Toxicology* 8 (1926): 466–80.

14. Sutherland, "Legislation and Pneumoconiosis."

15. McIvor and Johnston, *Miner's Lung*, 83.

16. Joseph Melling, "Beyond a Shadow of a Doubt? Experts, Lay Knowledge, and the Role of Radiography in the Diagnosis of Silicosis in Britain, c. 1919–1945," *Bulletin of the History of Medicine* 84 (2010): 424–66.

17. South Wales Miners' Federation, *The Prevention of Silicosis and Anthracosis*, 1.

18. E. M. Tansey, "Philip Montagu D'Arcy Hart (1900–2006)," *JLL Bulletin: Commentaries on the History of Treatment Evaluation* (www .jameslindlibrary.org). D'Arcy Hart was secretary of the Committee for the Study of Social Medicine. See also Edgar L. Collis and J. C. Gilchrist, "Effects of Dust upon Coal Trimmers," *Journal of Industrial Hygiene* 10 (1928): 101–10; Sutherland, "Legislation and Pneumoconiosis," 653; Philip D'Arcy Hart, "Chronic Pulmonary Disease in South Wales Coal Mines: An Eye-Witness Account of the MRC Surveys," *Social History of Medicine* 11 (1998): 459–68. While D'Arcy Hart refers to the "cooperation" of the unions, he ignores the unions' considerable agitation that led to the appointment of the committee. See McIvor and Johnston, *Miners' Lung,* and Bufton and Melling, "'A Mere Matter of Rock,'" for more on the MRC investigation. For an overview of the MRC in relation to industrial medicine, see A. Landsborough Thomson, *Half a Century of Medical Research*, vol. 1, *Origins and Policy of the Medical Research Council (UK)* (London: His Majesty's Stationery Office, 1974), 167–89; Helen Jones, "Industrial Health under the MRC," in *Historical Perspectives on the Role of the MRC*, ed. Joan Austoker and Linda Bryder (Oxford: Oxford University Press, 1989), 137–62.

19. Andy Ness, Lois Reynolds, and Tilli Tansey, *Population-Based Research in South Wales: The MRC Pneumoconiosis Research Unit and the MRC Epidemiology Unit*, vol. 13 of *Wellcome Witnesses to Twentieth-Century Medicine* (London: Wellcome Trust, 2002), 6; P. D'Arcy Hart and E. A. Aslett, *Chronic Pulmonary Disease in South Wales Coalminers*, vol. 1, *Medical Studies*

(London: His Majesty's Stationery Office, 1942). Coal trimmers who worked in the holds of ships were exposed to high levels of coal dust but not rock dust. Lung volumes and vital capacity were assessed on a subset of men with radiological disease. While both were reduced, "the wide scatter of the individual values around the means prevents lung volumes of being much use"; vital capacity was reduced (D'Arcy Hart and Aslett, *Chronic Pulmonary Disease in South Wales Coalminers*, vol. 1, *Medical Studies*, 111–21, 125).

20. Ness, Reynolds, and Tansey, *Population-Based Research in South Wales*, 12.

21. D'Arcy Hart and Aslett, *Chronic Pulmonary Disease in South Wales Coalminers*, vol. 1, *Medical Studies;* Ness, Reynolds, and Tansey, *Population-Based Research in South Wales;* Collis and Gilchrist, "Effects of Dust upon Coal Trimmers"; S. L. Cummins, "The Pneumoconioses in South Wales," *Journal of Hygiene* 36 (1936): 547–58.

22. Ness, Reynolds, and Tansey, *Population-Based Research in South Wales*, 7.

23. The debate over coal dust's contribution to bronchitis and emphysema in miners continued until 1992, when these two conditions were compensated. By this time, however, the industry was nearing its demise.

24. D'Arcy Hart and Aslett claimed that the rank of coal explained higher rates of disease in anthracite mines than in bituminous mines. Later work showed that anthracite mines were dustier because of poorer ventilation, power drills, and coal-cutting machinery (Ness, Reynolds, and Tansey, *Population-Based Research in South Wales*, 16). The belief persisted that tuberculosis contributed to complicated pneumoconiosis. See Heppleston, "Coal Workers' Pneumoconiosis."

25. P. Hugh-Jones and C. M. Fletcher, *Social Consequences of Pneumoconiosis among Coal Miners in South Wales*, Medical Research Council Memorandum, no. 25 (London: His Majesty's Stationery Office, 1951); Annual Report of the South Wales Area Council NUM, 1948–1949, 83, South Wales Miners' Library, hereafter SWML; John Gilson, Notes for an Address, "The Growth of Knowledge of Coal-Workers' Pneumoconiosis Related to Schemes for Its Compensation in Britain," 1955, 11, GC/237/C.1/3 Box 4, Archives and Manuscripts, Wellcome Library.

26. "Pneumoconiosis Conference," *Miner* 3 (February/March 1947): 5. The *Miner* was the official publication of the South Wales miners, SWML.

27. Ness, Reynolds, and Tansey, *Population-Based Research in South Wales*, 9.

28. "Conversation with Charles Fletcher," *British Journal of Addiction* 87 (1992): 529; Philip Hugh-Jones, "Obituary, Charles Fletcher," *British Medical Journal* 312 (1996): 117.

29. For more on the establishment of the unit, see Medicus [pseud.], "Organisation of Pneumokoniosis Research in South Wales Area under the Medical Research Council," *Miner* 3 (1947): 8–10; and Annual Reports of the South Wales Area Council NUM from 1947, SWML.

30. Fletcher's department consisted of nine physicians, four nonmedical scientists, eight technicians, and thirteen clerical workers ("Pneumoconiosis Conference," 2–6); "Charles Fletcher, Letter to Sir Christopher Booth," n.d. (circa November 17, 1986), Archives and Manuscripts, GC/D/4/2, Wellcome Library; "Oral Evidence of Charles Fletcher to the IIAC," June 6, 1951, PRO PIN 20/103.

31. Archibald L. Cochrane, *One Man's Medicine: An Autobiography of Pro-*

fessor Archie Cochrane, with Max Blythe (London: British Medical Journal, 1989), 129.

32. "Charles Fletcher, Letter to Sir Christopher Booth."

33. Cochrane, *One Man's Medicine*, 122. The Cochrane Collaboration, an international center that compiles systematic reviews, is named after Archie Cochrane.

34. Other important researchers in the early years included Owen Wade, who worked with the unit from 1948 to 1951. Wade collaborated with Gilson and Hugh-Jones on factors influencing lung function. See Owen L. Wade, *When I Dropped the Knife: The Joys, Excitements, Frustrations and Conflicts of a Life in Academic Medicine* (Edinburgh: Pentland Press, 1996), 50–56; and Ness, Reynolds, and Tansey, *Population-Based Research in South Wales*. Peter Oldham developed statistical techniques to analyze the epidemiologic and laboratory-based research data at the PRU.

35. Charles Fletcher, "Pneumoconiosis of Coal-Miners," *British Medical Journal* 1 (1948): 1016. By contrast, a chest physician writing about silicosis in the April 1958 edition of the *Bulletin of the National Association for the Prevention of Tuberculosis*, argued that "no one can be blamed for the situation" (34, in PRO MH 96/1972).

36. Alice Stewart, Idris Davies, Lynette Dowsett, F. H. Morrell, and J. W. Pierce, "Pneumoconiosis of Coal-Miners. A Study of the Disease after Exposure to Dust Has Ceased," *British Journal of Industrial Medicine* 5 (1948): 120–40.

37. "Charles Fletcher, Letter to Sir Christopher Booth."

38. At the Wellcome Witness Seminar, participants debated whether Alice Stewart even worked at the PRU. Her publication clearly identifies her affiliation with the PRU. For more on social medicine, see John Pemberton, "Social Medicine Comes on the Scene in the United Kingdom, 1936–1960," *Journal of Public Health Medicine* 20 (1998): 149–53; and Dorothy Porter, "Social Medicine and the New Society: Medicine and Scientific Humanism in Mid-Twentieth-Century Britain," *Journal of Historical Sociology* 9 (1996): 168–87. For a recent discussion of Alice Stewart, see Gayle Greene, "Richard Doll and Alice Stewart: Reputation and the Shaping of Scientific 'Truth,'" *Perspectives in Biology and Medicine* 54 (2011): 504–31.

39. Local institutions—such as the Welsh National Memorial Association for the Prevention, Treatment, and Abolition of Tuberculosis in Wales and Monmouthshire and Cardiff Medical School—had considerable expertise in industrial disease, but relations between the PRU and local experts were strained. See Ness, Reynolds, and Tansey, *Population-Based Research in South Wales*, 35; D. A. Powell and T. W. Davies, Report and Memorandum on Industrial Pulmonary Fibrosis (with special reference to silicosis in Wales), April 1940, RC 773 POW, SWML.

40. Michael Bloor, "The South Wales Miners Federation, Miners' Lung and the Instrumental Use of Expertise, 1900–1950," *Social Studies of Science* 30 (2000): 125–40.

41. Letter to the editor, "Dust Suppression and Ventilation," *Miner* 1 (December 1944): 13.

42. Medicus [pseud.], "Organisation of Pneumokoniosis Research in South Wales," 9.

43. Annual Reports of the NUM, SWML.
44. National Union of Mineworkers South Wales Area Council, *Agenda, Annual Report, and Balance Sheet for 1947–1948*, 44, SWML; Hywel Francis and David Smith, *The Fed: A History of the South Wales Miners in the Twentieth Century* (London: Lawrence and Wishart, 1980), 433; Bufton and Melling, "'A Mere Matter of Rock'"; Bloor, "The South Wales Miners Federation."
45. Charles Fletcher, interview by Max Blythe, *Interview 2* (Oxford, UK: Oxford Brooks University, 1984), video recording, Wellcome Library.
46. Ina Zweiniger-Bargielowska, *Austerity in Britain: Rationing, Controls, and Consumption 1939–1955* (Oxford: Oxford University Press, 2000).
47. The Ministry of Insurance administered the NIAA, now financed by workers, employers, and the state.
48. C. Fletcher to A. Massey, December 3, 1948, PRO PIN 20/82 1948–1960.
49. See McIvor and Johnston, *Miner's Lung*, for a discussion of the scant evidence for approved conditions.
50. C. M. Fletcher, K. J. Mann, I. Davies, A. L. Cochrane, J. C. Gilson, and P. Hugh-Jones, "The Classification of Radiographic Appearances in Coalminers' Pneumoconiosis," *Journal of the Faculty of Radiology* 1 (1949): 40–60.
51. National Union of Mineworkers, South Wales Area Council, Agenda, Annual Report and Balance Sheet for 1946–1947, 72, SWML.
52. Fletcher, "Pneumoconiosis of Coal-Miners," 1017.
53. For most of Fletcher's tenure as director, the unit was embattled with medical experts from the Pneumoconiosis Medical Panels that replaced the Silicosis Medical Panels.
54. See Gerald Markowitz and David Rosner, "The Illusion of Medical Uncertainty: Silicosis and the Politics of Industrial Disability, 1930–1960," *Milbank Quarterly* 67 (1989): 228–53.
55. C. M. Fletcher, "The Clinical Diagnosis of Pulmonary Emphysema—An Experimental Study," *Proceedings of the Royal Society of Medicine* 45 (1952): 577, 578.
56. J. C. Gilson and P. D. Oldam, "Lung Function Tests in the Diagnosis of Pulmonary Emphysema: The Use of Discriminant Analysis," *Proceedings of the Royal Society of Medicine* 45 (1952): 30–32.
57. "Instructions for the Use of the Questionnaire on Respiratory Symptoms," 1960, ALC/3/2/1, Archie Cochrane Archive, University Hospital. I thank Rosemary Soper for sending me this questionnaire.
58. See written evidence from Charles Fletcher to the Industrial Injuries Advisory Council about the problem of a pathological diagnosis, March 31, 1951, PRO PIN 20/103. Gilson and Hugh-Jones were more concerned with malingering than Fletcher.
59. Christopher Sellers, *Hazards of the Job: From Industrial Disease to Environmental Health Science* (Chapel Hill: University of North Carolina Press, 1997); Christopher Sellers and Joseph Melling, *Dangerous Trade: Industrial Hazards across a Globalizing World* (Philadelphia: Temple University Press, 2011).
60. Wade, *When I Dropped the Knife*, 54.
61. J. E. Cotes, "The Medical Research Council Pneumoconiosis Research Unit, 1945–1985: A Short History and Tribute," *Occupational Medicine* 50

(2000): 440–49; M. McDermott and T. J. McDermott, "Digital Incremental Techniques Applied to Spirometry," *Proceedings of the Royal Society of Medicine* 70 (1977): 169–71.

62. J. C. Gilson to E. A. Shearing, November 16, 1948, PRO PIN 20/82, 1948–1960; emphasis added.

63. National Union of Mineworkers South Wales Area Council, Agenda, Annual Report, and Balance Sheet for 1947–1948, 53, SWML.

64. MBC refers to the volume of air inhaled when breathing quickly and deeply for fifteen seconds (panting).

65. J. C. Gilson and P. Hugh-Jones, "The Measurement of the Total Lung Volume and Breathing Capacity," *Clinical Science* 7 (1949): 185–216. They classified X-ray abnormalities as (1) normal; (2) dust mottling but not of "certifiable degree"; (3) dust mottling "certified" by the Silicosis Board; and (4) advanced pneumoconiosis with massive shadows and emphysema.

66. J. C. Gilson and P. Hugh-Jones, *Lung Function in Coalworkers' Pneumoconiosis*, no. 290 in the Special Report Series of the Medical Research Council (London: Her Majesty's Stationery Office, 1955), 40; Basel Wright, "This Week's Citation Classic," *CC* 11 (March 16, 1981): 1; Wade, *When I Dropped the Knife*, 52; P. Hugh-Jones and A. V. Lambert, "A Simple Standard Exercise Test and Its Use for Measuring Exertion Dyspnoea," *British Medical Journal* 1 (1951): 65–71; B. M. Wright and C. B. McKerrow, "Maximum Forced Expiratory Flow Rate as a Measure of Ventilatory Capacity—with a Description of a New Portable Instrument for Measuring It," *British Medical Journal* 2 (1959): 1041–47; C. B. McKerrow, "A Simple Apparatus for Measuring the Maximum Breathing Capacity," *Journal of Physiology* 122 (1953): 3–4.

67. Gilson and Hugh-Jones, *Lung Function in Coalworkers' Pneumoconiosis*, 149.

68. C. L. Sutherland, "A Criticism of Dr. Fletcher's Written Evidence," October 4, 1951, and "Charles Fletcher's Oral Evidence," June 6, 1951, 3–6; 19, PRO PIN 20/103.

69. J. P. Lyons, R. Ryder, H. Campbell, and J. Gough, "Pulmonary Disability in Coal Works' Pneumononiosis," *British Medical Journal* 1 (1972): 713–16.

70. Cochrane, *One Man's Medicine*, 148.

71. Fletcher's oral evidence to IIAC, June 6, 1951; Fletcher, quoted in Cochrane, *One Man's Medicine*, 173n6.

72. Charles Fletcher, interview by Max Blythe; Cochrane, *One Man's Medicine*, 149.

73. C. B. McKerrow, M. McDermott, and J. C. Gilson, "A Spirometer for Measuring the Forced Expiratory Volume with a Simple Calibrating Device," *Lancet* 275 (1960): 149–51; P. Hugh-Jones, "Loss of Lung Function in Pneumoconiosis," *Pneumoniosis—Modern Trends: Reports of Meetings Held in Birmingham (April 1959) and in Glasgow (January 1960)*, vol. 1 (London: Chest and Heart Association, 1961), 38–48. The alternative American method used a simple spirometer with a recording kymograph. See E. A. Gaensler, "An Instrument for Dynamic Vital Capacity Measurements," *Science* 114 (1951): 444–46.

74. See John Craw, Dewi Davies, Julian Tudor Hart, Stephen Jones, and Michael Kennedy, *Coalworkers' Pneumoconiosis, Emphysema and Bronchitis: A Report to the National Union of Mineworkers* (London: Macdermott & Chant, 1978).

75. Reference Book for John Gilson's Tour through US, September 24, 1955–October 30, 1955, GC/237/C-1/2 Box 4, Archives and Manuscripts, Wellcome Library.

76. GCH, Director of the London Office of the ILO to the Secretary of the Welsh Board of Health, February 3, 1965, PRO MH 96/1972.

77. Gilson and Hugh-Jones, *Lung Function in Coalworkers' Pneumoconiosis*, 27.

78. Myers, *Vital Capacity of the Lungs*, 32–33.

79. This analysis is based on a large "systematic review" of 226 scientific articles on racial comparisons of lung function published between 1920 and 2008, which highlights the circulation of ideas among various countries and disciplines. A total of ninety-four different groups were compared to white/Europeans in the papers we examined. See Lundy Braun, Melanie Wolfgang, and Kay Dickersin, "Defining Race/Ethnicity and Explaining Difference in Research Studies on Lung Function," *European Respiratory Journal* 41 (2013): 1362–70.

80. J. E. Cotes and M. P. Ward, "Ventilatory Capacity in Normal Bhutanese," *Journal of Physiology* 186 (1966): 88–89; R. H. T. Edwards, G. J. Miller, C. E. D. Hearn, and J. E. Cotes, "Pulmonary Function and Exercise Responses in Relation to Body Composition and Ethnic Origin in Trinidadian Males," *Proceedings of the Royal Society B: Biological Sciences* 181 (1972): 407–20; G. J. Miller, J. E. Cotes, A. M. Hall, C. B. Salvosa, and A. Ashworth, "Lung Function and Exercise Performance of Healthy Caribbean Men and Women of African Ethnic Origin," *Quarterly Journal of Experimental Physiology and Cognate Medical Sciences* 57 (1972): 325–41; J. E. Cotes, M. J. Saunders, J. E. Adam, H. R. Anderson, and A. M. Hall, "Lung Function in Coastal and Highland New Guineans—Comparison with Europeans," *Thorax* 28 (1973): 320–30; J. E. Cotes, H. R. Anderson, and J. M. Patrick, "Lung Function and the Response to Exercise in the New Guineans: Role of Genetic and Environmental Factors," *Philosophical Transactions of the Royal Society of London B: Biological Sciences* 268 (1974): 349–61; J. E. Cotes, J. M. Dabbs, A. M. Hall, S. C. Lakhera, M. J. Saunders, et al., "Lung Function of Healthy Young Men in India: Contributory Roles of Genetic and Environmental Factors," *Proceedings of the Royal Society B* 191 (1975): 413–25; R. P. M. Jones, F. M. Baber, C. Heywood, and J. E. Cotes, "Ventilatory Capacity in Healthy Chinese Children: Relation to Habitual Activity," *Annals of Human Biology* 4 (1977): 155–61.

81. Indirect maximum breathing capacity was the FEV multiplied by 40.

82. J. C. Gilson, H. Stott, B. E. C. Hopwood, S. A. Roach, C. B. McKerrow, and R. S. F. Schilling, "Byssinosis: The Acute Effect of Ventilatory Capacity of Dusts in Cotton Ginneries, Cotton, Sisal, and Jute Mills," *British Journal of Industrial Medicine* 18 (1962): 16.

83. E. G. Bowen, "The Incidence of Phthisis in Relation to Race Type and Social Environment in South and West Wales," *Journal of the Royal Anthropological Institute* 58 (1928): 363–98; W. J. Martin, "Phthisis and Physical Measurement in Wales," *Journal of Hygiene* 36 (1936): 540–46.

84. J. E. Cotes and M. S. Malhotra, "Differences in Lung Function between Indians and Europeans," *Journal of Physiology* 177 (1965): 18P.

85. Cited one hundred times in the Web of Science ("Charles Fletcher, Letter to Sir Christopher Booth"); J. E. Cotes, C. E. Rossiter, I. T. T. Higgins, and J. C. Gilson, "Average Normal Values for the Forced Expiratory Volume in White Caucasian Males," *British Medical Journal* 1 (1966): 1016–19.

86. John E. Cotes, *Lung Function: Assessment and Application in Medicine,* 1st ed. (Oxford: Blackwell Scientific Publications, 1965), 325.
87. John E. Cotes, *Lung Function: Assessment and Application in Medicine,* 2d ed. (Philadelphia: F. A. Davis Company, 1968), 356–57.
88. John E. Cotes, *Lung Function: Assessment and Application in Medicine,* 3d ed. (Oxford: Blackwell Scientific Publications, 1975), 360.
89. John E. Cotes, *Lung Function: Assessment and Application in Medicine,* 4th ed. (Oxford: Blackwell Scientific Publications, 1979), 347–49.
90. Charles E. Rossiter and Hans Weil, "Ethnic Differences in Lung Function: Evidence for Proportional Differences," *International Journal of Epidemiology* 3 (1974): 55–61. Weil drew on the interdisciplinary nature of the unit when he established his department in the United States (John Gilson to Charles Fletcher, November 23, 1986, Archives and Manuscripts, GC/D/4/2, Wellcome Library).

7. Diagnosing Silicosis

1. Francis Wilson, *Labour in the South African Gold Mines 1911–1969* (Cambridge: Cambridge University Press, 1972), 14. In 1910, the colonies of the Transvaal, the Orange River Colony, the Cape Colony, and Natal formed the Union of South Africa as a dominion of the British Empire. In 1961, the Union of South Africa withdrew from the British Commonwealth to become the Republic of South Africa.
2. Ibid., 5.
3. L. G. Irvine, A. Mavrogordato, and Hans Pirow, "A Review of the History of Silicosis on the Witwatersrand Goldfields," *Silicosis Records of the International Silicosis Conference Held at Johannesburg 13–27 August 1930* (London: International Labour Organization, 1930), 178–207.
4. "Chamber of Mines of South Africa"; accessed August 17, 2012, http://www.bullion.org.za/.
5. Irvine, Mavrogordato, and Pirow, "A Review of the History of Silicosis on the Witwatersrand Goldfields." See also Edwin Higgins, A. J. Lanza, E. B. Leny, and George S. Rice, *Siliceous Dust in Relation to Pulmonary Disease among Miners in the Joplin District, Missouri,* prepared by the Bureau of Mines, Bulletin no. 132 (Washington, D.C.: U.S. Government Printing Office, 1917), 1–98.
6. Elaine Katz, *The White Death: Silicosis on the Witwatersrand Gold Mines, 1886–1910* (Johannesburg: Witwatersrand University Press, 1994); Jaine Roberts, *The Hidden Epidemic among Former Miners* (Westville, South Africa: Health Systems Trust, 2009). See also Jock McCulloch, *South Africa's Gold Mines and the Politics of Silicosis* (Suffolk: James Currey, 2012), published after this chapter was written.
7. Irvine, Mavrogordato, and Pirow, "A Review of the History of Silicosis," 182–83; Gerard Sluis-Cremer, "Pneumoconiosis Research in South Africa with Emphasis on Developments in the Last Quarter Century," *American Journal of Industrial Medicine* 22 (1992): 591–603. The term "miners' phthisis" was used to refer to both silicosis and silicosis complicated by tuberculosis.
8. Katz, *The White Death;* Jonathan E. Myers and Ian Macun, "The Sociologic Context of Occupational Health in South Africa," *American Journal of Public Health* 79 (1989): 213–21. White trade unionists supported the color bar and opposed blacks' legal right to strike throughout the twentieth century. For

details on the history of labor activity in South Africa, see Wilson, *Labour in the South African Gold Mines,* 171–79; and "Trade Unions Fear New Native Labour Bill," *Star,* April 14, 1952, 1.

9. Wilson, *Labour in the South African Gold Mines;* David Yudelman, *The Emergence of Modern South Africa: State, Capital, and the Incorporation of Organized Labor on the South African Gold Fields, 1902–1939* (Westport, Conn.: Greenwood Press, 1983). Labor activity among black workers has not been fully explored in this period. The Industrial Conciliation Act of 1924, passed in the wake of the Rand Rebellion Conflict, partly resolved conflict between white workers and the state at the expense of black workers.

10. The central bureau changed its name in response to legislation. First called the Miners' Phthisis Medical Bureau, it became the Silicosis Medical Bureau, the Pneumoconiosis Bureau, the Miners' Medical Bureau, and the Miners' Bureau of Occupational Disease.

11. For a commissioned history of health care on the mines, see A. P. Cartwright, *Doctors on the Mines: A History of the Mine Medical Officers' Association of South Africa* (Cape Town: Purnell, 1971).

12. This fact is almost never mentioned in publications on silicosis in South Africa. See Randall Packard, *White Plague, Black Labor: Tuberculosis and the Political Economy of Health and Disease in South Africa* (Berkeley: University of California Press, 1989).

13. The reality of the color bar differed underground, where, unrecognized and uncompensated, blacks performed skilled and semiskilled work.

14. Miners' Phthisis Act (No. 44) of 1916, 842; 32.44 percent of miners were from South Africa; 52.42 percent were from the United Kingdom; 11.06 percent were from other European countries (Italy, Greece, Austria, Russia, Montenegro, the Balkans, Sweden, Norway, and France); 3.06 percent were from Australia and New Zealand; and 1.02 percent were from Canada and the United States. See *Fourth Annual Report of the Miners' Phthisis Board for the Year Ended 31st July, 1916* (Cape Town: Cape Times Government Printers, 1917).

15. Shula Marks, "The Silent Scourge? Silicosis, Respiratory Disease and Gold Mining in South Africa," *Journal of Ethnic and Migration Studies* 32 (2006): 569–89. In our 2001 investigation of the extent of asbestos-related diseases in the Northern Cape and Northwest Province, community members consistently told us that they had little access to the compensation system (The Asbestos Collaborative, *Asbestos-Related Disease in South Africa: Opportunities and Challenges Remaining since the 1998 Parliamentary Summit,* presented to the South African Parliament, October 2001).

16. Quoted in Marks, "The Silent Scourge?" 579.

17. L. G. Irvine and W. Steuart, "The Radiology and Symptomatology of Silicosis," in *Silicosis. Records of the International Conference Held at Johannesburg 13–27 August 1930* (Geneva: P. S. King & Son for the International Labour Office, 1930), 288–89. See also Martin Cherniack, *The Hawk's Nest Incident: America's Worst Industrial Disaster* (New Haven: Yale University Press, 1989); David Rosner and Gerald Markowitz, *Deadly Dust: Silicosis and the Politics of Occupational Disease in Twentieth-Century America* (Princeton, N.J.: Princeton University Press, 1991).

18. *General Report of the Miners' Phthisis Prevention Committee* (Pretoria: Government Printing and Stationery Office, 1916), 14; A. W. S. Verster, "Some

Aspects of the Silicosis Problem in South Africa," *South African Medical Journal* 28 (1954): 843.

19. B. T. Tindall to Manager and Secretary of the Chamber of Mines, February 27, 1953, WLNA File 14, Pad 2: 1/1/51-28.2.53, TEBA archives, University of Johannesburg. In the legal settlement in South Africa between asbestos miners and Gencor, obtaining work records remains a serious problem; see Deed of Trust, creating the Asbestos Relief Trust, March 12, 2003.

20. *General Report of the Miners' Phthisis Prevention Committee, 9–14.*

21. Packard, *White Plague, Black Labor;* Randall Packard, "The Invention of the 'Tropical Worker': Medical Research and the Quest for Central African Labor on the South African Gold Mines, 1903–36," *Journal of African History* 34 (1993): 271–92.

22. L. G. Irvine, "The Present Position of Miners' Phthisis on the Rand," address delivered to the Association of Mine Managers, July 20, 1928, the National Library, Cape Town, South Africa.

23. Verster, "Some Aspects of the Silicosis Problem in South Africa," 842.

24. See Marais Malan, *The Quest for Health: The South African Institute for Medical Research, 1912–1973* (Johannesburg: Lowry Publishers, 1988), 354–72.

25. *Report upon the Work of the Miners' Phthisis Medical Bureau for the Twelve Months Ending July 31st, 1923* (Cape Times Limited, Government Printer, 1924), 2.

26. Harry W. Haynes, *Phthisis Commission Report: The Case for Miners' Phthisis Sufferers and Their Dependents* (Johannesburg, 1930), 7.

27. Pulmonary disability is not an exact English translation of *borkswaal*. *Borkswaal* refers to disease of the chest, not respiratory organs. This difference added confusion to the attempts to define pulmonary disability.

28. "Gold Mining Seen as Flywheel of S.A. Economy," *Star*, January 4, 1952, 3; "Remarkable Development of Welkom in Five Years," *Star*, January 8, 1952, 2.

29. "Meeting with Hon. Minister of Native Affairs, Dr. H. F. Verwoerd, 13th February 1953," 11, WLNA File 14, Pad 2: 1/1/51-28.2.53, TEBA archives, University of Johannesburg Library (hereafter referred to as TEBA archives).

30. "Report of a Meeting of the Sub-committee Held in Chamber of Mines Building, Feb 11, 1953," WLNA File 14, Pad 2: 1/1/51-28.2.53, TEBA archives.

31. Jock McCulloch, "Hiding a Pandemic: Dr. G. W. H. Schepers and the Politics of Silicosis in South Africa," *Journal of Southern African Studies* 35 (2009): 841.

32. *Report of the Commission of Enquiry regarding the Occurrence of Certain Diseases, Other Than Silicosis and Tuberculosis, Attributable to the Nature of Employment in and about Mines*, U.G. 22/1951 (Pretoria: Government Printer, 1951), 1; emphasis in the original (hereafter referred to as the *Allan Commission Report*).

33. McCulloch, "Hiding a Pandemic," 837.

34. Testimony from SAIMR physicians (one of whom was Director Cluver), the Gold Mines Employees' Provident Fund, physicians for the Mine Benefit Society, a chemist, the government mining engineer, chairman of the Silicosis Medical Bureau (SMB), and other experts from the Chamber of Mines provided "the evidence" for the final recommendations.

35. *Allan Commission Report*, 9.

36. Ibid., 13.

37. Silicosis Amendment Act (No. 63) of 1952, 949.

38. *Allan Commission Report*, 14.

39. "New Silicosis Bill Raises Benefits," *Star*, February 5, 1952, 3.

40. *Extraordinary Government Gazette*, February 11, 1953, 1.

41. The commission also considered the status of the doctors in the separate units, one containing general practitioners and the other specialists, a source of antagonism.

42. "Government Meets Miners' Demands," *Star*, January 30, 1954, 1.

43. "Commission Asks Miner to Walk Up and Down," *Star*, January 29, 1952, 2.

44. McCulloch, "Hiding a Pandemic."

45. *Report of the Commission of Enquiry into the Functioning of the Silicosis Medical Bureau and the Silicosis Medical Board of Appeal* (Pretoria: Government Printer, 1952), 7 (hereafter referred to as the *Beyers Commission Report*).

46. Ibid., 9, 14. The commission also called for more frequent exams, improved radiography, and submission of the reasons for rejections. See Extracts of Minutes of Gold Producer's Committee, Sub-committee of Group Medical Officers, November 4, 1952, 8, WLNA File 14, Pad 2: 1/1/51-28.2.53, TEBA archives.

47. "Transvaal Chamber of Mines, Memorandum, 26 Nov 1952 to the Manager and Secretary from the Legal Advisor John Schilling," WLNA File 14, Pad 2: 1/1/51-28.2.53, 12, TEBA archives. The stages of pulmonary disability included "reduction in capacity for exertion"—that is, the destruction of the pulmonary reserve.

48. *Beyers Commission Report*, 8.

49. *Extraordinary Government Gazette*, February 11, 1953, 1. In 1953, the PDC's physician members included Comyn Duther, G. R. McLeish, G. K. Sluis-Cremer, L. M. Wessels, and G. W. H. Schepers (chair). *Report upon the Work of the Silicosis Medical Bureau for the Two Years April 1951–March 1953* (Pretoria: Government Printer, 1953). The PDC had difficulty assembling resources, space, and equipment for its examinations. Any benefits of the new legislation to blacks would be an incidental by-product of anxieties over white labor.

50. "Doctor Alleges That No Staff Conferences Were Held," Star, January 29, 1952, 3; "Silicosis Inquiry Evidence," Star, February 1, 1952, 3; McCulloch, "Hiding a Pandemic," 847.

51. "Meeting of the Gold Producer Committee of the Chamber of Mines with the Secretary for Mines," Mr. V. H. Osborn, February 11, 1953, 4. WLNA File 14, Pad 2: 1/1/51-28.2.53, TEBA archives.

52. *Report of the Departmental Committee of Enquiry into the Relationship between Silicosis and Pulmonary Disability and the Relationship between Pneumoconiosis and Tuberculosis* (Pretoria: Government Printer, 1955), hereafter referred to as the *Oosthuizen Commission Report*. The committee members visited the United States, Canada, the United Kingdom, Sweden, Holland, Belgium, France, Germany, Switzerland, Austria, Italy, and Spain.

53. *Oosthuizen Commission Report*, 8.

54. Ibid., 12.

55. Ibid., 18.
56. Ibid., 34.
57. Ibid., 39.
58. Pneumoconiosis Act (No. 57) of 1956, 1411.
59. Margaret Becklake, "Occupational Lung Disease—Past Record and Future Trend Using the Asbestos Case as an Example," *Clinical and Investigative Medicine* 6 (1983): 305. Becklake became a renowned expert on lung function and asbestos-related diseases.
60. Ibid., 305. *Report of the Pneumoconiosis Bureau for the Period 1 August 1956 to 31 March 1958* (Pretoria: Government Printer, 1959–60), 9.
61. "Transvaal Chamber of Mines, Memorandum, 26 Nov 1952 to the Manager and Secretary from the Legal Advisor John Schilling."
62. *Director's Interim Report*, South African Council for Scientific and Industrial Research, Pneumoconiosis Research Unit, October 1956, 2.
63. "Extracts from Dr. B. Van Lingen's Memorandum," August 20, 1956, PRU.
64. *Progress Report of Work Carried Out in the Pulmonary Function Laboratory, Pneumoconiosis Bureau*, submitted to the director, Pneumoniosis Research Unit, n.d. (circa 1956).
65. Anonymous interview, Montreal, August 2011.
66. J. C. Theron, S. Zwi, and Maurice McGregor, "A Respiratory Valve of Low Resistance," *Lancet* 1 (1958): 415; anonymous interview, Montreal, August 2011.
67. Margaret R. Becklake and H.I. Goldman, "The Influence of Pulmonary Dead Space on Lung Mixing Indices," *South African Journal of Medical Science* 19 (1954): 21–27; Saul Zwi and Margaret R. Becklake, "Respiratory Function of Witwatersrand Gold-Miners," *British Journal of Industrial Medicine* 15 (1958): 258–61; H.I. Goldman and Margaret R. Becklake, "Respiratory Function Tests: Normal Values at Median, and the Prediction of Normal Results," *American Review of Tuberculosis and Pulmonary Disease* 79 (1959): 457–67.
68. Pierre Ernst, "A Conversation with Margaret Becklake," *Epidemiology* 15 (2004): 245–49; anonymous interview, Montreal, 2011.
69. Anonymous interview, Montreal, 2011.
70. Zwi and Becklake, "Respiratory Function of Witwatersrand Gold-Miners."
71. B. van Lingen, *Report of the Physiology Division for the Year 1957–1958*, PRU, 2.
72. The problem of staff is a recurrent issue in PRU reports during the 1950s and 1960s.
73. "Pneumoconiosis Body Replies to Its Critics," *Star*, April 27, 1961.
74. *Seventh Annual Report, 1962–63*, 6. This shift to physiology most likely was politically motivated. Christopher Wagner, who first identified mesothelioma in the Northern Cape, was a pathologist.
75. Ibid., 8.
76. Pneumoconiosis Compensation Act (No. 64) of 1962, 1067–69.
77. *Report of the Pneumoconiosis Bureau for the Period 1st April 1962 to 30th September 1962 and of the Miners' Medical Bureau for the Period 1st October 1962 to 31st March 1963*, 15.
78. *Seventh Annual Report, 1962–63*, 29.

79. B. van Lingen, *Report of the Physiology Division for the Year 1958–1959*, PRU, 5.

80. Between 1951 and 1959, Becklake published sixteen papers from her work in South Africa. In 1985–86, she returned to South Africa, writing two careful analyses of the sources of lung function variation, including socio-economic factors.

81. Sluis-Cremer trained numerous scientists in the epidemiology of lung function, including Patrick Hessel, who migrated to Canada, and Eva Hzido, who migrated to the United States to work at NIOSH.

82. Eric Bateman, *The Respiratory Clinic at Groote Schuur Hospital, 1965–1990: The First 25 Years* (Cape Town: University of Cape Town and Groote Schuur Hospital, 1990).

83. Anonymous interview, Cape Town, 2009; "South African Medical Research Council: Four New Medical Research Units," *South African Medical Journal* 2 (February 1974): 194; Andries Brink, "M.A. de Kock," *South African Medical Journal* 97 (2007): 1052–53.

84. Deborah Posel, "What's in a Name? Racial Categorisations under Apartheid and Their Afterlife," *Transformations* 47 (2001): 50–74. I thank Eugene Caincross for bringing this article to my attention.

85. Zofia M. Johannsen and Leslie D. Erasmus, "Clinical Spirometry in Normal Bantu," *American Review of Respiratory Disease* 97 (1968): 585. For a comprehensive review of the scientific literature on race and lung capacity, see L. Braun, M. Wolfgang, and K. Dickersin, "Defining Race/Ethnicity and Explaining Difference in Research Studies on Lung Function," *European Respiratory Journal* 41 (2013): 1362–70.

86. Web of Science, accessed March 1, 2013.

87. B.W. van de Wal, L.D. Erasmus, and R. Hechter, "Stem and Standing Heights in Bantu and White South Africans: Their Significance in Relation to Pulmonary Function Values," *South African Medical Journal* 45 (1971): 568–70, 568.

88. G.K. Sluis-Cremer, "Factors That Influence Simple Lung Function Tests with Special Reference to Ethnic Factors," *Proceedings of the Mine Medical Officers' Association of South Africa* 54 (1974): 15–20.

89. S.R. Benatar, "Pulmonary Function in Normal Children Aged 11–15 Years," *South African Medical Journal* 53 (1978): 543–46, 546.

90. J.B. Schoenberg, G.J. Beck, and J. Bouhuys, "Growth and Decay of Pulmonary Function in Healthy Blacks and Whites," *Respiratory Physiology* 33 (1978): 367–95.

91. Anonymous interviews, Cape Town, 2001, 2006.

92. A.J. Brink, "Opening Address," *Mechanisms of Airways Obstruction in Human Respiratory Disease*, Proceedings of the International Symposium, 1978, ed. M.A. de Kock, J.A. Nadel, and C.M. Lewis (Cape Town and Rotterdam: A.A. Balkema for the South African Medical Research Council, 1979), 2–3.

93. Myers would later direct the Occupational and Environmental Health Unit at the University of Cape Town's School of Public Health and Family Medicine.

94. The revitalization of black trade unionism occurred after a wave of strike activity in the 1970s. See Myers and Macun, "The Sociologic Context of Occupational Health in South Africa"; anonymous interview, Cape Town, 2009.

95. *Health of Workers in South Africa: Project on Poverty, Health and the State in Southern Africa,* proceedings of the Second Workshop, ed. Pippa Green (New York: Columbia University, January 1987), 84.
96. J.E. Myers, "Differential Ethnic Standards for Lung Functions, or One Standard for All?" *South African Medical Journal* 65 (1984): 768–72. Myers stresses that this is not an example of the healthy worker effect. Norms were generated from studies of selective populations of nonsmokers screened against respiratory disease, so the international norms should have been higher than those of the dockworkers exposed to asbestos.
97. S.W., anonymous interview, Cape Town, 2001.
98. Neil White, "An Investigation of Byssinosis among South African Textile Workers," MD thesis, University of Cape Town, 1985, 3.
99. J.C.A. Davies and Margaret R. Becklake, "Reference Values for Lung Function—More to Be Done," *South African Medical Journal* 66 (1984): 830.
100. S.C. Morrison and S.R. Benatar, "Differential Ethnic Standards for Lung Function," *South African Medical Journal* 66 (1984), 833.
101. Jonny Myers, "Differential Ethnic Standards for Lung Functions: Reply," *South African Medical Journal* 66 (1984): 833.
102. E.M., anonymous interview, Cape Town, 2006.
103. M.A. de Kock, W.R.S. Swiegers, T.J. van W. Kotze, and G. Joubert, "Cross-Sectional Study of Uranium Mine Workers to Develop Predictive Equations for Lung Functions with Reference to Chronic Obstructive Pulmonary Disease," *South African Medical Journal* (March 19, 1988): supplement, 1–20.
104. J. Myers, "Evaluation of Lung Function in Uranium Mine Workers," *South African Medical Journal* 75 (1989): 195.
105. Anonymous interview, Cape Town, 2006. Stellenbosch University was historically a flagship school of the Afrikaner elite. In the recent settlement with Gencor, some sites disabled race correction.
106. J.G. Goldin, S.J. Louw, and G. Joubert, "Spirometry of Healthy Adult South African Men. Part II. Interrelationship between Socio-Environmental Factors and 'Race' as Determinants of Spirometry," *South African Medical Journal* 86 (1996): 820–26; S.J. Louw, J.G. Goldin, and G. Joubert, "Spirometry of Healthy Adult South African Men. Part I. Normative Values," *South African Medical Journal* 86 (1996): 814–19.
107. Neil White, "'Ethnic Discounting' and Spirometry," *Respiratory Medicine* 89 (1995): 312–13. For empirical findings on secular trends, see Neil White, James Hanley, Umesh Lalloo, and Margaret Becklake, "Review and Analysis of Variation between Spirometric Values Reported in 29 Studies of Healthy African Adults," *American Journal of Respiratory and Critical Care Medicine* 150 (1994): 348–55. For secular trends in black African populations, see Khathatso Mokoetle, Magda de Beer, and Margaret Becklake, "A Respiratory Survey in a Black Johannesburg Workforce," *Thorax* 49 (1994): 340–46.
108. Rodney Ehrlich, Neil White, Jonny Myers, Mary-Lou Thompson, Gavin Churchyard, David Barnes, and D.B. Devilliers, "Development of Lung Function Reference Tables Suitable for Use in the South African Mining Industry," Draft Final Report, Safety in Mines Research Advisory Committee, SIMHEALTH 610A, May 7, 2000, 2.

Epilogue

1. Anonymous interviews: family medicine physician, Providence, Rhode Island; pulmonologist, South Africa, 2001; internal medicine resident, New York City, 2012; pulmonologist, London, 2009.

2. In his examination of clinical pathology, Christopher Crenner argues that the study of racial difference in normal values was not a major focus of study in the 1930s ("Race and Laboratory Norms," *Isis*, 2014).

3. S. Abramowitz, G.C. Leiner, W.A. Lewis, and M.J. Small, "Vital Capacity in the Negro," *American Review of Respiratory Disease* 92 (1964): 287–92. This paper has been cited forty-six times, including four times in the 1990s and twice in the 2000s.

4. See Lundy Braun, Melanie Wolfgang, and Kay Dickersin, "Defining Race/Ethnicity and Explaining Difference in Research Studies on Lung Function," *European Respiratory Journal* 41 (2013): 1362–70, for details on explanations for difference over time. The most influential papers were assessed using citation patterns from the Web of Science.

5. A. Damon, "Negro–White Differences in Pulmonary Function (Vital Capacity, Timed Vital Capacity, and Expiratory Flow Rate)," *Human Biology* 38 (1966): 381–93.

6. U.S. studies accounted for nearly half of the literature on racial comparisons —but more than three-fourths of the research that employed conventionally rigorous study designs. See Braun, Wolfgang, and Dickersin, "Defining Race/Ethnicity and Explaining Difference."

7. This claim is based on data on explanations collected from each of the 226 scientific papers and citation tracing.

8. See, for example, Jenny Reardon, *Race to the Finish: Identity and Governance in an Age of Genomics* (Princeton, N.J.: Princeton University Press, 2005); Snait B. Gissis, "When Is 'Race' a Race? 1946–2003," *Studies in the History and Philosophy of Biology and Biomedical Sciences* 39 (2008): 437–50.

9. Keith Wailoo, *How Cancer Crossed the Color Line* (Oxford: Oxford University Press, 2011), 49–60; Samuel K. Roberts, *Infectious Fear: Politics, Disease, and the Health Effects of Segregation* (Chapel Hill: University of North Carolina Press, 2009), 57–60.

10. Suzanne S. Hurd and Claude Lenfant, "NHLBI: Fifty Years of Achievement in Pulmonary Biology and Medicine," *American Journal of Critical Care Medicine* 157 (1998): S168–71.

11. George Leiner, Sol Abramowitz, and Maurice J. Small, "Pulmonary Function Testing: In Laboratories Associated with Residency Training Programs in Pulmonary Diseases," *American Review of Respiratory Disease* 100 (1969): 240–44.

12. Henry W. Glindmeyer III, "Predictable Confusion," *Journal of Occupational Medicine* 23 (1981): 845–49; Martha R. Becklake, "Concepts of Normality Applied to the Measurement of Lung Function," *American Journal of Medicine* 80 (1986): 1158–64.

13. Benajmin G. Ferris, "Epidemiology Standardization Project," *American Review of Respiratory Disease* 118 (1978): 1–120.

14. "ATS Statement—Snowbird Workshop on Standardization of Spirometry," *American Review of Respiratory Disease* 119 (1979): 831–38.

15. The statement did note that the "appropriateness depends on precision

in definition of race" (American College of Chest Physicians Scientific Section Recommendations, "Statement on Spirometry: A Report of the Section on Respiratory Pathophysiology," *Chest* 83 [1983]: 547–50). The conference was staffed by ATS.

16. Alan H. Morris, Richard E. Kanner, Robert O. Crapo, and Reed M. Gardner, *Clinical Pulmonary Function Testing: A Manual of Uniform Laboratory Procedures*, 2d ed. (Salt Lake City: Intermountain Thoracic Society, 1984), 97–98.

17. Glindmeyer, "Predictable Confusion," 848.

18. Geoffrey Bowker and Susan Leigh Star, *Sorting Things Out: Classification and Its Consequences* (Cambridge: MIT Press, 2000).

19. Andrew J. Ghio, Robert O. Crapo, and C. Gregory Elliott, "Reference Equations Used to Predict Pulmonary Function," *Chest* 97 (1990): 400–403.

20. P. H. Quanjer, "Standardization of Lung Function Tests," supplement, *European Respiratory Journal* S6 (1993): 27.

21. Akshay Sood, Beth K. Dawson, Joseph Q. Henkle, Patricia Hopkins-Price, and Clifford Qualls, "Effect of Change of Reference Standard to NHANES III on Interpretation of Spirometric 'Abnormality,'" *International Journal of Chronic and Obstructive Pulmonary Disease* 2 (2007): 361–67.

22. Personal communication, Lewis Weidman, Vitalograph.

23. Melissa Nobles, *Shades of Citizenship: Race and the Census in Modern Politics* (Stanford, Calif.: Stanford University Press, 2000).

24. Ann Morning, "Ethnic Classification in Global Perspective: A Cross-National Survey of the 2000 Census Board," *Population Research and Policy Review* 27 (2008): 258. See also Ann Morning, *The Nature of Race: How Scientists Think and Teach about Human Difference* (Berkeley: University of California Press, 2011).

25. Morning, "Ethnic Classification in Global Perspective," 255.

26. Pilar Ossorio and Troy Duster, "Race and Genetics: Controversies in Biomedical, Behavioral, and Forensic Sciences," *American Psychologist* 60 (2005): 115–28; Nancy Krieger, "Stormy Weather: Race, Gene Expression, and the Science of Health Disparities," *American Journal of Public Health* 95 (2005): 2155–60; Steven Epstein, *Inclusion: The Politics of Difference in Medical Research* (Chicago: University of Chicago Press, 2007); Dorothy Roberts, *Fatal Invention: How Science Politics and Big Business Re-create Race in the Twenty-First Century* (New York: New Press, 2011).

27. R. Kumar, M.A. Seibold, M.C. Aldrich, K. Williams, A.P. Riner, L. Colangelo, et al., "Genetic Ancestry in Lung-Function Predictions," *New England Journal of Medicine* 363 (2010): 321–30.

28. For a critique of AIMs, see Duana Fulwilley, "The Biologistical Construction of Race: 'Admixture' Technology and the New Genetic Medicine," *Social Studies of Science* 38 (2008): 695–735.

29. P.D. Scanlon and M.D. Shriver, "'Race Correction' in Pulmonary-Function Testing," *New England Journal of Medicine* 363 (2011): 386.

30. "Lung Function and Ethnicity," http://www.spirxpert.com/refvalueschild .htm, accessed January 17, 2013; see also "Deriving 'All Age' Reference Values for Spirometry," http://www.spirxpert.com/refvalues5.htm, accessed January 17, 2013.

31. J.M. Brehm, E. Acosta-Perez, L. Kiel, et al., "African Ancestry and Lung

Function in Puerto Rican Children," *Journal of Allergy and Clinical Immunology* 129 (2012): 1490.

32. Roberts, *Fatal Invention*, 58.

33. Fulwilley, "The Biologistical Construction of Race"; D.A. Bolchick et al., "The Science and Business of Genetic Testing," *Science* 318 (2007): 399–400; K.M. Weiss and B.W. Lambert, "Does History Matter? Do the Facts of Human Variation Package Our Views or Do Our Views Package the Facts?" *Evolutionary Anthropology* 19 (2010): 92–97; Troy Duster, *Backdoor to Eugenics*, 2d ed. (New York: Routledge, 2003), 133.

34. Joan Fujimura and Ramya Rajagopalan, "Different Differences: The Use of 'Genetic Ancestry' versus Race in Biomedical Human Genetic Research," *Social Studies of Science* 4 (2011): 5–30; Catherine Bliss, *Race Decoded: The Genomic Fight for Social Justice* (Stanford, Calif.: Stanford University Press, 2012). This, of course, raises the larger question as to what constitutes social justice.

35. Randall Packard, *The Making of a Tropical Disease: A Short History of Malaria* (Baltimore: Johns Hopkins University Press, 2007).

36. Wailoo, *How Cancer Crossed the Color Line*, 183.

37. Awori J. Hayanga, Steve B. Zeliadt, and Leah M. Backhus, "Residential Segregation and Lung Cancer Mortality in the United States," *JAMA Surgery* 148 (2013): 37–42.

38. P.A. Braveman, C. Cubbin, S. Egerter, S. Chideya, K.S. Marchi, M. Metzler, et al., "Socioeconomic Status in Health Research," *JAMA* 294 (2005): 2879–88.

39. Karl Figlio, "What Is an Accident?" in *The Social History of Occupational Health*, ed. Paul Weindling (London: Croom Helm, 1985), 200–201.

40. M. Steinberg and M.R. Becklake, "Socio-Environmental Factors and Lung Function," *South African Medical Journal* 70 (1986): 270–74.

41. For more on embodiment, see Troy Duster, "Race and Reification in Science," *Science* 307 (2005): 1050–51; Nancy Krieger, "Stormy Weather: Race, Gene Expression, and the Science of Health Disparities," *American Journal of Public Health* 95 (2005): 2155–60; Anne Fausto-Sterling, "Race and Bones," *Social Studies of Science* 38 (2008): 657–94.

42. M.J. Hegewald and R.O. Crapo, "Sociеconomic Status and Lung Function," *Chest* 132 (2007): 1608–14; N.W. White, J.H. Hanley, U.G. Lallo, and M.R. Becklake, "Review and Analysis of Variation between Spirometric Values Reported in 29 Studies of Healthy African Adults," *American Journal of Respiratory and Critical Care Medicine* 150, no. 2 (August 1994): 348–55; David Van Sickle, Sheryl Magzamen, and John Mullahy, "Understanding Socioeconomic and Racial Differences in Adult Lung Function," *American Journal of Respiratory and Critical Care Medicine* 184 (2011): 521–27; Peter Burney, "The Use of Ethnically Specific Norms for Ventilatory Function in African-American and White Populations," *International Journal of Epidemiology* 41 (2012): 782–90.

43. Dana B. Hancock et al., "Meta-Analyses of Genome-Wide Association Studies Identify Multiple Novel Loci Associated with Pulmonary Function," *Nature Genetics* 42 (2010): 45–52.

44. The NHLBI Working Group, "Respiratory Diseases Disproportionately Affecting Minorities," *Chest* 108 (1995): 1380–92; Charles Pilleer, Edmund

Sanders, and Robyn Dixon, "Dark Cloud over Good Works of Gates Foundation," *Los Angeles Times,* January 7, 2007.

45. W.J. Gauderman, R. McConnell, F. Gilliland, S. London, D. Thomas, E. Avol, et al., "Association between Air Pollution and Lung Function Growth in Southern California Children," *American Journal of Respiratory and Critical Care Medicine* 162 (2000): 1383–90; R. Morello-Frosch and B. Jesdale, "Separate and Unequal: Residential Segregation and Estimated Cancer Risks Associated with Ambient Air Toxics in U.S. Metropolitan Areas," *Environmental Health Perspectives* 114 (2006): 386–93.

46. William Checkley, Keith P. West, Robert A. Wise, Matthew R. Baldwin, Lee Wu, Steven C. LeClerq, et al., "Maternal Vitamin A Supplementation and Lung Function in Offspring," *New England Journal of Medicine* 362 (2010): 1784–94; Donald Massaro and Gloria DeCarlo Massaro, "Lung Development, Lung Function, and Retinoids," *New England Journal of Medicine* 362 (2010): 1829–31; T.J. Ong, A. Mehta, S. Ogston, and S. Mukhopadhyay, "Prediction of Lung Function in the Inadequately Nourished," *Archives of Diseases of Children* 79 (1998): 18–21.

47. I thank Susan Reverby for this insight.

48. Anonymous interview, Kimberley, South Africa, 2001.

Index

Gleitsmann, William, 53
Glindmeyer, Henry, 200
Goldin, Jonathan, 192
gold mining, 167–82, 169, 170
Gold Producers Committee (South
    Africa), 178–82
Goodwyn, Edmund, 4
Gould, Benjamin A., xxii, xxvi, xxvii,
    32–37, 40–41, 43–46, 51, 61, 62,
    102, 189, 192, 197, 202
Gould, Stephen Jay, xxii
Graham, Sylvester, 58
Greenleaf, Charles R., 102
Greenwood, Major, 121–22
Groote Shuur Hospital, South Africa,
    187
group differences, xxi–xxii; spirometry
    and, xxiii–xxiv. See also racial dif-
    ference
Guy, William Augustus, 14, 19
gymnasiums, 61, 86, 88
gymnastic apparatuses, 69, 87
gymnastics, 63, 67, 71, 85, 87, 89. See
    also exercise

Hacking, Ian, 15, 19
Haitians, 46–47
Haldane, John S., 169
Haley, Bruce, 1
Hall, C. R., 29
Hall, G. Stanley, 42
Haller, John S., 43
Hamberger, Georg Erhard, 11
Hamilton, Alice, 50–51
Hammersley (British officer), 89,
    229n16
Hankinson, John, 201
Hanna, Delphine, 79
Hartman, Saidiya, 27
Hartwell, Edward Mussey, 76
Harvard Annex, 78
Harvard Instrument Company, 81
Harvard Summer School of Physical
    Training, 69, 78–79
Harvard University, 57, 68–71, 73, 78,
    88, 100
Hastings, William, 74, 79
Hawksley of London, 94
health and fitness: of African Ameri-

cans, 28, 39–40, 44–46, 49; anthro-
    pometry and, 120–21; in Britain,
    2, 20–21, 85–89, 103–5, 104; class
    as factor in, 106; evolution and,
    84; of men, 67, 228n90; models of,
    104; race in relation to, 204; social
    conditions as factor in, 106, 126,
    135, 233n89; of soldiers, 31–41, 85,
    87–88, 105–6, 116–18; in South
    Africa, 126; spirometry's monitor-
    ing of, xxiv, xxvi, xxvii–xxviii, 2;
    in United States, 67, 75–79; vital
    capacity as indicator of, 80, 97–103,
    135; of whites, 75–77; of women, 67,
    78–79, 228n90; of workers, 2, 20,
    100, 106, 126, 132. See also exercise;
    physical culture
health reform movements, 58, 62,
    77–78
height: lung capacity in relation to,
    xxv–xxvi, 7, 12–13, 17, 19, 24–25,
    65, 113–14, 119, 122–23
Helmholt, Hermann, xxiii
Henson, G. F., 121
Higginson, Thomas Wentworth, 58–59
high-altitude flying, 117–18, 124
Hill, A. V., 121
Hill, Lucille, 79
Hispanic populations, 202
Hitchcock, Edward (Amherst presi-
    dent), 59, 60, 224n7
Hitchcock, Edward (doctor), xxvii,
    57–67, 69, 71–76, 100, 224n7; An
    Anthropometric Manual, 75
Hitchcock, Edward, Jr. (educator), 69,
    79, 224n7
Hobson, F. W., 119–20
Hoffman, Frederick, xxvi, 223n88;
    Race Traits and Tendencies of the
    American Negro, 42–51
Holland, George Calvert, 10
Home Office and Mines Department
    (Great Britain), 145
Hooker, John W., 57
hookworm, 131–33, 239n89, 239n90
Horner, Arthur, 151
Howell, Joel, 110, 111
Hsieh, P. L., 130–31
Hughes, Thomas, 58

Lundy Braun is Royce Family Professor in Teaching Excellence, professor of medical science and Africana studies, and a member of the program in Science and Technology Studies at Brown University.